FOUNDATIONS FOR
HEALTH PROMOTION

FIFTH EDITION

FOUNDATIONS FOR
HEALTH PROMOTION

JANE WILLS MA, MSC, PGCE

Professor of Health Promotion
London South Bank University
London

ELSEVIER

ISBN: 978-0-7020-8506-2

Content Strategist: Robert Edwards
Content Project Manager: Tapajyoti Chaudhuri
Design: Ryan Cook
Marketing Manager: Samantha Page

Printed in China by 1010 Printing International Ltd

Last digit is the print number: 9 8 7 6 5 4 3

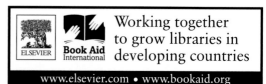

Working together
to grow libraries in
developing countries

www.elsevier.com • www.bookaid.org

CONTENTS

Since the first edition of this book the practice of health promotion has developed considerably. More practitioners are now engaged in health promotion as a core element of their role, and there has been an increase in specialist health promoters. Many graduate and undergraduate programmes in healthcare include health promotion, and specialist health promotion programmes exist across the world. Many countries have health promotion organizations providing a structural basis for activities, programmes and interventions in a variety of settings including schools, workplaces, universities and healthcare organizations. The context for health promotion has also changed dramatically in recent years. In the years since the Ottawa Charter (World Health Organization, 1986) that provided a framework for health promotion there has been a change in the burden of disease in developed countries, with more chronic conditions, a growing prevalence of violence and mental health problems and widening health inequalities. Alongside this are the worrying health effects of climate change, increasing antimicrobial resistance, and new emerging communicable diseases like COVID-19. Practitioners seeking to address these developments are aided by a revolution in communication technology, which increases their own and the public's access to knowledge and information to manage their health. It is now widely accepted that there is a key role in health and social care for prevention and population health management systems as well as people-centred approaches to the provision of care. This book sets out how we have moved from the first revolution of control of communicable diseases and the second revolution of managing some of the lifestyles associated with non-communicable diseases to what Kickbusch (2008) describes as the third revolution of health promotion.

When first published, this book sought to establish distinctive ways of thinking of health promotion based on social justice and empowerment, challenging the biomedical perspectives that underpin most healthcare. Health promotion is now a core aspect of the work of a wide range of healthcare workers and those engaged in education and social care. This book aims to provide a theoretical framework for health promotion, as this is vital to clarify practitioners' intentions and desired outcomes. It offers a foundation for practice which encourages practitioners to see the potential for health promotion in their work, to be aware of the implications of choosing from a range of strategies, and to be able to evaluate their health promotion interventions in an appropriate and useful manner.

This fifth edition of *Health Promotion: Foundations for Practice* has been comprehensively updated and expanded to reflect recent research findings and major organizational and policy changes. It includes new material on health protection and on the communication of risk, reflecting the devastating COVID-19 pandemic and the contribution of health promotion to individual behaviour change and disease management and to strengthening communities. This edition also includes a new chapter on evidence and the skills needed to access, appraise and apply evidence in practice.

The book is divided into four main parts. The first part provides a theoretical background, exploring the concepts of health, health education and health promotion. Part I concludes that health promotion is working towards the positive health and well-being of individuals, groups and communities. Health promotion includes health education and also acknowledges the social, economic and environmental factors which determine health status. Ethical and political values inform practice, and it is important for practitioners to reflect upon these values and their implications. Part I embraces the shift towards well-being rather than a narrow interpretation of health, and the move away from a simple focus on lifestyle changes as the goal of health promotion. Its aim is to enable readers to understand and reflect upon these theoretical drivers of health promotion practice within the context of their own work.

Part II explores strategies to promote health, and some of the dilemmas they pose. Using the Ottawa Charter (World Health Organization, 1986) framework to identify the range of strategies, the potential, benefits and challenges of adopting each strategy are discussed. Examples of interventions using the different strategies are presented. What is reflected here is how health services have not moved towards prioritizing prevention, although there is now much greater acceptance and support for empowerment approaches in work with individuals and communities. While policies that impact on health are still developed in isolation from each other, there is a recognition of the need for health to be taken into account in all policies, and for democratic working methods that engage with communities, as the way forward.

Part III focuses on the provision of supportive environments for health, identified as a key strategy in the Ottawa Charter (World Health Organisation, 1986). It explores how a range of different settings in which health promotion interventions take place can be oriented towards positive health and well-being. The settings discussed in Part III – schools, universities, workplaces, neighbourhoods, health services and prisons – have all been targeted by national and international policies as key settings for health promotion. Reaching specific target groups such as young people, adults or older people within these settings is also covered in Part III. There is much debate about the need for systems thinking and seeing such settings more broadly as environments where physical, social and economic drivers come together, and not just as places in which to carry out health education, lifestyle and behavioural interventions.

Part IV focuses on the implementation of health promotion interventions. Each chapter in this part discusses a different stage in the implementation process, from finding evidence and needs assessment, through planning and on to the final stage of evaluation. This part is designed to help practitioners to reflect on their practice through examining what drives their choice of implementation strategies. A range of real-life examples helps to illustrate the options available and the criteria that inform the practitioner's choice of approach. 'Checklist for Health Promotion Practice' identifies some of the key information that practitioners need in order to promote health and where this is discussed in the book.

This book is suitable for a wide range of professional groups, and this is reflected in the choice of examples and illustrative case studies, which have been completely updated for this edition. Each chapter has between 6 and 15 learning activities which encourage readers to engage with the text and extend their learning. Indicative feedback about the points that a reader or student might wish to consider is provided at the end of the chapter. Each chapter also includes at least one case study and research example to provide the reader with examples of practical application, and to encourage a focus on topics. New for this edition is the 'Reflection(s) on Practice' feature at the end of each chapter, which will be of particular interest to students on placements in vocational courses.

The book is targeted at a range of students, including those in basic and post-basic training and qualified professionals. By combining an academic critique with a readable and accessible style, this book will inform, stimulate and encourage readers to engage in ongoing enquiry and reflection regarding their health promotion practice. The intention, as always, is to encourage readers to develop their practice through considering its foundation in theory, policy and clear principles.

Jennie Naidoo
Bristol
Jane Wills
London

REFERENCES

Kickbusch, I., 2008. Healthy Societies: Addressing 21st Century Health Challenges. Available at: https://www.ilonakickbusch.com/kickbusch-wAssets/docs/Leavell-Lecture.pdf.

World Health Organization, 1986. Ottawa Charter for Health Promotion. Geneva. Available at: http://www.who.int/healthpromotion/conferences/previous/ottawa/en.

CHECKLIST FOR HEALTH PROMOTION PRACTICE

Topic	Key Information for Practice	Part and Chapter
Drivers of health promotion	What are the key drivers of health promotion practice?	Part I
	What is the relative contribution of scientific evidence versus theory and values?	
	What skills and competences are necessary for my health promotion practice?	
Theoretical frameworks and models	What is my vision for health promotion?	Chapters 1 and 5
	How do I take account of the culture and experience of clients, patients or the public that may impact on their perceptions and expectations of health and well-being?	Chapter 1
	What determines health?	Chapter 2
	Is addressing inequalities in health an important priority in my practice?	
	What information do I need to be able to deliver health promotion?	Chapter 3
	How can I know if I have promoted health and well-being successfully?	
	What informs my understanding of health promotion?	Chapters 4 and 5
	What principles underpin my practice?	Chapters 6 and 7
Strategies for promoting health	What are the key strategies used to promote health and well-being?	Part II
	What is my contribution as a health promoter during a pandemic?	Chapter 8
	How can I work collaboratively across sectors to promote health?	Chapters 9 and 12
	How am I able to influence policy?	Chapter 12
	How can I empower my patients, clients and the public to increase control over their health?	Chapters 10 and 11
	How can I best encourage behaviour change that promotes health and well-being?	
	How can I provide and communicate information to meet the needs of those with whom I work, whether clients, patients or the public?	Chapter 13
	How should I take account of the sources of information that are used by the public and patients?	
	Can I critically appraise national or international initiatives aimed at promoting health and well-being?	
Settings for Health Promotion	What should I take account of in a setting's features that could influence the ways in which health promotion is delivered?	Part III
	How can I create a supportive environment for health?	Chapters 14–19
Implementing health promotion	How do I know what the priorities should be for my practice?	Part IV; Chapter 20
	What are effective strategies for addressing priorities?	

Continued

Topic	Key Information for Practice	Part and Chapter
Research and evidence	Is my practice founded on evidence?	Chapter 21
	How robust is the evidence base for health promotion?	
	Where can I find appropriate sources of evidence to address issues?	
	How do I know if my practice is effective and value for money?	
	How do I know if my practice is acceptable?	
Planning and evaluating interventions	How can I best influence and shape service provision following the concerns and interests of those I work with?	Chapter 22
	How do I plan a health promotion intervention?	
	How are patients and the public involved and engaged in the design and delivery of an intervention?	
	How should I evaluate an intervention and report on its effects and make suggestions for its improvement?	Chapter 23

ACKNOWLEDGEMENTS

Jennie Naidoo is retiring from this fifth edition, and I want to pay tribute to her immense contribution to this book over the years. Her clarity and intellect helped both shape and maintain it as a core text for so many students and practitioners since its first publication in 1994. Readers have come to associate 'Naidoo and Wills' with the promise of an accessible but thought-provoking insight into the emerging discipline of health promotion – and this has been undeniably aided by Jennie's unfailing ability to communicate complex ideas with fluency and depth. On a personal level, I have deeply valued not only our friendship over many years but also this partnership in working together.

This current edition hosts a variety of features to engage the reader – which we pioneered in the first edition, and which arose out of our experience while teaching together on the first postgraduate specialist courses in health promotion. Students and colleagues at the University of the West of England, Bristol, and London South Bank University have, over the years, contributed much to the different editions through their ideas, debates and examples of practice – and we are grateful to them for ensuring that the book remains relevant.

To our children – Kate, Alice, Jessica and Declan – and families.

The Theory of Health Promotion

Part I explores the concepts of health, health education and health promotion. Health promotion draws upon many different disciplines, ranging from the scientific (e.g., epidemiology) and the social sciences (e.g., sociology and psychology) to the humanities (e.g., ethics). This provides a wealth of theoretical underpinnings for health promotion, ranging from the scientific to the moralistic. This in turn means that health promotion in practice may range from a scientific medical exercise (e.g., vaccination) or an educational exercise (e.g., sex and relationships education in schools) to a moral query (e.g., end-of-life options). An important first step for health promoters is to clarify for themselves where they stand in relation to these various different strategies and goals. Are they educators, politicians or scientists? In part, this will be determined by their background and initial education, but health promotion is an umbrella which encompasses all these activities and more. Working together, practitioners can bring their varied bodies of knowledge and skills to focus on promoting the health of the population, and achieve more significant and sustainable results than if they were operating on their own.

This first part of the book explores different understandings of the concept of health and well-being, and the ways in which health can be enhanced or promoted. The effect on health of structural factors such as income, gender, sexuality and ethnicity and the way in which social factors are important predictors of health status are explored in Chapter 2. The different ways in which health is measured reflect different views on health, from the absence of disease to holistic concepts of well-being, and these are discussed in Chapter 3. Chapters 4 and 5 debate what health promotion is, adopting an ecological model in which change in health is said to be influenced by the interaction of individual, social and physical environmental variables. Chapters 6 and 7 will help those who promote health to be clear about their intentions and how they perceive the purpose of health promotion. Is it to encourage healthy lifestyles? Or is it to redress health inequalities and empower people to take control over their lives?

1

Concepts of Health

LEARNING OUTCOMES

By the end of this chapter you will be able to:
- define the concepts of health, well-being, disease, illness and ill health, and understand the differences between them
- discuss the nature of health and well-being, and how culture and populism influence our definitions
- understand the elements of the medical model of health and how it influences healthcare practice.

KEY CONCEPTS AND DEFINITIONS

Biomedicine Focuses on the causes of ill health and disease within the physical body. It is associated with the practice of medicine, and contrasts with a social model of health.

Disease The medical term for a disorder, illness or condition that prevents an individual from achieving the full functioning of all their bodily parts.

Health The state of complete mental and physical well-being of an individual, not merely the absence of disease or illness.

Ill health A state of poor health when there is some disease or impairment, but not usually serious enough to curtail all activities.

Illness A disease or period of sickness that affects an individual's body or mind and prevents the individual achieving his or her optimal outputs.

Well-being The positive feeling that accompanies a lack of ill health and illness, and is associated with the achievement of personal goals and a sense of being well and feeling good.

IMPORTANCE OF THE TOPIC

Everyone engaged in the task of promoting health starts with a view of what health is. However, these views, or concepts, of health vary widely. It is important at the outset to be clear about the concepts of health to which you personally adhere, and recognize where these differ from those of your colleagues and clients. Otherwise, you may find yourself drawn into conflicts about appropriate strategies and advice that are actually due to different ideas concerning the end goal of health. This chapter introduces different concepts of health and traces the origin of these views. The scientific medical model of health is dominant, but is challenged by social and holistic models. Working your way through this chapter will enable you to clarify your own views on

the definition of health and locate these views within a conceptual framework.

DEFINING HEALTH, WELL-BEING, DISEASE, ILLNESS AND ILL HEALTH

Health

Health is a broad concept which can embody a huge range of meanings, from the narrowly technical to the all-embracing moral or philosophical. The word 'health' is derived from the Old English word for heal (*hael*) which means 'whole', signalling that health concerns the whole person and their integrity, soundness or well-being. There are 'common-sense' views of health which are passed through generations as part of a common cultural heritage. These are termed 'lay' concepts of health, and everyone acquires a knowledge of them through socialization into society. Different societies and different groups within one society have different views on what constitutes their 'common-sense' notions about health. Learning Activity 1.1 asks about what 'health' means to you.

 Learning Activity 1.1   What Does Health Mean to You?

What are your answers to the following?
- I feel healthy when ….
- I am healthy because ….
- To stay healthy I need ….
- I become unhealthy when ….
- My health improves when ….
- (An event) affected my health by ….
- (A situation) affected my health by ….
- … is responsible for my health.

Health has two common meanings in everyday use, one negative and one positive. The negative definition is the absence of disease or illness. This is the meaning of health within the scientific medical model, which is explored in greater detail later in this chapter. The positive definition of health is a state of well-being, interpreted by the World Health Organization in its constitution as 'a state of complete physical, mental and social well-being, not merely the absence of disease or infirmity' (World Health Organization, 1946). This moves the definition of health to one that is holistic and includes different dimensions, each of which needs to be considered. Holistic health means taking account of the separate influences and interaction of these dimensions. It is also presenting 'health' as a positive concept. Fig. 1.1 shows a diagrammatic representation of the dimensions of health.

The inner circle represents individual dimensions of health.
- Physical health concerns the body, for example, fitness, not being ill.
- Mental health refers to a positive sense of purpose and an underlying belief in one's own worth, for example, feeling good, feeling able to cope.
- Emotional health concerns the ability to feel, recognize and give a voice to feelings, and to develop and sustain relationships, for example, feeling loved.

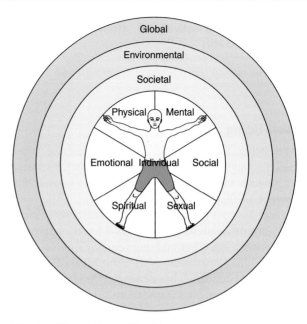

Fig. 1.1 Dimensions of health

- Social health concerns the sense of having support available from family and friends, for example, having friends to talk to, being involved in activities with other people.
- Spiritual health is the recognition and ability to put into practice moral or religious principles or beliefs, and the feeling of having a 'higher' purpose in life.
- Sexual health is the acceptance and ability to achieve a satisfactory expression of one's sexuality.

The three outer circles are broader dimensions of health which affect the individual. Societal health refers to the link between health and the way a society is structured. This includes the basic infrastructure necessary for health (such as shelter, peace, food, income) and the degree of integration or division within society. We shall see in Chapter 2 how the existence of patterned inequalities between groups of people harms the health of everyone. Environmental health refers to the physical environment in which people live, and the importance of good-quality housing, transport, sanitation and pure-water facilities. Global health involves caring for the planet and ensuring its sustainability for the future. The holistic model of health looks at the whole person, and Learning Activity 1.2 asks you to consider what are the implications of this conceptualization in professional practice.

Learning Activity 1.2   Holistic Model of Health

What are the implications of a holistic model of health for the professional practice of health workers?

Well-Being

'Well-being' is a term widely used to describe 'what makes a good life'. It is also used in healthcare discourse to broaden views on what health means beyond the absence of illness. Feeling good and functioning well are seen as important components of mental well-being. This, in turn, leads to better physical health, improved productivity, less crime and more participation in community life (Department of Health, 2010). The New Economics Foundation has developed the Happy Planet Index (New Economics Foundation, 2016) as a headline indicator of how nations compare in enabling long and happy lives for their citizens. In 2016:

- Costa Rica topped the rankings. Costa Ricans have higher well-being than the residents of many rich nations, including the USA and the UK, and live longer than people in the USA. This is achieved with a per capita ecological footprint that is just one-third the size of the USA.
- Six of the ten countries that are achieving the highest and sustainable well-being are in Latin America and the Caribbean.
- The highest-ranking Western European nation, Norway, is in 12th place.
- The USA is in 108th position out of 140 countries.

Similarly, the UNICEF (United Nations Children's Fund) index of child well-being (UNICEF, 2013) shows that well-being is greater in more egalitarian countries, such as Norway and other Scandinavian countries.

Evidence (Government Office for Science, 2008) suggests that there are five methods or steps that individuals can take to enable themselves to achieve well-being as shown in Fig. 1.2. Learning Activity 1.3 asks you to find evidence that these steps – learning, giving, noticing, being active and connecting – are beneficial for health.

Learning Activity 1.3   Five Steps to Well-Being

What evidence is there for each of the steps to well-being?

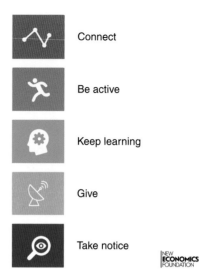

Fig. 1.2 Five ways to well-being (Adapted from New Economics Foundation, 2008. Five ways to wellbeing. London. Available at: https://neweconomics.org/2008/10/five-ways-to-wellbeing.)

Disease, Illness and Ill Health

Disease, illness and ill health are often used interchangeably, although they have very different meanings. Disease derives from *desaise*, meaning uneasiness or discomfort. Nowadays, disease implies an objective state of ill health, which may be verified by accepted canons of proof. In our modern society, these accepted canons are couched in the language of scientific medicine. For example, microscopic analysis may yield evidence of changes in cell structure, which may in turn lead to a diagnosis of cancer. Disease is the existence of some pathology or abnormality of the body which is capable of detection. Disease can be due to exogenous (outside the body, e.g., viral infection) or endogenous (inside the body, e.g., inadequate thyroid function) factors.

Illness is the subjective experience of loss of health. This is couched in terms of symptoms, for example, the reporting of aches or pains, or loss of function. One way that illness is given meaning is through the narratives we construct about how we fall sick. The process of making sense of illness is a task most sick people engage in to answer the question 'why me?' Illness and disease are not the same, although there is a large degree of coexistence. For example, a person may be diagnosed as having cancer through screening, even when there have been no reported symptoms; thus, a disease may be diagnosed in someone who has not reported any illness. When someone reports symptoms, and further investigations, such as blood tests, prove a disease process, the two concepts of disease and illness coincide. In these instances, the term ill health is used. Ill health is therefore an umbrella term used to refer to the experience of disease plus illness. Health is the normal functioning of the body as a biological entity. Health is both not being ill and the absence of symptoms.

Social scientists view health and disease as socially constructed entities. Health and disease are not states of objective reality waiting to be uncovered and investigated by scientific medicine; rather, they are actively produced and negotiated by ordinary people. Cornwell's (1984) study of London's East Enders used three categories of health problems.

1. Normal illness, for example, childhood infections.
2. Real illness, for example, cancer.
3. Health problems, for example, ageing, allergies.

Illness has often been conceptualized as deviance – as a different state from the healthy norm and a source of stigma. Goffman (1968) identified three sources of stigma.

1. Abominations of the body, for example, psoriasis.
2. Blemishes of character, for example, human immunodeficiency virus (HIV)/acquired immunodeficiency syndrome (AIDS).
3. Tribal stigma of race, nation or religion, for example, apartheid.

The subjective experience of feeling ill is not always corroborated by an objective diagnosis of disease. When this lack of corroboration happens, doctors and health workers may label sufferers 'malingerers', denying the validity of subjective illness. This can have important consequences. For example, a sick certificate, and therefore sick pay, may be withheld if a doctor is not convinced that someone's reported illness is genuine. The acceptance of reported symptoms as signs of an illness leads to a debate about how to manage the illness. Learning Activity 1.4 asks you to identify conditions, for example, chronic fatigue syndrome and repetitive strain injury, which have taken a long time to be recognized as legitimate illnesses.

 Learning Activity 1.4   The Medicalization of Health

What examples are there of a condition or behaviour where its medicalization has led to its acceptance or otherwise?

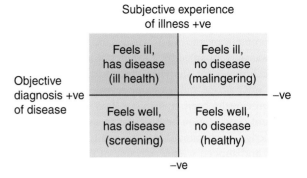

Fig. 1.3 The relationship between disease and illness

It is also possible for an individual to experience no symptoms or signs of disease, but to be labelled sick as a result of medical examination or screening. Hypertension and pre-cancerous changes to cell structures are two examples where screening may identify a disease even though the person concerned may feel perfectly healthy. Fig. 1.3 gives a visual representation of these discrepancies. The central point is that subjective perceptions cannot be overruled, or invalidated, by scientific medicine.

THE MEDICAL MODEL OF HEALTH

In modern Western societies, and in many other societies as well, the dominant professional view of health adopted by most healthcare workers during their training and practice is a biomedical one. Scientific medicine operates within a medical model using a narrow view of health, which is often taken to mean the absence of disease and/or illness. In this sense, health is a negative term, defined more by what it is not than by what it is.

This view of health is extremely influential, as it underpins much of the training and ethos of a wide variety of health workers. Its definitions become powerful because they are used in a variety of contexts, not just in professional circles. For example, the media often present this view of health, disease and illness in dramas set in hospitals or documentaries about health issues. By these means, professional definitions become known and accepted in society at large.

The scientific medical model arose in Western Europe at the time of the Enlightenment, with the rise of rationality and science as forms of knowledge. In earlier times, religion provided a way of knowing and understanding the world. The Enlightenment changed the old order, and substituted science for religion as the dominant means of knowledge and understanding. This was accompanied by a proliferation of equipment and techniques for studying the world. The invention of the microscope and telescope revealed worlds which had previously been invisible. Observation, calculation and classification became the means of increasing knowledge. Such knowledge was put to practical purposes, and applied science was one of the forces which accompanied the Industrial Revolution. In an atmosphere when everything was deemed knowable through the proper application of scientific method, the human body became a key object for the pursuit of scientific knowledge. What could be seen, and measured and catalogued, was 'true' in an objective and universal sense.

Health is viewed as located in the individual body, and the causes of ill health are biological or physiological in origin. Health is thus predominantly viewed as the absence of disease. This view sees health and disease as linked, as if on a continuum, so that the more diseases a person has, the further away they are from health and 'normality'. If disease or abnormality is not present, then the person is assumed to be healthy.

The pathogenic focus on finding the causes for ill health has led to an emphasis on risk factors, whether these are health behaviours or social circumstances.

Antonovsky (1993) called for a *salutogenic* approach which looks instead at why some people remain healthy. He identifies coping mechanisms which enable some people to remain healthy despite adverse circumstances, change and stress. An important factor for health, which Antonovsky labels a 'sense of coherence', involves the three aspects of understanding, managing and making sense of change. These are human abilities which are in turn nurtured or obstructed by the wider environment.

The medical model focuses on aetiology and the belief that disease originates from specific and identifiable causes. The causes of contemporary long-term chronic diseases in developed countries are often 'social'. Medicine and medical practice thus recognize that disease and the diseased body must be placed in a social context. Nevertheless, the professional training of many healthcare workers provides an exaggerated view of the benefits of treatment and pays little attention to prevention. In part, this is due to the dominant concern of the biomedical model with the organic appearance of disease and malfunction as the causes of ill health.

Table 1.1 shows the characteristics of the medical model of health and points out its critique.

1. The role of medicine in determining health:

   The view that health is the absence of disease and illness, and that medical treatment can restore the body to good health, has been criticized.

TABLE 1.1	The Medical Model of Health	
Characteristic	**Description**	**Critique**
Biomedical	Health is assumed to be the property of biological beings.	A narrow and simplistic view of health.
Reductionist	States of being, such as health and disease, may be reduced to smaller and smaller constitutive components of the biological body.	Explanations for health and ill health also caused by social and environmental factors.
Mechanistic	Conceptualizes the body as if it were a machine in which all the parts are interconnected but capable of being separated and treated separately.	Holistic definitions see dimensions (including social and mental) as interconnected and health as subjectively experienced.
Pathogenic	Focuses on why people become ill.	Salutogenesis focuses on the origins of health and why some people are resilient. Medicine leads to a focus on risk factors.
Dualistic	The mind and the body can be treated as separate entities.	Mental and physical health are interconnected and of equal importance, and there should be 'parity of esteem'.
Scientific expertise	The understanding of health and ill health is through science.	Lay understandings and knowledge are important, and approaches are about working with people to facilitate change.

The distribution of health and ill health has been analysed from a historical and social science perspective. It has been argued that medicine is not as effective as is often claimed. The medical writer Thomas McKeown (1976) showed that most of the fatal diseases of the 19th century had disappeared before the arrival of antibiotics or immunization programmes. McKeown concluded that social advances in general living conditions, such as improved sanitation and better nutrition made available by rising real wages, have been responsible for most of the reduction in mortality achieved during the last century. Although his thesis has been disputed, there is little disagreement that the contribution of medicine to reduced mortality has been minor when compared with the major impact of improved environmental conditions. Learning Activity 1.5 asks you to consider what other reasons might there be for reductions in mortality rates.

Learning Activity 1.5   The Impact of Medicine

- What effects do medical advances in knowledge have on death rates?
- What other reasons could account for declining death rates?

The rise of the evidence-based practice movement (see Chapter 21) is attributed to Archie Cochrane (1972). His concern was that medical interventions were not trialled to demonstrate effectiveness prior to their widespread adoption. Instead, many procedures rest on habit, custom and tradition rather than rationality. Cochrane advocated greater use of the randomized controlled trial as a means to gain scientific knowledge and the key to progress.

2. The role of social factors in determining health:

Most countries are characterized by profound inequalities in income and wealth, and these in turn are associated with persistent inequalities in health (see Chapter 2). The impact of scientific medicine on health is marginal when compared to major structural features such as the distribution of wealth, income, housing and employment. It has been estimated that restricted access to medical care accounted for about 10% of premature deaths in high-income countries and behavioural factors accounted for between 16% and 65% (Kaplan and Millstein, 2019). Chapter 2

shows, the distribution of health mirrors the distribution of material resources within society. In general, the more equal a society is in its distribution of resources, the more equal, and better, is the health status of its citizens (Wilkinson and Pickett, 2009).

3. Medicine as a means of social control:

Social scientists argue that medicine is a social enterprise closely linked with the exercise of professional power. Foucault (1975) argues that power is embedded in social organizations, expressed through hierarchies and determined through discourses. Medical power derives from its role in legitimizing health and illness in society and the socially exclusive and autonomous nature of the profession. The medical profession has long been regarded as an institution for securing occupational and social authority. Access to such power is controlled by professional associations that have their own vested interests to protect (Freidson, 1986). The Medical Act 1858 established the General Medical Council, which was authorized to regulate doctors, oversee medical education and keep a register of qualified practitioners. The Faculty of Public Health Medicine opened membership to non-medically qualified specialists in 2003, becoming the Faculty of Public Health.

Medicine is a powerful means of social control, whereby the categories of disease, illness, madness and deviancy are used to maintain a status quo in society. Doctors who make diagnoses are in a powerful position. The role of the patient during sickness as conceptualized by Parsons (1951) is illustrated in Table 1.2.

Increasingly, too, doctors are involved in decisions relating to the beginning and ending of life (terminations, assisted reproduction, neonatal care, euthanasia). The encroachment of medical decisions into these stages of life subverts human autonomy and,

TABLE 1.2 **The Sick Role**	
Rights	**Responsibilities**
- Patient is relieved of normal responsibilities and tasks - Patient is given sympathy and support - Patient has the right to a diagnosis, examination and treatment	- Patient must want to recover as soon as possible and only then can they be seen as 'sick' - Patient must seek professional advice and comply with treatment

it is argued, gives to medicine an authority beyond its legitimate area of operation (Illich, 1975).

4. Medicine as surveillance:

Public health medicine has been concerned with the regulation and control of disease. Historically this included the containment of bodies, such as those infected with the plague, tuberculosis or venereal disease. Mass-screening programmes have given rise to what has been called medical surveillance. The wish to identify the 'abnormal' few with 'invisible' disease justifies monitoring the entire target population. Another critique of the pervasive power of medicine suggests the mapping of disease and identification of risk have subtly handed responsibility of health to individuals. This may invite new forms of control in the name of health, for example, random drug testing or linking deservingness for surgery to lifestyle factors. The ability to identify risk also means there can be a moral discourse in which reducing one's risk factors, for example, eating 'sensibly' and living 'well', is seen as a good thing.

5. Medicine as harm:

According to Illich (1975), doctors and health workers contribute to ill health and create harm (iatrogenesis).

- Clinical iatrogenesis is ill health caused by medical intervention, for example, side-effects caused by prescribed medicine, dependence on prescribed drugs and cross-infection in medical settings such as hospitals.
- Social iatrogenesis is the loss of coping and the right to self-care which have resulted from the medicalization of everyday life.
- Cultural iatrogenesis is the loss of the means whereby people cope with pain and suffering, which results from the unrealistic expectations generated by medicine.

The social model of health, in contrast, views health as influenced by a range of factors outside of the physical body. It views health as a social construct and therefore individual differences can arise due to lifestyle, access to health services, identity and structural or environmental factors such as poverty.

BIOPSYCHOSOCIAL MODEL

Another way of looking at health is to integrate the social, psychological and medical aspects of health.

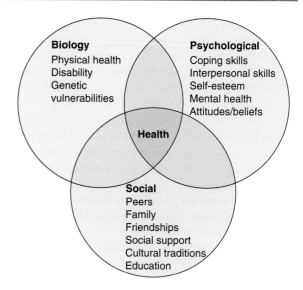

Fig. 1.4 The biopsychosocial model of health

This model is holistic with a focus on the whole individual. Fig. 1.4 shows how this model might explore the relationship of biology (e.g., genetics and physiological factors), social and environmental factors (e.g., relationships, employment, income) and psychological factors (e.g., personality, self-esteem, coping) to explain mental health and well-being.

LAY CONCEPTS OF HEALTH

For people concerned with the promotion of health, there is another problem with the dominance of scientific medicine: the focus within medicine on illness and disease, and the neglect of health as a positive concept in its own right. Many researchers have studied the general public's beliefs about health or lay concepts of health. The findings present an interesting picture, where there are continuities in definitions but also differences attributable to age, sex and class.

Blaxter (1990) identified five common concepts of health.

1. 'Health as not-ill', health is the absence of symptoms or medical input, is widely used by all groups.
2. 'Health as physical fitness', health as having energy and strength, is mostly used by younger men.
3. 'Health as social relationships' is mostly used by women.

RESEARCH EXAMPLE 1.1
Caregivers' Health

An ageing population means that caring for the elderly will become a more common experience for younger adults or even children. This has significant implications for the health of the population as a whole. Research studies have reported a clear association between caring and caregivers' poor mental and physical health, emotional distress and increased mortality. A more intense caring role (e.g., having to provide 24-hour cover, or caring for someone with both mental and physical ill health) is associated with poorer health outcomes on the part of the carer. Yet evidence also shows that not all carers report poor health. Indeed, caring has the opposite effect on some carers, conferring positive benefits through feelings of altruism, fulfilment of familial obligations and personal growth. It is likely that the impact of caring on the health of carers will be to some extent dependent on the existence, or lack, of a supportive environment, including, for example, community activities and respite opportunities. It also seems likely that the existence of a person's religious and faith beliefs is associated with improved health and caring as religion provides an overarching rationale for existence, even if this is compromised by poor health. Religious centres often provide supportive and caring activities for members of their faith, enabling carers to cope better with their burden of care, and providing some respite care for people with disabilities.

See, for example, Awad and Voruganti, 2008; Rigby et al., 2009; Vellone et al., 2008.

Author (interviewer)
'Do you think that living here has affected your health either positively or negatively?'
Mary (interviewee)
'No, I don't think that's, I think my health problems are just my health problems [diabetes and angina] and that's it, I think. I think that the diabetes was because of my weight, and the heart condition was a combination of the diet and possibly the passive smoking. I wouldn't say that, that it was the environment that's caused my problems.'
Airey (2003, p. 1320)

 Learning Activity 1.6   Moral Identities and Health
How do morality and moral identities influence the ways in which people experience health and ill health?

---

4. 'Health as function', health as the ability to carry out tasks and activities, is mostly used by older people of both sexes.
5. 'Health as psychosocial well-being' is less used by young men, mostly used by higher socio-economic groups.

The concepts of 'control' and 'release' are also commonly found in lay accounts. Release is the taking of known risks (e.g., binge drinking), whereas control is the management of health. Researchers have found these issues of control and release in many accounts of health, together with a moral view about taking risks. Participants consistently describe behavioural contributors to poor health, such as high alcohol consumption, drug use, unhealthy diets and smoking, as 'coping' mechanisms or forms of escapism. They also may blame themselves as shown in this extract:

There is often a difference between lay and professional concepts of health. The gap between the two has been identified by health workers as a problem, giving rise to concern. The concern centres around two issues:

1. the perceived lack of communication or poor communication between health worker and client and
2. clients' lack of compliance with prescribed treatment regimens.

However, there is also a crossover between lay and professional beliefs about health. Health workers acquire their professional view of health during training. These beliefs overlie their original views of health adopted at an early age from family and society, so professionals are familiar with both. The general public is also aware of, and operates with, both sets of beliefs. In searching for meaning, lay patients frequently adopt professionals' explanations and interpretations about health and illness. So, the two sets of beliefs, scientific medicine and lay public, are not discrete entities but overlap each other and exist in tandem.

Cornwell (1984) describes how people operate with both official and lay beliefs about health. Her study of London's East Enders found that accounts of health were either public or private. Public accounts are couched in terms of scientific medicine and reflect these dominant beliefs. Health and illness are related to medical diagnosis and treatment, and medical terms and events are used to explain health status. These public accounts were offered first in Cornwell's interviews. What she terms 'private accounts' reflect lay views of health, which typically use more holistic and social concepts to explain health and illness. For example, private accounts related health to general life experiences, such as employment, housing and perceived stress. Private accounts were offered in subsequent interviews, when a relationship had been established between Cornwell and the women she was interviewing. Cornwell suggests that people are therefore aware of both systems of beliefs and can use either when asked to talk about health. In encounters with strangers who are perceived as professionals, people use public accounts; in more informal settings, they use private accounts.

CULTURAL VIEWS OF HEALTH

We are able to think about health using the language of scientific medicine because that is part of our cultural heritage. We do so as a matter of course, and think it is self-evident or common sense. However, other societies and cultures have their own ideas of common sense and ways of talking about health which are very different. Different belief systems may view disease as the outcome of malign human or supernatural agencies, and diagnosis is a matter of determining who has been offended. Treatment includes ceremonies to propitiate these spirits as an integral part of the process. Ways of thinking about health and disease reflect the basic preoccupations of a society, and dominant views of the society and the world. Anthropologists refer to this phenomenon as the cultural specificity of notions of health and disease.

In any multicultural society, a variety of cultural views coexist at any one time. For example, traditional Chinese medicine is based on the dichotomy of yin and yang, female and male, hot and cold, which is applied to symptoms, diet and treatments, such as acupuncture and Chinese herbal medicine. Complementary therapists offer therapies based on these cultural views of health and disease alongside (or increasingly within) the National Health Service, which is based on scientific medicine.

Research Example 1.3 describes some of the beliefs that people have about food and its contribution to their health. Learning Activity 1.7 probes you to think about your practice and examples of how you have acknowledged and incorporated people's own explanations for their health or illness.

RESEARCH EXAMPLE 1.2
Orthodox Judaism and Screening in Maternity Care

Religious communities such as Orthodox Jews believe that alongside an individual's obligation to take care of one's health as commanded in the religious book, the Torah, so will the trust in God be a reason to not screen (Gross and Shuval, 2008; Tkatch et al., 2014). For Orthodox Jews, the objective assessment of risk held by healthcare professionals is a counter to the invoking of religious faith and fatalism. Women in pregnancy or going through cancer treatment have been found to rely on rabbinic involvement as 'socially sanctioned' in the health decision-making process. Such views are summed up by a participant in a study of low vaccination uptake amongst the community in London (Henderson et al., 2008) who stated:

> When you don't know what to do, when there's a risk involved both ways, then there's no need to put yourself in the danger of doing one of them. By not doing it (we) trust that God will help you out of these things.

For healthcare professionals, it is important to understand that risks are perceived and managed in accordance with principles that exist within different forms of social organization. Thus, Orthodox Judaism, with its confidence in divine intervention, holds a different set of principles, what Douglas (2004) calls 'cosmology', than is generally accepted in biomedicine.

IMPLICATIONS FOR HEALTH PROMOTION

Is there any unifying concept of health which can reconcile these different views and beliefs? Attempts at such a synthesis have come from philosophers such as Seedhouse (1986) and from organizations concerned with health, such as the World Health Organization.

- *Health as an ideal state* provides a holistic and positive definition of health. It is important in showing the interrelationship of different dimensions of health. A medical diagnosis of ill health does not necessarily coincide with a sense of personal illness or feeling unwell. Equally, a person free from disease may be isolated and lonely.
- *Health as mental and physical fitness* is a perspective developed by Talcott Parsons (1951), a functional sociologist. It suggests that health is when people can fulfil their everyday tasks and roles expected of them.

Understandings About Food and Meals Across the Lifespan and Genders

Food is as much related to identity and social relations as it is to nutrition. In the UK, there is still considerable emphasis placed on the shared meal, especially on Sunday, as reflective of the family. Stead et al. (2011), for example, found that young people saw food choices as a way of signifying their identity; healthy choices conflicted with the types of food they felt would help them fit in with their peer group. De Wit et al. (2015) found that children from families who ate together and saw mealtimes as communal occasions were more likely to eat healthy food and be able to self-regulate their eating. The work of planning and preparing food can often reflect heteronormative gendered expectations. Carrington's (2012) study of lesbian and gay families found that ideas of gender still influenced attitudes, with food-associated domestic work being seen as feminine. Carrington found that lesbian couples were careful not to imply that the partner who did less food work had a reduced feminine identity, whereas male gay couples did not want the partner who did the majority of food work being seen as a 'housewife'. Food therefore became a territory within which couples managed identity. Food is also a marker of cultural identity that affirms, in shared patterns of consumption and shared notions of edibility, difference from others that is frequently illustrated in the experience of immigrants and refugees.

From Burch, S., 2022. Cultural studies and anthropology and health. In: Naidoo, J., Wills, J. (eds.), Health Studies: An Introduction, fourth edn. Springer, Singapore.

? Learning Activity 1.7   Understanding Health Beliefs

People's explanations for their health and illness are complex. Why is it important for health promoters to understand the health beliefs of those with whom they work? How might they do this?

- *Health as a commodity* leads to unrealistic expectations of health as something which can be purchased. Health cannot be guaranteed by paying a higher price for healthcare.
- *Health as a personal strength* is a view which derives from humanistic psychology and suggests that an individual can become healthy through self-actualization and discovery (Maslow, 1970).

? Learning Activity 1.8   Theories of Health

Fig. 1.5 shows four theories of health.
1. Health as an ideal state.
2. Health as mental and physical fitness.
3. Health as a commodity.
4. Health as a personal strength.
   What problems can you identify with each of these four views of health?

Seedhouse (1986) suggests that these four views can be combined in a unified theory of health as the foundation for human achievement (Fig. 1.5). Health is thus a means to an end rather than a fixed state to which a person should aspire.

> *[Health is] the extent to which an individual or group is able, on the one hand, to realize aspirations and satisfy needs; and, on the other hand, to change or cope with the environment. Health is, therefore, seen as a resource for everyday life, not an object of living; it is a positive concept emphasizing social and personal resources, as well as physical capacities.*
>
> ### World Health Organization (1984)

Provided certain central conditions are met, people can be enabled to achieve their potential. The task of health practitioners is to create these conditions for people to achieve health:

- basic needs of food, drink, shelter and warmth;
- access to information about the factors influencing health;
- skills and confidence to use that information.

This definition acknowledges that people have different starting points, which set limits for their potential for health. It encompasses a positive notion of health that is applicable to everyone, whatever their circumstances. However, it could be argued that this definition does not acknowledge the social construction of health sufficiently. People as individuals have little scope to determine optimum conditions for realizing their potential.

> *By health I mean the power to live a full, adult, living, breathing life in close contact with what I love…. I want to be all that I am capable of becoming.*
>
> ### Mansfield (1977, p. 278)

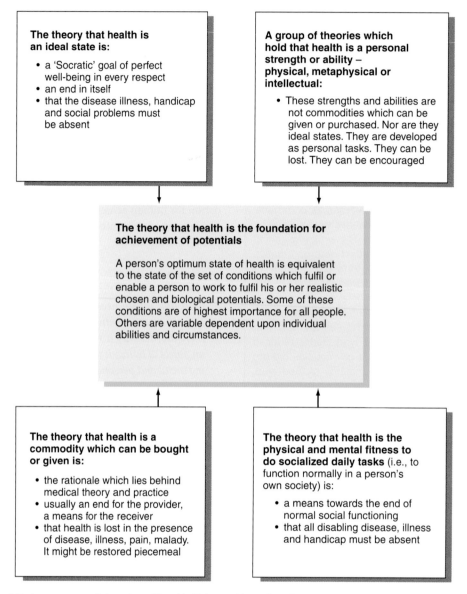

Fig. 1.5 A summary of theories of health (Adapted from Seedhouse, D., 1986. Health: Foundations for Achievement. John Wiley, Chichester.)

The view of health as personal potential is attractive because it is so flexible, but this very flexibility causes problems. It leads to relativism (health may mean a thousand different things to a thousand different people), which makes it impracticable as a working definition for health promoters.

Health is regarded by the World Health Organization as a fundamental human right, and there are certain prerequisites for health, which include peace, adequate food and shelter, and sustainable resource use.

Looking at health this way establishes it as a social as well an individual product, and it emphasizes its dynamic and positive nature. Health is viewed as both a fundamental human right and a sound social investment. This view was publicly affirmed by the Jakarta Declaration, which linked health to social and economic development (World Health Organization, 1997). This definition provides a variety of reasons for supporting health which are likely to meet the concerns of a range of groups. It establishes a broad consensus for prioritizing health and legitimizes a range of activities designed to promote it. For example, in addition to the more acceptable strategies of primary healthcare and personal skills development, the World Health Organization also identified in the Ottawa Charter the more radical strategies of community participation and healthy public policy as essential to the promotion of health (World Health Organization, 1986). However, it could still be argued that such a broad definition makes it difficult to identify practical priorities for health promotion activities.

There is no agreement on what is meant by health. Health is used in many different contexts to refer to many different aspects of life. Given this complexity of meanings, it is unlikely that a unified concept of health which includes all its meanings will be formulated.

CONCLUSION

There are no rights and wrongs regarding concepts of health. Different people are likely to hold different views of health and may operate with several conflicting views simultaneously. Where people are located socially, in terms of socio-economic status, gender, ethnic origin and age, will affect their concept of health. The medical model has dominated Western thinking about health, yet its value for health promotion is limited.

- It relies on a concept of normality that is not widely accepted.
- It ignores broader societal and environmental dimensions of health.
- It ignores people's subjective perceptions of their own health.
- The focus on pathology and malfunction leads to practitioners responding to ill health rather than being proactive in promoting health.

There is such a range of meaning attached to the notion of health that in any particular situation it is important to find out what views exist. Clarifying what you understand about health, and what other people mean when they talk about health, is an essential first step for the health promoter.

REFLECTIONS ON PRACTICE

- How would you describe your own concept and understanding of health?
- What have been the most important influences on your views?
- How might this be different from those you work with in practice, for example, a person living with a long-term condition, a person with severe mental illness, a woman in labour?
- Person-centred care means understanding what is important for the individual as a person, not just a patient with a condition. What questions would you ask a person living with a long-term condition, a person with severe mental illness, a woman in labour?

SUMMARY

Definitions of health arise from many different perspectives. While scientific medicine is the most powerful ideology in the West, it is not all-embracing. Social sciences' perspectives on health produce a powerful critique of scientific medicine and point to the importance of social factors in the construction and meaning of health. Lay concepts of health derived from different cultures coexist alongside scientific medicine. Attempts to produce a unified concept of health appear to be founded through overgeneralization and vagueness.

FURTHER READING AND RESOURCES

Barry, A., Yuill, C., 2016. Understanding the Sociology of Health: An Introduction, fourth edn. Sage Publications, London.
An accessible introduction to the sociology of health and illness exploring key concepts and the social structures that shape and pattern health.
Lupton, D., 2012. Medicine as Culture: Illness, Disease and the Body in Western Societies, third edn. Sage Publications, London.
An interesting account of the dependence on, and disillusionment with, medicine.
Naidoo, J., Wills, J., (eds.), 2022. Health Studies: An Introduction, fourth edn. Springer, Singapore.
An accessible introduction to different disciplinary perspectives on health including sociology, culture and anthropology and biology.

➤ FEEDBACK TO LEARNING ACTIVITIES

1.1. Health is a complex concept that encompasses different dimensions, including physical, mental, social and emotional. Some theorists suggest there is a hierarchy of health, whereby physical health needs are the most basic, and it is only once these needs have been met that people can move on to identify and meet mental, social and emotional health needs. Maslow (1943) identified a hierarchy of needs (often represented as a pyramid), with the most basic need (at the base of the pyramid) being physiological, moving through safety, belonging and esteem to self-actualization (at the tip of the pyramid).

1.2. A holistic model of health implies that professional health workers can only address some aspects or causes of health or ill health (and not necessarily the most basic or important causes). Many of the most important factors affecting health, such as social equality or environmental quality, are beyond the remit of health workers. A holistic model of health also implies that health workers need to work collaboratively with others (e.g., social workers or environmental health officers) in order to achieve optimum results.

1.3. Evidence suggests that a small improvement in well-being can help to decrease some mental health problems and also help people to flourish. The New Economics Foundation (2008), on behalf of Foresight, presented a document which sets out five actions to improve personal well-being based on this evidence.

- Connect: Having social support and relationships is beneficial to well-being and acts as a buffer against mental ill health.
- Be active: Regular physical activity is associated with a greater sense of well-being and possibly delays cognitive decline.
- Take notice: Being aware of sensations, thoughts and feelings enhances well-being. Being in a state of mindfulness (being attentive to, and aware of, what is taking place in the present) is positive.
- Give: Mutual cooperation is associated with feelings of regard. Active participation in social and community life is associated with positive affect.
- Keep learning: Learning is important in social and cognitive development, enhances self-esteem and encourages interaction.

1.4. According to Hart and Wellings (2002), homosexuals, formerly considered to be sinners, were labelled as ill up to the late 1970s in the USA. Commitments to mental institutions, hormonal treatments and castrations were used to deal with their unwanted sexual behaviour. In 1973 the American Psychiatric Association redesignated homosexuality as non-pathological. Mental health is probably the most medicalized aspect of human life such that if several symptoms are present, a mental disorder is said to exist. Foucault (1975) considered the process of indefinite medicalization to be one of the main features of society.

1.5. There were few effective medicines or therapies available to combat infectious diseases before the mid-1930s, so medical care did not play an important role during this period. Historical epidemiologists, such as McKeown (1976), observed that a large share of the decline in infectious disease mortality during the 20th century preceded the advent of medical treatments, and concluded that rising living standards, better nutrition and public health measures that improved water supplies, sanitation systems and household hygiene were responsible for the drop in mortality rates. Since the late 20th century, the principal causes of mortality have been attributed to 'lifestyles', and medical advances such as the treatment of hypertension and diabetes and the medical and surgical treatment of coronary artery disease have contributed to increased life expectancy.

1.6. Moral identity, such as strength of character and personal control, is frequently cited in lay accounts of health. In a survey of disadvantaged areas, Popay et al. (2003) and Smith and Anderson (2017) both found that some respondents suggested that stress mediated the relationship between the experience of disadvantage and poor health. As you will find in Chapter 2, psychosocial pathways provide an important conceptual link within lay understandings to the moral framework within which explanations for health and illness are 'constructed'. Individual resilience and strength of character are seen as the means to avoid ill health.

1.7. There is often a gulf between healthcare professionals' and patients' knowledge, expectations and values regarding illness and healthcare. Healthcare professionals often assume their prioritization of Western scientific medicine and associated values is universal and shared by all their patients. However, this is not the case. Patients' and clients' cultural values vary widely and have a significant impact on their understanding of medical diagnoses and prescribed care, as well as their ability to manage illness, disability and death. Gender and position within the family may also impact on patients' ability to understand and cope with ill health. Cultural values impact on all stages of ill health, from receiving and understanding a diagnosis, through management of illness and treatment, to coping with death and bereavement.

1.8. Definitions of health.
  • The definition of health as a complete state of well-being is unrealistic and does not help health professionals or lay people set practical or achievable goals. The requirement for complete health means that most people are unhealthy most of the time. This view therefore supports the tendencies of the medical technology and drug industries, in association with professional organizations, to redefine diseases, detect more and more abnormalities through screening, and thus expand the scope of the healthcare system (see Huber et al., 2011).
  • The definition of health as normal social functioning ignores the fact that people can be contented and healthy but unable to fulfil social roles (e.g., employee) due to factors such as chronic illness or disability.
  • The definition of health as something that can be acquired (e.g., through medicine) suggests health can be slotted into different activities which have a price. However, this is not how people experience health and illness.
  • The definition of health as individually defined strength ignores the fact that health and ill health are created within a social context. It is this social context, as much as the individual, which determines what is perceived and recognized to be health and ill health.

REFERENCES

Airey, L., 2003. 'Nae as nice a scheme as it used to be': lay accounts of neighbourhood incivilities and well-being. Health Place 9 (2), 129–137.

Antonovsky, A., 1993. The sense of coherence as a determinant of health. In: Beattie, A., Gott, M., Jones, L. (eds.), Health and Wellbeing: A Reader. Macmillan/Open University, Basingstoke, pp. 202–214.

Awad, A.G., Voruganti, L.N., 2008. The burden of schizophrenia on caregivers: a review. Pharmacoeconomics 26, 149–162.

Blaxter, M., 1990. Health and Lifestyles. Tavistock/Routledge, London.

Carrington, C., 2012. Feeding lesbigay families. In: Counihan, C., Van Esterik, P. (eds.), Food and Culture: A Reader. Routledge, London, pp. 187–210.

Cochrane, A.L., 1972. Effectiveness and Efficiency. Nuffield Provincial Hospitals Trust, London.

Cornwell, J., 1984. Hard-Earned Lives. Tavistock, London.

De Wit, J.B.F., Marijn Stok, F., Smolenski, D.J., de Ridder, D.D.T., de Vet, E., et al., 2015. Food culture in the home environment: family meal practices and values can support healthy eating and self-regulation in young people in four European Countries. Appl. Psychol. Health Well-Being 7 (1), 22–40.

Department of Health, 2010. Healthy Lives, Health People: Our Strategy for Public Health. HM Government, UK. Available at: https://assets.publishing.service.gov.uk/government/uploads/system/uploads/attachment_data/file/216096/dh_127424.pdf.

Douglas, M., 2004. Natural Symbols: Explorations in Cosmology. Routledge, Abingdon, Oxfordshire.

Freidson, F., 1986. Professional Powers: A Study of the Institutionalization of Formal Knowledge. University of Chicago Press, Chicago.

Foucault, M., 1975. Discipline and Punish: The Birth of the Prison. Vintage Books, New York.

Goffman, E., 1968. Stigma: Notes on the Management of a Spoiled Identity. Penguin, Harmondsworth.

Government Office for Science, 2008. Foresight Report: Mental Capital and Wellbeing. Government Office for Science, London. Available at: https://www.gov.uk/government/uploads/system/uploads/attachment_data/file/292450/mental-capital-wellbeing-report.pdf.

Gross, S.E., Shuval, J.T., 2008. On knowing and believing: prenatal genetic screening and resistance to 'risk-medicine'. Health Risk Soc. 10 (6), 549–564.

Hart, G., Wellings, K., 2002. Sexual behaviour and its medicalisation: in sickness and in health. Br. Med. J. 324, 896–900.

Henderson, L., Millett, C., Thorogood, N., 2008. Perceptions of childhood immunization in a minority community: qualitative study. J. R. Soc. Med. 101 (5), 244–251.

Huber, M.I., Knottnerus, J.A., Green, L., van der Horst, H., Jadad, A.R., et al., 2011. How should we define health? Br. Med. J. 343 (4163), 235–237.

Illich, I., 1975. Medical Nemesis, Part One. Calder and Boyers, London.

Kaplan, R.M., Millstein, A., 2019. Contributions of health care to longevity: a review of 4 estimation methods. Ann. Fam. Med. 17 (3), 267–272.

Mansfield, K., 1977. In: Stead, C.K. (ed.), The Letters and Journals of Katherine Mansfield: A Selection. Penguin, Harmondsworth.

Maslow, A.H., 1943. A theory of human motivation. Psychol. Rev. 50 (4), 370–396.

Maslow, A.H., 1970. Motivation and Personality, second edn. Harper and Row, New York.

McKeown, T., 1976. The Role of Medicine: Dream, Mirage or Nemesis? The Nuffield Provincial Hospitals Trust, Oxford. Available at: https://www.nuffieldtrust.org.uk/files/2017-01/1485273106_the-role-of-medicine-web-final.pdf.

New Economics Foundation, 2008. Five ways to wellbeing. London. Available at: https://neweconomics.org/uploads/files/five-ways-to-wellbeing-1.pdf.

New Economics Foundation, 2016. The Happy Planet Index. Available at: https://www.happyplanetindex.org.

Parsons, T., 1951. The Social System. Free Press, Glencoe, IL.

Popay, J., Bennett, S., Thomas, C., Williams, G., Gatrell, A., et al., 2003. Beyond 'beer, fags, egg and chips'? Exploring lay understandings of social inequalities in health. Sociol. Health Illn. 25 (1), 1–23.

Rigby, H., Gubitz, G., Phillips, S., 2009. A systematic review of caregiver burden following stroke. Int. J. Stroke 4, 285–292.

Seedhouse, D., 1986. Health: Foundations for Achievement. John Wiley, Chichester.

Smith, K., Anderson, R., 2017. Understanding lay perspectives on socioeconomic health inequalities in Britain: a meta-ethnography. Sociol. Health Illn. 40 (1), 146–170.

Stead, M., McDermott, L., MacKintosh, A.M., Adamson, A., 2011. Why healthy eating is bad for young people's health: identity, belonging and food? Soc. Sci. Med. 72, 1131–1139.

Tkatch, R., Hudson, J., Katz, A., Berry-Bobovski, L., Vichich, J., et al., 2014. Barriers to cancer screening among Orthodox Jewish women. J. Community Health 39 (6), 1200–1208.

UNICEF, 2013. Report Card 11, Child Well-Being in Rich Countries. Available at: https://www.unicef.org.uk.

Vellone, E., Piras, G., Talucci, C., Cohen, M., 2008. Quality of life of caregivers of people with Alzheimer's disease. J. Adv. Nurs. 61, 222–231.

Wilkinson, R., Pickett, K., 2009. The Spirit Level: Why Equality is Better for Everyone? Penguin, London.

World Health Organization, 1946. Constitution, first edn. World Health Organization, Geneva. Available at: http://www.who.int/governance/eb/who_constitution_en.pdf.

World Health Organization, 1984. Health Promotion: A Discussion Document on the Concept and Principles. World Health Organization Regional Office for Europe, Copenhagen. Available at: http://apps.who.int/iris/bitstream/10665/107835/1/E90607.pdf.

World Health Organization, 1986. Ottawa Charter for Health Promotion. J. Health Promot. 1, 1–4. Available at: http://www.euro.who.int/en/publications/policy-documents/ottawa-charter-for-health-promotion,-1986.

World Health Organization, 1997. 4th International Conference on Health Promotion. New Players for a New Era: Leading Health Promotion into the 21st Century. World Health Organization, Jakarta. Available at: http://www.who.int/healthpromotion/conferences/previous/jakarta/declaration/en/index1.html.

2

Influences on Health

LEARNING OUTCOMES

By the end of this chapter you will be able to:
- identify and critically discuss the social factors influencing health and the mechanisms by which they do so
- understand the associations between socio-economic status and health, gender and health, and ethnicity and health
- have a critical understanding of theories of social determinants of health and explanations for health inequalities
- describe the range of policy interventions to address health inequalities aimed at individuals and populations.

KEY CONCEPTS AND DEFINITIONS

Health inequalities The avoidable and unfair differences in health status between groups of people who are united by their shared socio-economic status or gender rather than by any health-related attributes, for example, medical conditions such as diabetes.

Inequity A lack of equity or fairness.

Social class A group of people united through having the same educational, social or economic status, for example, the working class.

Social determinants Economic and social factors (e.g., income, social class, gender) that have a profound effect on health. These differences are not natural, but are created and maintained by social and economic policies and legislation.

IMPORTANCE OF THE TOPIC

Chapter 1 showed that there is a wide range of meanings attached to the concept of health, and different perspectives are offered by the scientific medical model and social science. It emphasized the importance of social factors in the construction and meaning of health. This chapter shows how the major influences on mortality and morbidity are social and environmental factors. It summarizes the considerable body of research suggesting that the existence of inequalities in health status between groups of people reflects structural inequalities linked to social class, gender and ethnicity.

Reducing health inequalities is a key priority for those working in health and social care because of:
- the economic burden from lost production due to high rates of ill health, the higher welfare payments for those who are sick and the higher burden of disease in deprived neighbourhoods that costs the National Health Service (NHS),
- the unfairness and injustice of avoidable differences in health across the population and between different groups in society,
- the legal and institutional requirements on clinical commissioning groups and local authorities to reduce health inequalities.

DETERMINANTS OF HEALTH

Since the decline in infectious diseases in the 19th and early 20th centuries, there have been considerable changes in the major causes of sickness and death. One hundred years ago, bronchitis was the leading cause of death, killing more than 39,000 people, and tuberculosis and pneumonia were among the 10 leading causes. Ten years ago, cancers (30%), circulatory disease, including coronary heart disease (CHD) and stroke (29%), and respiratory disease (14%) were the major burdens of disease and mortality (Office for National Statistics, 2013). In 2018 the leading cause of death in the UK was dementia and Alzheimer's disease, accounting for 12.7% of all deaths registered, as people live longer and this disease is identified as a cause of death. In England, in July 2020 COVID-19 was the eighth most frequent underlying cause of death, accounting for 2.6% of all deaths.

In the UK, increased longevity with the current average lifespan of 82 years for women and 79 years for men accounts for the increase in degenerative diseases in the population as a whole. Despite the increase in life expectancy, epidemiologists who study the pattern of diseases in society have found that not all groups have the same opportunities for increased longevity and good health, and that there are population patterns which make it possible to predict the likelihood of people from different groups dying prematurely.

As well as differences within countries, there are also differences across countries (www.healthdata.org).

- A child born in Malawi can expect to live for only 47 years, whereas a child born in Japan could expect to live for as long as 83 years.
- Nigeria and Myanmar have about 4 physicians per 10,000, while Norway and Switzerland have 40 per 10,000.
- The maternal mortality ratio in Afghanistan, Somalia and Chad is over 1000 (out of 100,000 live births) while the average figure for the WHO European Region is 21.

In trying to determine what affects health, social scientists and epidemiologists seek to compare at least two variables: firstly, a measure of health, or rather ill health, such as mortality or morbidity; and secondly, a factor such as gender or occupation that could account for the differences in health. Of course, effects on health can be due to several variables interacting together. For example, research into CHD has linked the disease with a large number of factors, including high levels of

---

CASE STUDY 2.1
Differences in Health in the UK

There are differences in health in relation to life expectancy and the prevalence of health conditions, access to healthcare and treatments, quality and experience of care, behavioural risks and social determinants of health, for example, quality of housing. Such differences can be experienced by people in different socio-economic groups, regions, having specific characteristics protected in the law such as sex, ethnicity or disability, or socially excluded groups, for example, those experiencing homelessness or misusing drugs. There are also interactions between these factors which can exacerbate the inequalities experienced.

- Women live around four years longer than men, but the gap has been shrinking and is expected to shrink further over time.
- Men living in deprived areas can expect to live 9.4 years less than men living in less deprived areas.
- People in the most deprived areas spend around a third of their lives in poor health, twice as long as is spent by those in the least deprived areas.
- Black women are five times more likely than White women to experience perinatal mortality.
- Three times as many men as women commit suicide, and rates are particularly high for younger men aged 25 to 44.
- Evidence suggests that lesbian, gay, bisexual and transgender people may have an increased risk of attempted suicide.
- Children from ethnic minorities are up to twice as likely as White children to be involved in road traffic accidents while walking or playing.

Based on Kings Fund, 2020. What are Health Inequalities? Available at: https://www.kingsfund.org.uk/publications/what-are-health-inequalities?utm_source=facebook&utm_medium=social&utm_term=thekingsfund.
Mothers and Babies: Reducing Risk Through Audits and Confidential Enquiries (MBBRACE) report (https://www.npeu.ox.ac.uk/mbrrace-uk/reports).

---

blood cholesterol, high blood pressure, obesity, cigarette smoking and low levels of physical activity. Other research indicates there may be links between CHD and psychosocial factors, such as stress and lack of social support, depression and anger (Marmot and Wilkinson, 2006). Many studies have tried to establish whether there is a coronary-prone personality that is competitive, impatient and hostile (known as type A). We also know that mortality from CHD is higher among lower

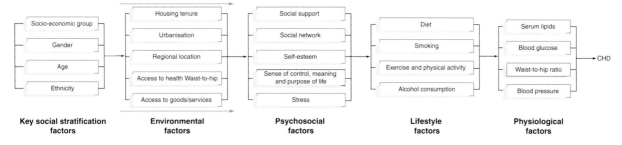

Fig. 2.1 Factors influencing the development of coronary heart disease (*CHD*)

socio-economic groups, among men rather than women and among South Asians (British Heart Foundation, 2012). Fig. 2.2 illustrates in a simple form how health status can be accounted for not by one variable, but by many factors interacting together. It shows that some factors have an independent effect on health while others may be mediated by intervening variables. While physical inactivity, smoking and raised blood cholesterol are the major risk factors for CHD, it is important to look 'upstream' and understand the causes of these risk factors and their roots in the social context of people's lives. Fig. 2.1 shows some of these physiological, social, behavioural and environmental causal pathways to CHD.

What is clear is that ill health does not happen by chance or through bad luck. A report by Lalonde (1974) published in Canada, was influential in identifying four fields which have a major impact on health:

1. Genetic and biological factors which determine an individual's predisposition to disease.
2. Lifestyle factors and health behaviours, such as smoking, which contribute to disease.
3. Environmental factors, such as housing and pollution.
4. The extent and nature of health services.

Genetic factors remain largely unalterable, and what limited scope there is for intervention lies in the medical field. Chapter 1 outlined McKeown and Lowe's (1974) work showing that medical interventions in the form of vaccination had remarkably little impact on mortality rates. This suggests that factors other than the purely biological determine health and well-being, and that probably the greatest opportunities to improve health lie in the environment and individual lifestyles. Fig. 2.2 shows the estimated relative contribution of different factors to health and ill health. Learning Activity 2.1 asks you to generate a list of factors that influence a lifestyle such as eating behaviour or physical activity.

 Learning Activity 2.1   Influences on Health

Lifestyles are frequently the focus of health promotion interventions. Figs. 2.1 and 2.2 show a whole range of factors that may influence behaviour. Take one of the lifestyle factors implicated in CHD, for example, physical activity, and identify the influences on that health behaviour.

Dahlgren and Whitehead (1991) identify 'layers of influence on health' that can be modified (Fig. 2.3):
- personal behaviour and lifestyles, and the knowledge, awareness and skills that can enable change, for example, in diet or physical activity
- support and influence within communities which can sustain or damage health
- living and working conditions, and access to facilities and services
- economic, cultural and environmental conditions, such as pollution levels, standards of living or the labour market.

The specific features and pathways by which societal conditions affect health are termed the social determinants. The social determinants of health refer to factors determined by social policies which affect health, for example, working conditions, housing and the physical environment. The medical model of health, as outlined in Chapter 1, tends to focus on individuals and their biological bodies rather than socially patterned behaviours. For example, an unhealthy diet is linked to many causes of ill health and premature mortality, and most advice is focused on trying to persuade individuals to change their dietary behaviour. Yet social forces are heavily implicated in unhealthy dietary choices, for example, advertising, pricing and availability of healthy products.

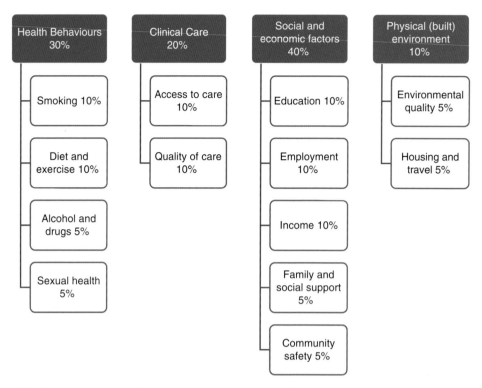

Fig. 2.2 The relative contribution of factors that contribute to population health (Adapted from McGovern, L., Miller, G., Hughes-Cromwick, P., 2014. Health Affairs/RWJF Health Policy Brief. Health Affairs, Princeton, NJ. Available at: https://www.healthaffairs.org/do/10.1377/hpb20140821.404487/full/healthpolicybrief_123.pdf.)

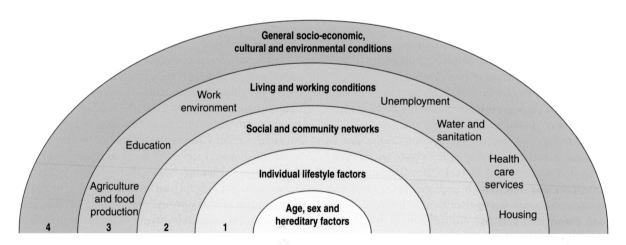

Fig. 2.3 The main determinants of health (Adapted from Dahlgren, G., Whitehead, M., 1991. Policies and Strategies to Promote Social Equity in Health. Institute for Future Studies, Stockholm, p. 23.)

TABLE 2.1   Types of Health Inequalities

Inequality	Example
Determinants of health	Education, employment, income, housing, geographic location
Health outcomes	Life expectancy, quality of life
Access to healthcare services	GP services
Protected characteristic	Age, sex, race, sexual orientation and disability

TABLE 2.2   Social Class Classification

Class	Example
Higher managerial and professional	Company director, bank manager, doctor, lawyer, teacher
Lower managerial and professional	Nurse, police officer, military, creative
Intermediate	Secretary, clerk, assistant
Small employers, own account workers	Taxi driver, restaurant owner, publican, farmer
Lower supervisory, craft and related occupations	Printer, plumber, train driver
Semi-routine occupation	Shop assistant, hairdresser, traffic warden
Routine occupation	Cleaner, courier, road sweeper, waiter
Never worked and long-term unemployed	

From Office for National Statistics, 2020. National Statistics socio-economic classification. Office for National Statistics, Newport. Available at: https://www.ons.gov.uk/methodology/classificationsandstandards/otherclassifications/thenationalstatisticssocioeconomicclassificationnssecrebasedonsoc2010.

There is a large body of research supporting the link between socio-economic status and health in all countries (Commission on Social Determinants of Health, 2008). This research shows there is an undisputed link between lower socio-economic status and poorer health. While describing and documenting health inequalities which are now a key topic in research and policy, addressing such inequalities requires a distinction between inequality and inequity. Inequalities refer to differences between groups which are largely avoidable. If these differences are deemed inequitable, this implies a judgement that they are not only avoidable but also unfair and unjust. Table 2.1 lists some of the types of inequalities in health.

SOCIO-ECONOMIC STATUS AND HEALTH

Most research in the UK which has sought to identify the major determinants of health and ill health has focused on the links between social class and health. The terms social class, social disadvantage, socio-economic status and occupation are often used interchangeably. The classification of social class derives from the Registrar General's scale of five occupational classes, ranging from professionals in class I to unskilled manual workers in class V. This was largely unchanged from 1921 (although class III was divided into manual and non-manual work in 1971). Since 2001 the National Statistics Socio-Economic Classification (NS-SEC) has been used for all official statistics and surveys as shown in Table 2.2.

A report was published of a Department of Health and Social Security working group on inequalities in health (Townsend and Davidson, 1982). Known as the Black Report after the group's chairman, Sir Douglas Black, it provided a detailed study of the relationship between mortality and morbidity and social class. A later government inquiry (Marmot, 2010) drew together data which show that, far from ill health being a matter of bad luck, health and disease are socially patterned, with the more affluent members of society living longer and enjoying better health than disadvantaged social groups. Although the health of the whole population has steadily improved, there is still a strong relationship between socio-economic group and health status.

A wealth of research has examined this relationship between socio-economic status and health status in most Western countries. Simply put, people from lower socio-economic groups have much worse health than those in higher groups. This is known as the social gradient in health and exists in all countries.

Fig. 2.4 shows the stepwise social gradient in health in Europe whereby the poorest have the worst health and the richest enjoy the best health. In general, and in all countries, the lower an individual's socio-economic position, the worse is their health. This health gradient is evident in death rates as well as in reports of ill health. It is also evident across a range of indicators that include infant mortality, disease prevalence, life expectancy and mental health.

Although infant deaths (deaths under 1 year) are declining, an inverse association between the risk of infant death and socio-economic status has been demonstrated across countries. Children from manual

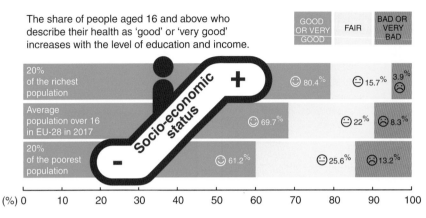

Fig. 2.4 Self-reported health and socio-economic status in Europe (From World Health Organization, 2019. Healthy, Prosperous Lives for All: The European Health Equity Status Report. Available at: http://www.euro.who.int/en/publications/abstracts/health-equity-status-report-2019.)

backgrounds are more likely to die in the first year of life. One of the United Nations Millennium Development Goals was to reduce child mortality by two-thirds between 1990 and 2015. According to this, the UK should have reduced the 1990 infant mortality rate of 7.9 deaths per 1000 live births to 2.6 by 2015. The UK only managed to reduce its infant mortality rate by half, to 3.9 deaths per 1000 live births, so did not meet this target.

Although it is common to talk of 'diseases of affluence', such as CHD, being the major killers in contemporary Europe, most disease categories are more common among lower socio-economic groups. Particularly, large differentials have developed for respiratory disease, lung cancer, accidents and suicide. An exception to this is the death rate from breast cancer, which is evenly distributed across all social groups. Measures of mental health and well-being also reflect a social gradient, as shown in Fig. 2.5.

The pathways by which members of different socio-economic status groups are at risk of such exposures and vulnerabilities are often due to political and economic forces and social stratifications in society as described in Chapter 7. The past decade, the 2010s, has also seen a huge impact on inequalities from firstly, the global financial crisis of 2008, followed by the COVID-19 pandemic (Table 2.3).

INCOME AND HEALTH

Better health is strongly associated with higher income levels. The UK is the world's sixth-largest economy, yet one in five of the UK population live below the official poverty line, meaning that they experience life as a daily struggle and their income is insufficient to meet their needs. The Marmot Review 10 Years On (Institute of Health Equity, 2020) highlighted poverty, particularly child poverty, as a direct risk to health leading, for example, to children not having enough to eat, being unable to heat the home or having limited access to food outlets. Those in better health are more likely to gain and maintain employment and have more options such as having physically active pastimes. Episodes of poverty accumulated over the life course are associated with worse health outcomes.

In low-income countries, infectious diseases such as diarrhoeal illness and malaria are associated with lack of income resulting in lack of access to clean water, food and medical services. Disease then further impoverishes the poor, preventing people from working and incurring high medical costs.

HOUSING AND HEALTH

Frank Dobson, briefly health minister in 1997, remarked: 'everyone with a grain of sense knows that it's bad for your health if you don't have anywhere to live'. The issues of housing stock, dampness, inadequate heating and energy efficiency are recognized as key determinants of health. There is clear evidence of negative physical health effects of toxins within the home, damp and mould, cold indoor temperatures, overcrowding and lack of safety factors and also of negative mental health effects arising from cold indoor temperatures, noise, overcrowding/lack of personal space, and damp and mould (World Health Organization, 2018).

For example, there are 40,000 excess winter deaths (deaths which would not be expected if the average

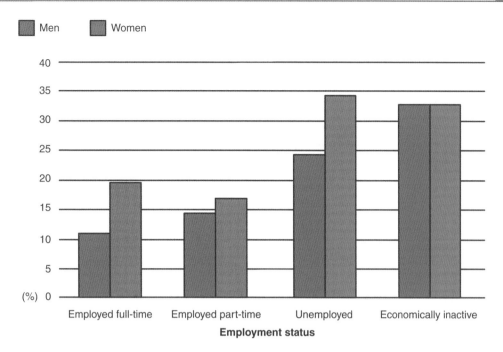

Fig. 2.5 The social gradient of mental ill health (From Mental Health Foundation, 2016. Mental health statistics: poverty. Available at: https://www.mentalhealth.org.uk/statistics/mental-health-statistics-poverty.)

TABLE 2.3   **The Impact of COVID-19 Pandemic on Inequalities**

- Unequal risk of becoming seriously ill or dying from COVID-19 (age, gender, ethnicity, socio-economic status)
- Unequal impact of measures introduced to control the pandemic (children and young people – education and skills)
- Unequal impact on employment prospects (youngest and oldest owners)
- An unequal economic impact (those already economically vulnerable)
- Lockdown – estimated 8% loss of income
- Employees in lower income jobs are more likely to have been placed on furlough (28% in lower quintiles compared to 17% in top quintile)
- Doubling in food parcels
- Sharp increases in non-payment of bills
- 3 million applications for universal credit

From Health Foundation, 2020. Will Covid 19 be a watershed moment for health inequalities? Available at: https://www.health.org.uk/publications/long-reads/will-covid-19-bea-watershed-moment-for-health-inequalities#lf-section59576-anchor. Tinson, A., 2020. Living in Poverty Was Bad for Your Health Before COVID-19. Health Foundation, London.

death rate for the rest of the year applied in winter) each year in the UK. These are attributable to:

- energy efficiency
- level of occupancy
- income
- cost of fuel.

Cold and damp housing has been shown to contribute to illness. Children living in damp houses are likely to have higher rates of respiratory illness, symptoms of infection and stress. These will be exacerbated by overcrowding. The high accident rates of children in lower socio-economic groups are associated with high-density housing where there is a lack of play space and opportunities for parental supervision. Psychological and practical difficulties accompany living in high-rise flats and isolated housing estates, which may adversely affect the health of women at home and older people.

EMPLOYMENT AND HEALTH

Work as a social determinant of health is important to consider because:

- it determines income levels
- it affects self-esteem
- the type of employment may directly affect health.

RESEARCH EXAMPLE 2.1
Children, Poverty and Health

A systematic review of 34 studies, mainly from America but including some British research, found a strong causal link between household income and children's achievements in education, their well-being and positive behavioural outcomes. Children in richer households were more likely to do better in all spheres of life, including education and health. The link between household income and childhood well-being appears to be due to money rather than any other confounding factors such as parental expectations. While a parent's level of education, attitude towards bringing up children and other parental factors have a bearing, research shows that having more money has a direct positive impact on children's social and behavioural development and educational achievement. The evidence is strongest for a link between income and educational outcomes. Conversely, reductions in family income, including benefit cuts, are likely to have wide-ranging negative effects. Money seems to have more of an effect among low-income families.

Research evidence supports two theories as to why income matters so much. The family stress model focuses on the stress and anxiety caused by low income, while the investment model focuses on parental ability to invest in services and goods that support child development. Research findings are more supportive of the family stress model than the investment model.

Based on Cooper, K., Stewart, K., 2013. Does Money Affect Children's Outcomes? Joseph Rowntree Foundation. Available at: https://www.jrf.org.uk/report/does-money-affect-children%E2%80%99s-outcomes.

The traditional focus of occupational health has been to consider how particular types of employment carry high occupational health risks. This may be because of the risk of accidents (e.g., in mining), exposure to hazardous substances or stress. Some occupations encourage lifestyles which may be damaging to health, for example, publicans are at high risk of developing cirrhosis.

There has been considerable interest in how the psychosocial work environment can affect health (Marmot et al., 2006). Most research has identified high demands and low control over work decisions contributing to job stress and cardiovascular risk. These factors, together with the amount of social support people get at work, have been confirmed in workplace studies in many developed countries (see Chapter 15 for further discussion). There is also a considerable body of evidence, mostly gathered in the 1980s, that unemployment can damage health (McLean et al., 2005). It is, however, uncertain whether unemployment itself leads to a deterioration in health or whether it is the poverty associated with unemployment which contributes to the poor health of the unemployed. Learning Activity 2.2 asks you to consider how and in what ways being unemployed and high rates of unemployment affect individual health and the health of populations.

 Learning Activity 2.2   Unemployment and Health

Consider the following evidence concerning the effects of unemployment on health. What could account for this relationship?

- The unemployed report higher rates of mental ill health, including depression, anxiety and sleep disturbance.
- Suicide and parasuicide rates are twice as high among the unemployed as among the employed.
- The death rates among the unemployed are at least 20% higher than expected after adjustment for social class and age.
- The unemployed have higher rates of bronchitis and ischaemic heart disease than the employed.
- Over 60% of unemployed people smoke, compared to 30% of employed people.

GENDER AND HEALTH

Gender refers to the social categorization of people as men or women, and the social meaning and beliefs about sexual difference. Some of the sex differences in morbidity have been viewed as an artefact of measurement of the use of health services. Women are more likely to report illness, as they are less likely to be in full-time employment and have easier access to primary care, or because they are more inclined to take care of their health, resulting in increased consultation rates (Wang et al., 2013). Nor is there a consistent pattern of women's greater willingness to consult, for example, women are no more likely than men to visit their general practitioners (GPs) for musculoskeletal, respiratory or digestive problems.

There are several explanations for these differences:

- biological explanations focusing on reproductive roles
- materialist and structural explanations focusing on different social roles

---

RESEARCH EXAMPLE 2.2
The Whitehall Studies

The Whitehall studies are important because they have followed employees of the British Civil Service over a number of years and have shed light on the causation of ill health among employees. The original Whitehall study began in 1967 and studied the careers and health of 18,000 men. The study found that premature death was more prevalent among men in the lowest employment grades. Furthermore, it appeared to be the lower employment status rather than any other confounding factors (such as smoking) that was responsible for the increased mortality rate. The second Whitehall study, started in 1985, recruited over 10,000 employees, including women, and has collected data from 10 cohorts of civil servants. The study sought to clarify risk factors for ill health and premature mortality. Consistent findings are that psychosocial factors (e.g., work-related stress and conflict, unfairness at work, domestic conflict) make a significant contribution to poor health outcomes. The study also found that environmental changes were more effective than targeting individuals employees to change their behaviour, for example, to quit smoking. The Whitehall studies support the view that social hierarchy is an important factor impacting on health, and that the more subordinate individuals lower down in the hierarchy suffer increased ill health and premature death due to their low status. The impact of social position is greater than that of individual risk behaviours such as smoking.

More details are available at: https://www.ucl.ac.uk/epidemiology-health-care/research/epidemiology-and-public-health/research/whitehall-ii.

- social constructionist explanations focusing on expectations and behaviours associated with masculinity and femininity.

The biological explanation suggests that women are more resistant to infection and benefit from the protective effect of oestrogen, accounting for their lower mortality rates. Paradoxically, female hormones and the female reproductive system are claimed to render women more liable to physical and mental ill health. But biological explanations are unable to account for the social class difference in women's health, whereby women in professional and managerial social classes experience better health than women in lower socio-economic groups. It is also important to note that greater female longevity only arose in the 20th century, and is mostly attributable to the dramatic decline in infectious disease mortality and a decline in the number of births. It is not evident in low-income countries.

Lifestyle explanations argue that women are socialized to be passive, dependent and sick. Women readily adopt the sick role because it fits with preconceived notions of feminine behaviour. Men, by contrast, are encouraged to be aggressive and risk-taking, both at work and in their leisure time. The higher rates for accidents and alcoholism among men are cited as evidence for this. Men are far less likely to take part in weight-management programmes or the national bowel cancer screening programme, or to set quit dates for smoking cessation. Learning Activity 2.3 probes you to find some explanations why men are less likely to engage with primary care.

Learning Activity 2.3 Men's Health

What could account for why men under the age of 45 visit their GPs only half as often as women (www.menshealthforum.org.uk)?

More recently, the focus has been on the distinct roles and behaviours of men and women in a given culture, dictated by that culture's gender norms and values, and how these give rise to gender differences in health. Globally, there is considerable concern about how women, because of gender norms, are disempowered from, for example, receiving healthcare because they cannot travel alone to a clinic or protecting themselves against HIV because of their male partners' promiscuity or refusal to use a condom.

In most societies, women, when compared with men, tend to have:
- lower status
- lower income
- lower power
- limited access to financial and other assets
- lower educational status
- lower levels of participation in legal and political institutions, and hence less influence on decision-making
- limited access to work
- increased likelihood of being victims of domestic violence.

Yet women often have greater health needs (e.g., during pregnancy and child-related care). In most cases, women take the leading role in caring for children and dependants, and are also expected to look after the house and work in the fields producing food.

CASE STUDY 2.2

Gender-Based Interventions: Football Fans in Training

The prevalence of obesity in men in the UK is among the highest in Europe, but men are less likely than women to use existing weight-loss programmes. Developing weight-management programmes which are appealing and acceptable to men is a public health priority. Football Fans in Training (FFIT), a men-only weight-management programme delivered to groups of men at top professional football clubs, encourages men to lose weight by working with, not against, cultural ideals of masculinity. The setting enabled men to join a weight-management programme in circumstances that felt 'right' rather than threatening to them as men. FFIT is an example of how to facilitate health promotion activities in a way that is consistent with, rather than challenging, common ideals of masculinity.

Based on Wyke, S., Hunt, K., Gray, C.M., Elisabeth, F., Christopher, B., et al., 2015. Football Fans in Training (FFIT): a randomised controlled trial of a gender-sensitised weight loss and healthy living programme for men – end of study report. Available at: https://www.ncbi.nlm.nih.gov/books/NBK273998/.

HEALTH OF ETHNIC MINORITIES

Race commonly refers to a biological marker of difference assigned to a group of people who are recognized as sharing common physical or physiognomic characteristics and/or a common lineage of descent, such as 'Asian' or 'Chinese'. Essentialist racism emphasizes race difference in hierarchical terms of biologic inequality, and 'scientific' categories such as the Aryan superiority assumed by the Nazis over the Jews. A racial logic becomes a system of differentiation based upon the ascription of people to specific categories on the basis of assumed biological, physiognomic or cultural differences, usually bestowing privilege to one group. It becomes a means of exclusion and subordination, and a way of making a group of people inferior within society. In extreme cases this is demonstrated by extermination, for example, in Rwanda and Nazi Germany.

The concept of race was largely discredited in Europe and replaced by reference to ethnicity, defined as the group a person belongs to because of culture, language, diet, country of origin or religion. Ethnicity can be actively constructed through self-identification but may also be combined with racial meanings, for example, 'White Irish'. In the UK public discourse refers to BAME groups,

meaning Black, Asian and Minority Ethnic groups, as a way of distinguishing the experience of these groups as different from that of White groups. A government website recommends when writing about ethnicity not to use the term BAME, but rather 'people from a Black Caribbean background' which was preferred in user research (https://www.ethnicity-facts-figures.service.gov.uk/style-guide/writing-about-ethnicity).

There are significant challenges relating to completeness and consistency of data on ethnicity and health outcomes. Ethnicity is inconsistently recorded in hospitals and primary care, and ethnic group was not recorded on death certificates in England until October 2020, in response to COVID-19. Public Health England (2018) outline some evidence on ethnicity and health outcomes which are also represented in an infographic by the NHS Race and Health Observatory (https://www.nhsrho.org/publications/ethnic-health-inequalities-in-the-uk/).

- **General poor health:** Some groups, notably individuals identifying as Gypsy or Irish Traveller, and to a lesser extent those identifying as Bangladeshi, Pakistani or Irish, stand out as having poor health across a range of indicators. By contrast, Chinese people have better rates of health than White British people.
- **Poor self-rated health:** A study of adults aged over 60 in the UK found that minority ethnic groups are more likely than White people to report limiting health and poor, self-rated health, after accounting for social and economic disadvantage.
- **Type 2 diabetes:** National Institute of Health and Care Excellence (NICE) concluded that people from BAME groups are at an equivalent risk of type 2 diabetes, other health conditions or mortality, at a lower body mass index (BMI) than the White European population.
- **Cardiovascular disease:** The associations between cardiovascular disease and ethnicity in the UK is complex; a 2017 study (Patel et al., 2017) found as expected, based on previous studies, a substantial predominance of CHD presentations in South Asian people and a predominance of stroke presentations in Black patients.
- **Mental health:** BAME people are over-represented in mental health inpatients.
- **Maternity:** Asian women are more than twice as likely as White women to die during or soon after pregnancy. Black women are five times more likely than White women to experience perinatal mortality (Mothers and Babies Reducing Risk through Audits

and Confidential Enquiries (MBBRACE) reports at https://www.npeu.ox.ac.uk/mbrrace-uk).

That particular diseases, poor perceived health or premature deaths are more common in ethnic minority groups is a complex issue found in many countries such as Australia, New Zealand, South Africa, Brazil, the USA and the UK. In the past, explanations tended to focus on simple differences in culture.

The factors influencing ethnic health inequalities were summarized by Bhopal (2014) as:

- genetic and biological factors, for example, birth weight, body composition
- culture, for example, diet
- social education and economic status, for example, knowledge of biology and health influences, languages spoken and read, poverty, employment
- environmental, for example, before and after migration
- lifestyle, for example, behaviours in relation to diet, alcohol and tobacco
- access to and concordance with healthcare advice, willingness to seek health and social services, and use of complementary/alternative methods of care or treatment.

Socio-economic factors have a profound impact, but it is important not to put all members of ethnic minorities into one disadvantaged category. More data would enable us to find out how many people from ethnic minority groups are disadvantaged, and in what way. It would also then be possible to determine whether the poor health of Black and ethnic minority groups is associated with the low-income, poor working conditions or unemployment and poor housing shared by those in lower social classes, or whether there is, in addition, ill health resulting from other factors, known as intersectionality. Racism in service delivery, either directly or through the ethnocentrism of services which are based on the needs of the majority, is also often invoked as the explanation for health inequalities. Learning Activity 2.4 tries to reflect on your practice, personal experience or your reading about whether healthcare differs in its delivery according to the patient's race or ethnicity.

Learning Activity 2.4   Healthcare and Ethnicity

In your experience or reading, do you think that healthcare differs according to the ethnicity of the patient?

CASE STUDY 2.3
Racial and Ethnic Inequalities and COVID-19

The pandemic in the UK exposed substantial differences between people of different ethnic origins, both within and between groups.

People who may be disadvantaged by an inability to self-isolate include Gypsies, seasonal migrants in communal accommodation and asylum seekers and refugees. Black and minority ethnic groups have the following characteristics (Public Health England, 2020):

- **High employment rates in the NHS and other key worker organizations**, which may increase the risk of infection to individuals and their families and also create additional anxieties around childcare, for example, 26.4% Transport for London (TfL) staff, 45% of NHS staff in London and 67% of staff providing social care for adults are from Black and minority ethnic groups.
- **Higher likelihood of multi-generational households**, which could have some positive impacts in terms of social isolation and mental health, but may also increase the risk of infection. Twenty-five percent of over 70s live with another adult under 60.
- **Higher rates of underlying illnesses**, especially diabetes and cardiovascular disease, which may mean there are higher numbers in shielded groups and may indicate a need for some specialized advice and support.
- **Barriers to effective communication in health and social care settings, because of language, stigma, prejudice or cultural differences**, are likely to lead to negative outcomes. This is particularly the case when people are attending primary care settings unaccompanied by family or friends. This may require tailored action such as translation services and translated materials, including in easy-read formats.
- **Support for ethnic minority groups**; people from ethnic minorities were more likely than indigenous White people to say that they did not have support in times of crisis.

PLACE AND HEALTH

In the 1980s mortality rates increased steadily in the UK, moving from south-east to the north-west, with a north–south divide for most diseases. This divide seemed to be associated with poverty and disadvantage. For example, Glasgow's Shettleston, a poor and deprived area, had twice the national average mortality rate. In the UK, Danny Dorling has written extensively on the impact of place on health (http://www.dannydorling.org/?page_id=70). One obvious explanation for geographic differences in death rates might be differences in the distribution of socio-economic groups with areas with high mortality rates having a greater proportion of people in lower socio-economic groups. Increasingly, the effect of place on health has been seen as more complex, including not only the socio-economic characteristics of individuals concentrated in particular places but also the local physical and social environment and the shared norms and traditions that might promote or inhibit health.

Fig. 2.6 shows the ways in which different factors discussed in this chapter impact on health and how these factors stem from the wider determinants of health and interact and reinforce each other. The report from Public Health England (2019) emphasizes the importance of place-based approaches that address these wider determinants at a local level.

EXPLAINING HEALTH INEQUALITIES

In the context of health and healthcare, the term 'inequalities' is mainly used to refer to differences that arise from socio-economic factors, including income, work,

housing and location of residence. The documented differences are sometimes also attributed to the adoption of unhealthy lifestyles. You may believe that people in lower socio-economic groups choose more unhealthy ways of living, or you may believe they have low incomes which prevent them from adopting a healthy lifestyle and cause them to live in unhealthy conditions. There is a continuing debate over this question, and no simple answer. Explanations for health inequalities focus on cultural/behavioural, materialist/structural and psychosocial explanations which suggest that adverse environmental conditions at different points in the life course can lead to ill health.

Health Inequalities as a Consequence of Lifestyles

This argument suggests that the social distribution of ill health is linked to differences in the prevalence of risk behaviours. These risk behaviours – smoking; high alcohol consumption; lack of exercise; and high-fat, high-sugar and high-salt diets – are more common among lower socio-economic groups. For example, although smoking has decreased in all social classes over the last 20 years, there are still major differences in the proportion of

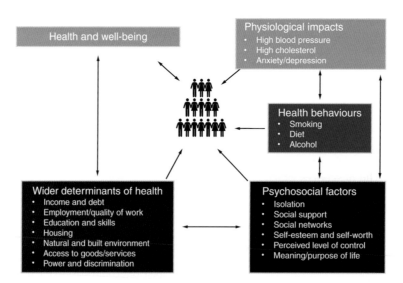

Fig 2.6 The causes of health inequalities (From Public Health England, 2019. Place based approaches for reducing health inequalities. Available at: https://www.gov.uk/government/publications/health-inequalities-place-based-approaches-to-reduce-inequalities/place-based-approaches-for-reducing-health-inequalities-main-report.)

smokers in each socio-economic group: in 2019, 25.4% of those in manual occupations smoked compared to 10.2% smokers from managerial and professional backgrounds (Office for National Statistics, 2019).

Behaviour cannot, however, be separated from the social context in which it takes place. Many studies on smoking have shown how the decision to smoke is a coping strategy to deal with the stress associated with poverty and isolation (Hiscock et al., 2012). The decision to smoke *is* a choice, but it is not taken through recklessness or ignorance; it is rather a choice between 'health evils' – stress versus smoking.

As spending on tobacco consumes a relatively high proportion of the household income for smokers with low incomes, tobacco addiction can lock people into poverty. Almost half of all the children living in poverty in the UK – around 1.1 million children – live with at least 1% who smokes (Belvin et al., 2015). Those from higher socio-economic groups also find it easier to quit smoking: 68.6% compared to 50.9% for those from lower socio-economic groups (Office for National Statistics, 2019). Although raising the price of tobacco is an effective measure for reducing smoking rates, it also has the most impact on those who are already poor and may continue to smoke. Learning Activity 2.5 reflects on your attitudes towards patients or clients who smoke. Understanding your own unconscious biases is important because they can affect your interactions with a patient or client or the priorities you set for interventions.

 Learning Activity 2.5   Attitudes to Lifestyle Inequalities

Smoking is the biggest single cause of the differences in death rates between rich and poor people. Which of the following views comes closest to your own?

'Poor people bring ill health upon themselves. They don't care about their health. If they are so poor, how can they afford to smoke and drink and eat junk food?'

'People's use of tobacco and alcohol is to a large extent determined by their social relations and networks, which in turn affect their self-esteem and levels of stress. Tobacco offers a prop of sorts.'

Some writers claim that there are cultural differences between social groups in their attitudes towards health and protecting their health for the future. Thus, giving up cigarettes, a form of deferred gratification, is more likely to appeal to middle-class people who, as we saw in Chapter 1, may have a stronger locus of control and are more likely to believe that they determine the course of their lives. People in lower socio-economic groups, who may struggle to get by each day, focus on current needs over long-term plans, and may have a fatalistic view of health, believing it to be a matter of luck. These attitudes are passed on from generation to generation. This phenomenon is referred to as the 'culture of poverty' or 'cycle of deprivation'. According to such views, ill health can be explained in terms of the characteristics of poor people and their inadequacy and incompetence. In 1986 Edwina Currie, a newly appointed health minister, caused a storm of controversy by suggesting that the high levels of premature death, permanent sickness and low birth weights in the northern regions were due to ignorance and people failing to realize that they had some control over their lives.

A behavioural explanation, which sees lifestyles and cultural influences determining health, has considerable appeal to any government that wants to reduce public expenditure. If individuals are seen as responsible for their own health, government inactivity is legitimized. Such viewpoints, which are particularly associated with neoliberal governments (see Chapter 7), have been widely criticized as victim-blaming, in that people are seen as being responsible for factors which disadvantage them but over which they have no control.

Health Inequalities as a Consequence of the Life Course

This explanation for health inequalities suggests that early life circumstances predict future morbidity and mortality rates. There are cumulative effects of both material and psychosocial hazards over the life course of an individual that explain observed differences in health and life expectancy, as shown in Fig. 2.7.

- The early life environment has a significant impact on the later health of the adult, regardless of other health-related factors. For example, foetal exposure to passive smoking (due to maternal smoking or maternal exposure to passive smoking) may impact on foetal health and result in low birth weight. Low birth weight is linked to poorer health outcomes (e.g., greater mortality from CHD, stroke and respiratory disease) in adult life.

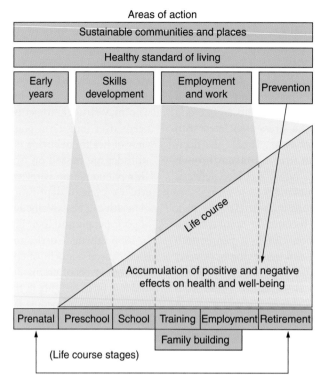

Areas of action

Sustainable communities and places

Healthy standard of living

| Early years | Skills development | Employment and work | Prevention |

Life course

Accumulation of positive and negative effects on health and well-being

| Prenatal | Preschool | School | Training | Employment | Retirement |

Family building

(Life course stages)

Fig. 2.7 The social gradient of health across the life course (From Marmot, M., 2010. Fair Society, Healthy Lives. DH-Publisher, London, p. 31; © The Marmot Review, Marmot Review Secretariat, Department for Epidemiology and Public Health. University College, London.)

- The early life environment of an individual is linked to later lifestyle factors which have a direct impact on health. For example, a lower socio-economic family background is associated with poorer educational attainment and poorer housing, job security and work opportunities. Early interventions can change this association. Interventions in the early years can help individuals achieve better educational, work and social outcomes (e.g., home ownership, higher incomes), which in turn are associated with better health outcomes.

- The environment to which individuals are exposed is also an important factor in determining their health status. Exposure to a health-damaging environment, for example, smoky indoor areas, will have a cumulative effect on an individual's health. The intensity and duration of the exposure are directly linked to later outcomes, for example, mortality from cancer, CHD, strokes or respiratory illness.

The 1958 birth cohort study, which follows a group of individuals from childhood to adulthood,

demonstrates that socio-economic status is linked to factors such as low birth weight and height. Childhood development in all spheres (physical, psychological, social and intellectual) is sensitive to the wider environment and is an important determinant of health status in later life (Graham and Power, 2004). Learning Activity 2.6 asks you to consider how your physical and mental health has been influenced throughout your life, what were the important factors or events and when they took place. Consider also whether there were any opportunities for enhancing or improving your health and well-being.

 Learning Activity 2.6   The Life Course and Health

Chart your own life course in relation to health
- Are there any external factors which influenced your and your family's health?
- Were there any personal events which affected your physical and psychological well-being?

Health Inequalities as a Consequence of Psychosocial Factors

There is a growing body of evidence demonstrating that it is relative inequalities in income and material resources, coupled with the resulting social exclusion and marginalization, which are linked to poor health (Wilkinson, 1996; Wilkinson and Pickett, 2010). The key evidence on this comes from international data on income distribution and national mortality rates. In high-income countries, it is not the richest nations which have the best health, but the most egalitarian, such as Sweden. While the exact mechanisms linking social inequality to ill health are uncertain, it is likely that social cohesion – as measured by levels of trust – provides the causal link between the two. The most plausible explanation for income inequality's apparent effect on health and social problems is 'status anxiety'. This suggests that income inequality is harmful because it places people in a hierarchy which increases status competition and causes stress, leading to poor health and other negative outcomes (Wilkinson and Pickett, 2010). Healthy egalitarian societies are more socially cohesive and have a stronger community life with greater social capital.

The degree to which an individual is integrated into society and has a social support network has been shown to have a significant impact on health. Wilkinson and Pickett (2010) demonstrate that people with stronger social relationships are half as likely to die as those with weaker social ties. Indicators of social relationships and networking, such as marital status, feeling lonely, size of social network and participation in social activities, are as important to health as smoking, and much more important to survival than heavy drinking, physical activity or obesity. There are lots of different views about what constitutes a healthy society from access to services to the quality of the environment. Learning Activity 2.7 asks you to consider and discuss what are the characteristics of living in a healthy society.

 Learning Activity 2.7   Characteristics of a Healthy Society

The quality of the social life of a society is one of the most powerful determinants of health (and this, in turn, is very closely related to the degree of income equality)

Wilkinson (1996, p. 5)

Which of the following, in your view, reflects the characteristics of life in a healthy society?

1. High level of civic activities.
2. High gross national product.
3. Low crime rates.
4. High percentage of adults receiving a university education.
5. High levels of employment.
6. Narrow differences in income.
7. Sense of social solidarity and cohesion.

The negative emotional experience that arises from living in an unequal society is illustrated in the second Whitehall study (Marmot et al., 2006), a longitudinal study of civil servants and their experience of ill health (described in Research Example 2.2). Irrespective of health behaviour, those in control of their working lives (those in higher grades) are less likely to suffer from CHD, diabetes and metabolic syndrome.

Health Inequalities as a Consequence of Material Disadvantage

This explanation argues that the distribution of health and ill health in the population reflects a profoundly unequal distribution of resources in society. Thus those who experience ill health are those who are lower in the social hierarchy, are least educated, and have least money and fewest resources. Low income may be the result of unemployment or ill-paid hazardous occupations. It can lead to poor housing in polluted and unsafe environments with few opportunities to build social support networks; in turn such conditions lead to poor health. Lack of money can make it difficult for households to implement what they may know to be healthy choices.

- People on low incomes eat more processed foods, which are much higher in saturated fats and salt.
- They also eat a smaller variety of foods, due to the need to buy cheaper in bulk and from fear of potential waste.
- People living on state benefits eat less fruit and vegetables, which are less widely available and relatively expensive.

Absolute poverty is the inability to meet basic human needs such as access to food, shelter, warmth and safety. More than a billion people worldwide live in such extreme poverty. Relative poverty is determined by the standards of the rest of the society in which the individual lives. Although a person's basic needs may be met, relative poverty means they may be unable to afford any social participation and are then more likely to suffer from a range of physical health problems, for example, CHD, as well as social and emotional health problems such as stress and depression, marital breakdown and addiction to drugs or alcohol.

CASE STUDY 2.4
Food Banks

Across Europe there has been a huge rise in the number of people relying on food banks for emergency supplies. According to the Trussell Trust, nearly two million people, including nearly 400,000 children, received at least three days' emergency food in 2019. Germany's Tafel network of 940 food banks gave food to 1.65 million people. In France, the Restos du Coeur gave out 130 million meals. It is estimated that 2.8% of households in the UK are severely food insecure with adults skipping meals so children can eat. In all European countries, the reliance on emergency food is said to be triggered by low wages and limited welfare with no crisis payments. Although there are widespread efforts to ensure that food reaching expiration dates is given to those who need it, the UN's former Special Rapporteur on the right to food and 57 other prominent academic and nongovernmental organization voices have warned we should never get used to the idea of 'leftover' food for 'left behind people'.

Trussell Trust, 2019. State of Hunger: A Study of Poverty and Food Insecurity in the UK. Available at: https://www.stateofhunger.org/wp-content/uploads/2019/11/State-of-Hunger-Report-November2019-Digital.pdf.

Poverty is just one aspect of socio-economic disadvantage, and is associated with other factors:

- having a family to provide for
- being unable to work due to incapacity or illness
- being geographically isolated from services or supports
- being a young person leaving the care system
- being a single parent
- living in substandard housing or experiencing homelessness
- lacking skills.

Health Inequalities as a Consequence of Limited Healthcare

A common response to the evidence of health inequalities is to see these as a consequence of restricted access to services. The intention of the NHS – to provide a universal service freely available to all – might have been expected to reduce inequalities in health status. Yet in the early 1970s a GP writing in *The Lancet* put forward the radical view that good healthcare tends to vary inversely with the needs of the population:

In areas with most sickness and death, GPs have more work, larger lists, less hospital support and

inherit more clinically ineffective traditions of consultation than in the healthiest areas; and the hospital doctors shoulder heavier caseloads with less staff and equipment, more obsolete buildings and suffer recurrent crises in the availability of beds and replacement of staff. These trends can be summed up as the Inverse Care Law: that the availability of good medical care tends to vary inversely with the needs of the population served.

Tudor Hart (1971)

Equality of access requires that, for different communities:

- travel distance to facilities is equal
- transport and communication services are equal
- waiting times are equal
- patients are equally informed about the availability and effectiveness of treatments
- charges are equal (with equal ability to pay)
- the quality of services offered does not vary between groups or locations.

Ensuring that everyone can access services is a key priority, and Learning Activity 2.8 asks you to find explanations for the inequalities that exist.

 Learning Activity 2.8   Equality of Access to Healthcare Services

Even in the UK, where services are universally available and not dependent on the ability to pay, some groups are more able to access services than others. Why is this?

There is evidence of variation in the quality and quantity of care available to people in different social groups, and between regions and different ethnic groups (House of Commons Health Committee, 2009). However, since medical care has had little impact on the overall death rate from heart disease or cancers, and probably only about 5% of deaths are preventable through medical treatment, it must be concluded that differences in health status are not wholly attributable to variations in the amount and type of care received.

REDUCING INEQUALITIES IN HEALTH

As we have seen in this chapter, health inequalities are unjust and preventable health differences that occur between groups. The fundamental causes of health inequalities lie in the varied distribution of resources that result in differences in the quality and availability of housing, access to services and social and cultural resources. These are usually described in terms of socio-economic status but can also arise from other characteristics such as age, race and sex. Taken together these shape individual exposure to factors which damage health and accumulate over time. This results in the effects described – the unequal and unfair distribution of health, ill health (morbidity) and death (mortality). Less equal societies, with greater differences in the distribution of income, power and wealth across the population, are associated with doing less well over a range of health and social outcomes including violence and homicide, teenage pregnancy, drug use and social mobility (Wilkinson and Pickett, 2010).

In England, the Marmot Review, *Fair Society, Healthy Lives* (Marmot, 2010), emphasizes the 'causes of the causes' of health inequalities, and the need to address these wider determinants. To tackle inequalities and reduce the steepness of the social gradient, the Marmot Review recommends actions of sufficient scale and intensity to be universal but also proportionately targeted. Strategies need to target those at the lower end of the gradient as well as throughout the whole of society, according to the level of disadvantage.

The report specifically proposed action on six policy objectives.
1. Give every child the best start in life.
2. Enable all children, young people and adults to maximize their capabilities and have control over their lives.
3. Create fair employment and good work for all.
4. Ensure a healthy standard of living for all.
5. Create and develop healthy and sustainable places and communities.
6. Strengthen the role and impact of ill-health prevention.

While health inequalities are shown in the social gradient across the whole population, focusing on improving the health of the most disadvantaged groups by improving social conditions, reducing risk factors and improving life opportunities is the commonly adopted approach. Place-based initiatives are often used to target low-income households or specific groups such as people who are homeless. However, place-based approaches may actually miss reaching the most disadvantaged individuals, as many low-income households and unemployed people do not live in the most disadvantaged areas.

Interventions to tackle health inequalities need to address the complexity of how health inequalities are created and perpetuated. For example, efforts to tackle inequalities of health status associated with behavioural risks (such as poor diets) should address the wider network of factors that influence these behaviours at:
• the structural level, for example, trade policy, food-labelling regulations, advertising restrictions, food fortification
• the local/community level, for example, access to affordable healthy food through food gardens, free fruit and vegetables in school, cooperative food outlets
• the individual/family level, for example, nutrition education in school or during pregnancy; mass-media campaigns, for example, to reduce salt, weight-loss programmes.

Proportionate universal approaches are interventions that are delivered to the whole population, with the 'intensity' adjusted according to the needs of specific groups (for example, some groups may need more frequent help and advice). This type of approach can help to reduce the social gradient of ill health and benefit everybody (Macdonald et al., 2014). Learning Activity 2.9 asks you to find or suggest indicators or measures that would show the successful tackling of inequalities. A good indicator is relevant to the issue, measures what it claims to measure (is valid)and has available data.

 Learning Activity 2.9   Indicators for Tackling Health Inequalities

Give an indicator for the successful tackling of each of the following:
• education
• economic stability
• social and community context
• health and healthcare
• neighbourhood and the built environment.

Although many health promoters may feel powerless to effect change at a macro-structural level, it is possible to address health inequalities in planning health promotion interventions, as the previous examples illustrate. One of the central tasks for health promoters is to acknowledge socio-economic factors as crucial in determining individual and population health. The last learning activity (Learning Activity 2.10) in this chapter poses a challenge by asking you to consider and discuss what, in your view, would bring about the greatest public health improvement.

 Learning Activity 2.10   What Improves Health?

In your experience, what long-term social policy initiatives would be most effective in bringing about an improvement in the health of your clients or patients, or people you know?

CONCLUSION

Health promotion is not a purely technical activity. As we have seen, even identifying the causes of ill health will lead to political judgements being made. In any area of work or discipline, there will always be debate about what constitutes good practice. It is important to clarify your thinking and where you stand, because it will affect your views on the purpose of health promotion and what would be appropriate health promotion activities. It is also important that you share these thoughts with colleagues and clients to reach a common understanding of the ideals upon which health promotion activities are based.

In practice, behavioural and structural explanations are often aligned to the right or left of the political spectrum, and have become linked with very different policies and approaches to health promotion. The behavioural approach, which focuses on individual lifestyles, has informed much of health education because it suggests that information, advice or mass-media messages can change behaviours such as smoking or sexual activity. A structural approach, which sees health as determined by social and economic conditions which reflect the unequal distribution of power and resources in society, requires the health promoter to become involved in political activity.

There are three main reasons why reducing inequalities is part of the practice of all health promoters (Public Health England, 2019).

1. Because inequalities are a burden on society, costing society £31 billion in lost production and costing the NHS an additional 22% per woman and 16% per man in the most deprived areas.
2. Because reducing inequalities is a legal requirement of Clinical Commissioning Groups and Local Authorities and is also part of the NHS Long-Term Plan.
3. Because reducing inequalities is a moral imperative: the gap in life expectancy and quality of life between the most affluent and poorest people is unjust and preventable.

REFLECTIONS ON PRACTICE

- Why is improving health equity so central to the practice of those working in public health and health promotion?
- What actions to improve health equity in clinical practice and at the community level have you seen?
- How would you assess the impact of such actions in relation to:
  - patients' perceived health
  - social support
  - social outcomes?

SUMMARY

This chapter has reviewed the evidence concerning health differences in the population and the physical, social and environmental variables that are implicated in ill health: poverty, unemployment, inadequate housing, stressful and dangerous working conditions, lack of social support and air and water pollution. It has considered the ways in which risk factors associated with personal behaviour, for example, smoking, nutrition and exercise are influenced by the social environment.

Several explanations for inequalities in health have been discussed. None offers a complete explanation, but the chapter concludes that there is sufficient evidence to point to social and economic factors determining health. It argues that disadvantage can give rise to, or exacerbate, health-damaging behaviours such as smoking or poor nutrition, and so health behaviours should not be separated from their social context.

FURTHER READING AND RESOURCES

Commission on Social Determinants of Health (CSDH), 2008. Closing the Gap in a Generation: Health Equity Through Action on the Social Determinants of Health. Final Report of the Commission on Social Determinants of Health. World Health Organization, Geneva. Available at: http://apps.who.int/iris/bitstream/10665/43943/1/9789241563703_eng.pdf.

Marmot, M., Wilkinson, R.G. (eds.), 2006. Social Determinants of Health, second edn. Oxford University Press, Oxford.
An overview of the factors known to affect health including unemployment, work and social support.

Useful websites include

The Institute of Health Equity. Available at: http://www.instituteofhealthequity.org.

The Black Report. Available at: http://www.sochealth.co.uk/history/black.htm.

Fair Society Healthy Lives (The Marmot Review). Available at: http://www.instituteofhealthequity.org/resources-reports/fair-society-healthy-lives-the-marmot-review.

The Marmot Review 10 Years On. Available at: http://www.instituteofhealthequity.org/resources-reports/marmot-review-10-years-on.

FEEDBACK TO LEARNING ACTIVITIES

2.1. Lifestyle behaviours are often viewed as being individual choices. While on one level this is true, many other factors influence individual behaviours. Taking the example of physical activity, it can be argued that individual motivation and willpower are all that is necessary. However, many factors will impact on the likelihood and ease of taking more physical activity, for example, availability of suitable facilities, access to facilities and social norms depicted in the mass media.

2.2. It seems that unemployment has a profound effect on mental health, damaging a person's self-esteem and social structure. Employment, as well as providing wages which provide for people's material needs, is also often part of someone's self-identity. The higher incidence of smoking amongst unemployed people appears paradoxical given the cost involved, but smoking is often used as a psychological prop. Unemployment also means lower income and material disadvantage, as well as social isolation (McLean et al., 2005).

2.3. There are several reasons why men under the age of 45 do not visit their GPs as often as women. The obvious reason is that they suffer less ill health and disease than women, but this is not corroborated by medical statistics. Some issues, for example, contraception, are seen as being women's responsibility. Pregnancy and childbirth will also contribute significantly to women's use of GPs. The sick role and its associated features, for example, dependency, are typically viewed as more feminine than masculine, and therefore women may feel more at ease reporting ill health and using their GPs than men. There are therefore both medical and social reasons why women visit their GPs more frequently than men.

2.4. Healthcare is a cultural as well as a medical activity and is based on various premises, for example, that the doctor knows best, and that the patient should be passive and cooperate with medical advice and treatment. Sometimes patients from minority ethnic groups may have different expectations about their role and treatment. If there is a disparity between the expectations and role behaviours of health staff and patients, healthcare may suffer.

2.5. The first comment suggests that individuals must take full responsibility for their health-related behaviour. The second comment recognizes that behaviours take place in social contexts, and that many factors impact on individual behaviours. While behaviour is an individual attribute, its causes, meanings and significance are all socially determined. While it is logical to think poor people should smoke less, because of the cost of cigarettes, the social reality is that smoking is often used for social bonding and as a marker of individual identity, which are both rendered precarious by poverty.

2.6. Reflecting on your own life course to date in this way will illuminate the variety of factors that have impacted on your health. These factors will probably include both external factors, for example, the impact of economic recession or growth, and personal events, for example, unemployment, migration or sickness. While we are encouraged to believe that we forge our own destinies, many other familial, social and societal factors and events have a profound impact on our lives.

2.7. It could be argued that all the listed factors reflect a healthy society. Several factors (1, 6 and 7) are characteristic of egalitarian societies with a high level of social capital or networking, which is arguably a bedrock of good health. Other factors (2 and 5) are indicative of a thriving economy which, while it does not guarantee good health for all, provides a supportive backdrop. Factors 3 and 4 suggest a society investing in education and the next generation.

2.8. Accessing services, even when they are free and universally available, requires some initiative and confidence on the part of the user. To access NHS services, people need to negotiate with medical staff and make their needs known. This requires a degree of confidence, and such communication is much easier if the service user and service provider share a common cultural background, i.e., the user comes from the same social class as the medical staff.

2.9. There is a wide variety of indicators that could be used, including government statistics, for example, increasing number of young people in higher education or increasing percentage of students achieving pass grades in exams; lay people's feedback and views, for example, the percentage of people who feel their neighbourhood is safe; and service users' views, for example, the percentage of patients who report feeling well cared for by the NHS.

2.10. Effective long-term social policy initiatives are varied, and include extending educational and business opportunities for young people (e.g., through apprenticeships), provision for older people with chronic ill health (e.g., nursing homes) and ensuring that everyone has sufficient income to meet their needs (e.g., welfare benefits).

REFERENCES

Belvin, C., Britton, J., Holmes, J., Langley, T., 2015. Parental smoking and child poverty in the UK: an analysis of national survey data. BMC Public Health 15, 507.

Bhopal, R.S., 2014. Migration, Ethnicity, Race and Health in Multicultural Societies. Oxford University Press, Oxford.

British Heart Foundation, 2012. Coronary Heart Disease Statistics 2012. British Heart Foundation. Available at: http://www.bhf.org.uk/publications/view-publication.aspx?ps=1002097.

Commission on Social Determinants of Health, 2008. Closing the gap in a generation: health equity through action on the social determinants of health. Final Report of the Commission on Social Determinants of Health. World Health Organization, Geneva. Available at: http://apps.who.int/iris/bitstream/10665/43943/1/9789241563703_eng.pdf.

Dahlgren, G., Whitehead, M., 1991. Policies and Strategies to Promote Social Equity in Health. Institute for Future Studies, Stockholm.

Dobson, F., 1997. Healthy Houses for Healthy Lives: Address to National Housing Federation 16/10/97. Department of Health Press Release 97/282.

Graham, H., Power, C., 2004. Childhood Disadvantage and Adult Health: A Life Course Framework. Health Development Agency, London.

Hiscock, R., Bauld, L., Amos, A., Fidler, J., Munafo, M., 2012. Socioeconomic status and smoking: a review. Ann. N. Y. Acad. Sci. 1248, 107–123.

House of Commons Health Committee, 2009. Health Inequalities: Third Report of Session 2008–2009. Stationery Office, London.

Institute of Health Equity, 2020. Health Equity in England. The Marmot Review 10 Years On. Available at: http://www.instituteofhealthequity.org/resources-reports/marmot-review-10-years-on/the-marmot-review-10-years-on-full-report.pdf.

Lalonde, M., 1974. A New Perspective on the Health of Canadians. Ministry of Supply and Services, Ottawa.

Macdonald, W., Beeston, C., McCullough, S., 2014. Proportionate Universalism and Health Inequalities. NHS Health Scotland, Edinburgh. Available at: http://www.healthscotland.com/uploads/documents/24296-ProportionateUniversalismBriefing.pdf.

Marmot, M., 2010. Fair Society, Healthy Lives. DH-Publisher, London. Available at: http://www.instituteofhealthequity.org/resources-reports/fair-society-healthy-lives-the-marmot-review.

Marmot, M., Siegrist, J., Theorell, T., 2006. Health and the psychosocial environment at work. In: Marmot, M., Wilkinson, R. (eds.), The Social Determinants of Health, second edn. Oxford University Press, Oxford, pp. 97–131.

Marmot, M., Wilkinson, R. (eds.) 2006. The Social Determinants of Health, second edn. Oxford University Press, Oxford.

McKeown, T., Lowe, C.R., 1974. An Introduction to Social Medicine. Blackwell Science, Oxford.

McLean, C., Carmona, C., Francis, C., Wohlgemuth, C., Mulvihill, C., et al., 2005. Worklessness and Health: What Do We Know about the Causal Relationship?

Health Development Agency, London. Available at: http://www.employabilityinscotland.com/media/83147/worklessness-and-health-what-do-we-know-about-the-relationship.pdf.

Office for National Statistics, 2013. The 21st century mortality files. Office for National Statistics, London. Available at: https://www.ons.gov.uk/peoplepopulationandcommunity/birthsdeathsandmarriages/deaths/datasets/the21stcenturymortalityfilesdeathsdataset/current.

Office for National Statistics, 2019. Adult smoking habits in the UK: 2019. Office for National Statistics, London. Available at: https://www.ons.gov.uk/peoplepopulationandcommunity/healthandsocialcare/healthandlifeexpectancies/bulletins/adultsmokinghabitsingreatbritain/2019#:~:text=In%202019%2C%20the%20proportion%20of,falling%20smoking%20prevalence%20since%202011.

Patel, N., Ferrer, H.B., Tyrer, F., Wray, P., Farooqi, A., et al., 2017. Barriers and facilitators to healthy lifestyle changes in minority ethnic populations in the UK: a narrative review. J. Racial Ethn. Health Disparities 4 (6), 1107–1119.

Public Health England, 2018. Understanding and Reducing Ethnic Inequalities in Health. Available at: https://assets.publishing.service.gov.uk/government/uploads/system/uploads/attachment_data/file/730917/local_action_on_health_inequalities.pdf.

Public Health England, 2019. Place Based Approaches for Reducing Health Inequalities. Available at: https://www.gov.uk/government/publications/health-inequalities-place-based-approaches-to-reduce-inequalities/place-based-approaches-for-reducing-health-inequalities-main-report

Public Health England, 2020. Disparities in the Risk and Outcomes of COVID-19. Available at: https://assets.publishing.service.gov.uk/government/uploads/system/uploads/attachment_data/file/908434/Disparities_in_the_risk_and_outcomes_of_COVID_August_2020_update.pdf.

Townsend, P., Davidson, N., 1982. Inequalities in Health: The Black Report. Penguin, Harmondsworth.

Tudor Hart, J., 1971. The inverse care law. The Lancet 1, 405–412.

Wang, Y., Hunt, K., Nazareth, I., Freemantle, N., Petersen, I., 2013. Do men consult less than women? An analysis of routinely collected UK general practice data. BMJ Open 3 (e003320). doi: 10.1136/bmjopen-2013-003320.

Wilkinson, R., 1996. Unhealthy Societies: The Afflictions of Inequality. Routledge, London.

Wilkinson, R., Pickett, K., 2010. The Spirit Level: Why Equality Is Better for Everyone? Penguin, London.

World Health Organization, 2018. WHO Housing and Health Guidelines. World Health Organization, Geneva. Available at: https://apps.who.int/iris/bitstream/handle/10665/276001/9789241550376-eng.pdf.

3

Measuring Health

IMPORTANCE OF THE TOPIC

Chapter 1 discussed how people define health in different ways, and Chapter 2 identified different determinants of health. This suggests that measuring health is not a simple task. This appears to be borne out by the existence of a number of ways of measuring health, and a lack of clear agreement about which are the best ways to do this and which sources of information are most useful. This chapter looks first at why we might want to measure health. It goes on to investigate the different means of measuring health currently in use, and unpacks some of their underlying assumptions. Finally, how the different kinds of measures are used is explored. The practical context of measuring health is discussed

further in Chapters 20, 22 and 23 on needs assessment, programme planning and evaluation, respectively.

WHY MEASURE HEALTH?

Finding a means to measure health is an important practical task for health promoters. There are several reasons why this is so.
- To establish priorities: Collecting and evaluating information about the health status and health problems of a community are important ways of identifying needs.
- To assist planning: Health promoters need information to assist the planning and evaluation of health promotion programmes. It is important to establish

baseline data in order to plan priorities and have a standard against which health promotion interventions can be evaluated.

- To justify resources: Health promotion often competes with other activities for scarce resources. To justify a claim for resources and prove the effectiveness of their activities, health promoters need information on the evolving health status of populations.
- To assist the development of the profession: Measurements of health gain are important to the professional development of health promoters. Unless there is a means of measuring the effect of health promotion, it will remain invisible, underfunded and of low priority. By demonstrating the efficacy of health promotion interventions, it is possible to argue for resources, prioritization and funding.

WAYS OF MEASURING HEALTH

Depending on the purpose, different measures of health may be used or developed. How one measures health depends on one's definition of health. If health is about physical functioning, then measures of physical fitness will be an adequate measure of health. If health is defined as the absence of disease, the incidence of disease may be used (in reverse) as a measure of health. If however health is more broadly defined as including positive social and mental aspects, specific measurements of health will need to be developed.

Learning Activity 3.1 asks you to consider or discuss how you would describe the health of your neighbourhood. This is the first of several learning activities in this chapter that ask you to consider or discuss the availability of valid and reliable data used in the analysis of population health and that are used in decision-making and priority setting. This learning activity will probe you to consider the assets or health-enhancing aspects that exist where you live or work, and also how you will gather the relevant information in order to describe it.

 Learning Activity 3.1   Describing the Health of Populations

If you wanted to describe the health of the people where you live or work, what information would you need?

Community health workers who profile their communities have many different ways of building a picture of their area. Some of these are described in Chapter 19 on needs assessment. In this chapter we look at sources of information available to describe a community's health. A great deal of information is available online. For example, in the UK you can find out about your local area at uklocalarea.com. Case Study 3.1 outlines a profile of the borough of Tower Hamlets in London. It is an example of how a place may be described using a variety of indicators, most of which can be obtained from the Office of National Statistics (ONS).

We look next at the contribution of epidemiology to negative measurements of health and then consider positive measurements of health. Negative measurements of health mean measuring the opposite to health (e.g., disease or death) and using these results to infer the degree

 CASE STUDY 3.1
Describing Tower Hamlets in London

Tower Hamlets is a densely populated and ethnically diverse London borough. It is the third most deprived borough in London and one of the 20% most deprived districts/unitary authorities in England. About 29% (15,400) of children live in low-income families. Life expectancy for both men and women is lower than the average for England. The ONS estimated the usual resident population of Tower Hamlets to be 308,000 as at 30 June 2017. In the year to June 2017, the borough gained an estimated 7000 additional residents, equivalent to 20 additional residents every day over the year.

Tower Hamlets is ranked the 16th most ethnically diverse local authority borough in England. More than two thirds of residents belong to minority ethnic groups, the largest being the Bangladeshi population who comprise 32% of the borough's population. More than four in ten residents (43%) were born outside the UK and 38% of residents are Muslim – the highest proportion in the UK.

The borough's employment rate has risen considerably over the last decade, from 56% during 2005–2008 to 68% in 2014–17, bringing it closer to the national rate for Great Britain (74%). The proportion of residents who rely on unemployment benefits has also seen a sharp fall over the last decade, dropping from 16% to 9% between 2007 and 2016. Despite these improving trends, inequalities exist within the labour market.

Tower Hamlets has a relatively young population compared with the rest of the country. The median age in 2017 was 31.0 years which was the fourth youngest median age out of all local authorities in the UK.

of health. Health is therefore defined in negative terms (health is not being ill or dead), rather than in positive terms (health is positive well-being).

MEASURING HEALTH AS A NEGATIVE VARIABLE

Epidemiology is the study of the occurrence and spread of diseases in the population. It is concerned with the health status (or, more usually, the ill-health status) of populations. Health promoters use epidemiological evidence to identify health problems, at-risk groups and the effectiveness of preventive measures.

The most common means of assessing a population's health are mortality and morbidity rates. This reflects the reductionist model of health, which reduces health to not being ill. Thus data on deaths and illnesses are often used as surrogate measures of health. There are clearly shortcomings to this approach. Measuring conditions which limit health, such as illness, is not the same as measuring health itself. Measuring mortality rates does not reflect the extent of illness in the population, nor does it say anything about the quality of health experienced by people when they were alive. Conditions such as arthritis or schizophrenia cause considerable suffering and pain, but do not lead to premature death and so are not mentioned in mortality rates. Later in this chapter we discuss the Quality of Life Year (QALY) measurement, which does take account of pain and suffering.

Statistics concerning mortality are readily obtainable in developed countries. A death certificate is submitted to the registrar of births, deaths and marriages and the director of public health in every health authority. The total number of deaths, geographic and population variations and the causes of death are all collated in each district's annual public health report. These statistics can also be used in international comparisons because most countries have some form of database on deaths and disease rates.

All countries have systems of collecting data on the health status of their population and the public's use of health services. Although these statistics are often presented as if they were objective facts, it is important to remember that statistics are devised by people in a social context, and are subject to assumptions, bias and error. At every stage of the data-collecting process, decisions are taken which help shape the final data and information that are presented. For example, the recording of deaths due to COVID-19 differed across countries, with some only recording deaths in hospitals.

Learning Activity 3.2 asks you to consider the reliability and validity of mortality rates as indicators of health.

 Learning Activity 3.2   Mortality Rates and Food Hygiene as an Indicator of Health Status

If you wished to develop a health promotion intervention to improve food hygiene and sanitation, why would mortality rates be a poor indicator of its priority?

- How else could you find out about the extent of poor food hygiene in your area?
- Why might mortality statistics be a good indicator of the necessity of health promotion concerning food hygiene in a low-income country?

MORTALITY STATISTICS

There are several different ways of expressing death rates. The crude death rate is the number of deaths per 1000 people per year. However, this figure is affected by the age structure of the population, which may vary over time and regions. An area with a high proportion of older people, such as an English south-coast retirement town, would have consistently higher death rates than a more deprived area with a higher percentage of premature deaths but a younger population, such as an inner-city area. The standardized mortality ratio (SMR) is a measure of the death rate which takes into account differences in populations' age structure. The SMR is the number of deaths experienced within a population group (which may be defined by geographic or socio-economic factors) compared to what would be expected for this group if national averages applied, taking age differences into account. The overall average for England and Wales is 100, so SMRs of below 100 indicate a lower than average mortality rate, whereas SMRs of more than 100 indicate higher than average mortality rates. Information on mortality from different diseases as we see in Learning Activity 3.2 is an important tool in population health decision-making.

Learning Activity 3.3 asks you to consider and discuss the well-established International Classification of Diseases and some of its limitations when there are multiple contributing intermediate or immediate causes of death.

The infant mortality rate (IMR), another commonly used statistic, is the number of deaths in the first year of life per 1000 live births. The IMR is strongly associated with adult mortality rates and reflects maternal health, particularly nutrition and the provision of social care and child welfare. The IMR can therefore be used as an indicator of the general health of the population, particularly when comparisons between countries are being drawn. The perinatal mortality rate is the number of stillbirths and deaths in the first 7 days after birth per 1000 births. The neonatal death rate is the number of deaths occurring in the first 28 days after birth per 1000 live births. Both the SMR and the IMR are readily available statistics, and therefore easy to use as surrogate measures of health.

Table 3.1 illustrates the marked inequalities across countries as shown by health indicators. There has been some progress: for example, since 2000, measles vaccines have averted over 14 million deaths. But four out of every five deaths of under-5-year-olds occur in sub-Saharan Africa or Southern Asia. Improving education for girls and women is a priority, as children of educated mothers – even mothers with only primary schooling – are more likely to survive than children of mothers with no education.

Learning Activity 3.4 asks you to interpret some simple data on established health indicators.

TABLE 3.1 Key Health Indicators Worldwide, 2019			
Country	Life expectancy (years) Men	Women	Infant mortality rate (IMR) (per 1000 live births)
Belgium	79	84	3.4
Canada	80	84	4.9
UK, the	79	83	4.2
USA, the	76	81	6.5
Zimbabwe	59	63	31.9
China	76	79	7.9
Brazil	71	79	11.0
Sweden	80	84	2.6
India	68	71	37.8
Australia	80	84	3.6

From Organisation for Economic Co-operation and Development, 2019. Health at a Glance 2019: OECD Indicators. Paris. Available at: https://www.oecd-ilibrary.org/sites/4dd50c09-en/1/2/1/index.html?itemId=/content/publication/4dd50c09-en&_csp_=82587932df7c06a6a3f9dab-95304095d&itemIGO=oecd&itemContentType=book.

Death rates are also available broken down by gender and cause (and, in the UK, by social class and occupation). People in lower socio-economic groups have higher than average death rates at all ages and for virtually all causes. These differences show no sign of diminishing. Indeed, inequalities in IMRs and life expectancy continue to grow, although there are some signs of progress, for example in child poverty and housing indicators. It may well take some time for any strategies currently being implemented to have an impact on mortality indicators. Reductions in mortality due to selected causes among targeted groups constitute the majority of targets in public health strategies.

A health indicator is a construct of public health surveillance that defines a measure of health such as mortality, or a disease or a factor associated with health such as smoking. Learning Activity 3.5 continues the discussion on the quality of such health data.

Learning Activity 3.5   Data Collection in Low-Income Countries

In low-income countries, mortality statistics may not be complete. Can you think of reasons why this might be the case?

MORBIDITY STATISTICS

Statistics measuring illness and disease are more difficult than mortality statistics to obtain. This is due in part to the difficulty in establishing a hard-and-fast line between health and disease. There is no one source of data for the whole population concerning disease and illness; instead, there are a number of different sources of relevant information. These are summarized below in Case Study 3.2.

CASE STUDY 3.2
Sources of Health Information in the UK

Sources of these data may be accessed from public health departments, hospital-based datasets, Public Health England, primary care consultation rates, local delivery plans, local surveys and the ONS. Useful websites include www.statistics.gov.uk (ONS) for local information and health trends, Public Health England (fingertips.phe.org.uk) for non-communicable disease information and www.gov.uk/government/organisations/public-health-england for communicable disease information.

Mortality
- death by cause, age, sex and area of residence
- infant deaths (in children under 1 year)
- perinatal deaths (after 28th week of pregnancy and in the first 7 days after birth)
- neonatal deaths (within the first 28 days of birth)

Morbidity
- General Household Survey (annual survey of health behaviour and experience of illness)
- health service records on consultation and treatment episodes in hospital and general practice, for example hospital episodes statistics available from National Health Service (NHS) Digital (digital.nhs.uk)
- registers for specific conditions such as cancers, disability, blindness and partial sight, people at risk of harm and drug addiction
- notification systems for infectious (communicable) diseases
- National General Practice Morbidity Survey, conducted by the ONS and the Royal College of General Practitioners
- surveys on mental health and psychiatric morbidity (for England, Scotland and Wales), since 1993
- data regarding incidence of disease obtained from screening programmes, for example for cervical cancer
- notifiable congenital malformations

Health and safety and accidents
- Reporting of Injuries, Diseases and Dangerous Occurrences Regulations (RIDDOR) data, available from the Health and Safety Executive (HSE).

Information on health status and behaviour
GP records on diagnoses, and communicable and respiratory disease monitoring, for example PRIMIS+ (primary care information services):
- dental health records
- child health surveillance records
  - child measurement (of obesity) from 5 to 11
- National surveys for the ONS, for example the annual Health Survey for England, the Living Costs and Food Survey, Smoking, Drinking and Drug Use Among Young People in England, the Infant Feeding Survey and occasional surveys, for example Active People Survey (Sport England). The Health and Social Care Information Centre (HSCIC) has links to the major national surveys at http://www.hscic.gov.uk/public-health.

Demographic data
- Census information on the whole population is collected every 10 years. Information includes numbers in household by age, sex, marital status, place of birth, occupation, ethnicity (since 1991), educational level, house type and tenure, accommodation and facilities. Information on self-reported health is collected
- register of births, including birth weight and mother's occupation, and deaths
- claimants of unemployment benefit, free school meals, housing benefit and income support

Environmental indicators and deprivation indices
- services available
- levels of pollution: air, water and noise
- crime statistics
- type of housing
- leisure facilities
- road traffic accidents
- education, skills and training
- employment

The health services collect routine data on the use of their services and activity rates. These data can be used to express the disease experience of different populations, but there are several problems with adopting this approach. The main problem with using many of the health authority measurements is that they were developed primarily for administrative, planning or management tasks, and reflect available services and their use rather than health itself. Health authority data are primarily collected as a management tool. To some extent, this determines what data are collected. Routinely available morbidity data represent only the tip of the illness iceberg. Many people who are ill do not seek help from primary care services or hospitals. However, the advantage of using data of this kind is that they are routinely collected, consistent across regions and easily accessed.

Learning Activity 3.6 continues the discussion about the value of health data by considering Hospital Episode Statistics (HES).

 Learning Activity 3.6   Hospital Episode Statistics as an Indicator of Health Status

Hospital Episode Statistics (HES) is a patient-based dataset that contains all finished episodes of hospital care by diagnosis and treatment (https://digital.nhs.uk/data-and-information/data-tools-and-services/data-services/hospital-episode-statistics).

- What will these data tell you about the health status of the local population?
- What do these data not tell you?
- Why do you think data are collected in this way?

The Health Survey for England (http://healthsurvey.hscic.gov.uk/data-visualisation/data-visualisation/explore-the-trends/general-health.aspx) includes questions on people's experience of illness, both long term (chronic) and within the last fortnight (acute). The data are difficult to use comparatively over time, as the wording of the questions changes occasionally. The following are examples of questions used:

- Over the last 12 months would you say your health has on the whole been good, fairly good or not good?
- Do you have any long-standing illness, disability or infirmity? By long-standing I mean anything that has troubled you over a period of time or that is likely to affect you over a period of time.

- Now I'd like you to think about the 2 weeks ending yesterday. During those 2 weeks, did you have to cut down on any of the things you usually do (about the house, at work or in your free time) because of (any chronic condition cited earlier in the interview) or some other illness or injury?

The survey is useful in providing information on people's subjective experience of illness, because it relies on self-reported illness rather than use of services. It also collects information on people's health-related behaviour, such as smoking, drinking and exercise. For example, one question asks: 'Do you smoke cigarettes at all nowadays?'

 Learning Activity 3.7   Indicators of Health

The following are used to describe the health of populations. Which are good indicators of health?
- standardized mortality rates
- IMRs
- life expectancy
- General Certificate of Secondary Education (GCSE) rates
- childhood obesity rates
- smoking prevalence
- depression rates
- happiness rates

These measures of mortality and morbidity are inadequate for assessing people who are not ill but have some limited function which affects their everyday life. With a growing burden of long-term chronic illness, different health indicators or health outcome measures have been developed to assist in the analysis of the consequences of disease:

- Healthy life expectancy (HLE) is the average number of years a new-born baby is expected to live in good health.
- Years of life lost (YLLs). This composite indicator combines morbidity and mortality to provide a quantitative measure of the impact of premature mortality (in Europe, taken as under 75 years) due to particular diseases.
- Quality-adjusted life years (QALYs). The QALY measures years of survival weighted for the quality of life which people may expect to have in the context of different states of illness.
- Disability adjusted life years (DALYs). The DALY combines years of healthy life lost due to disability

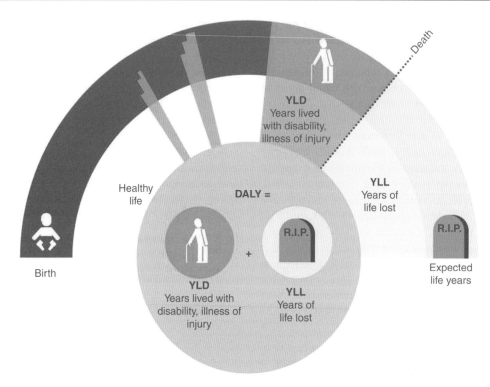

Fig. 3.1 Disability adjusted life (From Public Health England, 2015. The Global Burden of Disease: England. Public Health England, London. Available at: https://assets.publishing.service.gov.uk/ government/uploads/system/uploads/attachment_data/file/460518/Global_Burden_of_Disease_ England_infographics.pptx.)

with those lost due to premature death. DALYs were calculated for over 100 specific diseases for eight demographic regions worldwide. The measure is based on the incidence and duration of conditions resulting in non-fatal outcomes and weighted according to the severity of the disability and its impact (Fig. 3.1).

MEASURING DISEASE IN POPULATIONS

The Global Burden of Disease (GBD) study is a comprehensive regional and global assessment of mortality and disability from major diseases, injuries and risk factors (available at the Institute for Health Metrics http:// www.healthdata.org/gbd/publications). It allows for inter country comparisons and analysis of changes in risk factors. It shows, for example, the huge increase in YLL worldwide due to obesity and high blood pressure. The GBD for the UK from the latest study in 2019 shows

an increase over the past 20 years in the contribution to premature mortality of Alzheimer's disease and prostate and pancreatic cancer. COVID-19 was the most frequent underlying cause of death in 2020 in the UK. Compared with other countries, the UK had lower rates of road injury and diabetes, but significantly higher rates for depression and chronic obstructive pulmonary disease. The leading risk factor in the UK was tobacco, followed by increased blood pressure and high body mass index (BMI). The GBD does not show intra-country variations. For example, whilst life expectancy is rising in Australia as in most other countries, there are significant disparities between Aboriginal and Torres Strait Islander Australians, who on average live to 71.6 years for males and 75.6 years for females. Life expectancy at birth for non-Indigenous Australians was 80.2 years for males and 83.4 years for females (Australian Institute of Health and Welfare, 2020). The GBD study concludes that the rise in exposure to key risk factors worldwide, including air

TABLE 3.2	The Application of Epidemiology to Public Health	
Distribution	**Determinant**
How many diseases are there?	Why do diseases happen?
How often do diseases happen (frequency)?	What determines/causes diseases/health-related events?
Where do they happen (places)?	What works to reduce the burden or risk of the disease? What is effective?
When do they happen or how do they change over time?	Is there a relationship between the disease and factors surrounding people's lives? Which factors are associated with a higher risk of getting the disease?
Who has them and who does not (which population groups are at higher risk)?	How much higher is the risk associated with these factors?
	What kind of factors (e.g., genetic or lifestyle) determine which populations are at risk and which populations are relatively immune?

pollution, high blood pressure, high blood sugar, BMI and elevated cholesterol, combined with rising deaths from cardiovascular disease in some countries (e.g., the USA and the Caribbean), suggests that we might be approaching a turning point in life expectancy gains.

Epidemiological studies examine the distribution and patterns of health and disease in populations (Table 3.2). Epidemiological data help to build up a picture in the following ways:
- showing the scale of the problem
- showing the natural history and aetiology of the condition
- showing causation and association
- identifying risk.

Scale of the Problem
- Incidence. The number of people developing a disease over a specified period, for example in 2017 in the UK there were 54,700 cases of breast cancer diagnosed in women of which 17% were in women under 50 (breastcanceruk.org).
- Prevalence. The number of people with a condition or characteristic at a specified time, for example in 2019 in UK 14.1% of adults were smokers, amounting to 6.9 million people (ons.gov.uk).
- How the condition is distributed by gender, age, socio-economic status (SES), ethnicity, etc., for example data from the National Child Measurement Programme show that obesity is more common in young children aged 5 years from Black African and Black Other ethnic groups, and in boys from the Bangladeshi ethnic group (https://digital.nhs.uk/data-and-information/publications/statistical/national-child-measurement-programme/2016-17-school-year).

Natural History and Aetiology of the Condition
- Indicate if primary prevention is possible.
- Show severity of the problem and ways in which individuals, families or communities may be affected.

Causation and Association
- Show if there is evidence that exposure to a particular environmental, lifestyle or socio-economic factor contributes to ill health. There is a difference between causation (without which the ill health would not have occurred) and association (which links a socio-economic factor with ill health) (Fig. 3.2).

Identifying Risk
- Assessing the chance or probability of a disease or condition occurring.
- Assessing how much illness is due to a particular factor (the attributable risk).

Epidemiologists assess risk in terms of the statistical probability of adverse events or death occurring. The link between these events and identified contributory factors varies from negligible to high. Lay people, by contrast, assess risk in the light of their personal experience. This difference in focus (whole populations vs specific individuals at a specific time) is problematic for health promoters. Rose (1981) called this the 'prevention paradox': for one person to benefit, many people have to change their behaviour, even though they will not benefit from so doing. Public awareness of this paradox can become a barrier to behaviour change.

Epidemiological studies of mortality, illness, disease and disability are often used to talk about health. Such

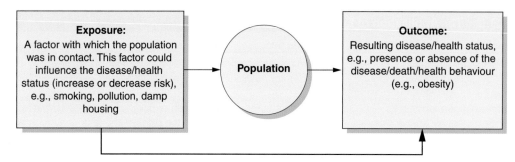

Fig. 3.2 The association of exposure to outcomes

usage reinforces, albeit in an indirect way, the definition of health as 'not disease'. But the advantage of such statistics is that they are already collected, relatively consistent and readily available. Recognizing the limitations of such measures has prompted health promoters to develop new means of measuring health as an independent phenomenon distinct from illness or disease. These measures may be conveniently divided into those describing health as an objective quality which is an attribute of people or environments, and those describing health as a subjective reality which is socially produced.

MEASURES OF HEALTH AS AN OBJECTIVE ATTRIBUTE

There are a number of ways of measuring health as an objective factor, including:

- health measures
- health behaviour indicators
- socio-economic or deprivation indicators
- environmental indicators.

Health Measures

There are various measures of the health status of people, including vital statistics such as height, weight and dental health (the decayed, missing and filled teeth, or DMF, index). Floud (1989) argues that the average height of a population may be taken as a measure of health, as it represents a proxy for nutritional status and therefore welfare. The Health Survey for England 2019 (NHS Digital, 2019 at https://digital.nhs.uk/data-and-information/publications/statistical/health-survey-for-england/) includes height and weight measurements for this reason. In the same way, the percentage of low-birth-weight babies is used as an indicator of health status as it indicates whether a child has a 'healthy start' – and also serves as a health outcome related to maternal health risk.

Health Behaviour Indicators

Measurements of people's behaviour are used as a measure of health. For example, the number of people smoking, the proportion of children who are overweight or obese, the percentage of the population who do more than 150 minutes of exercise a week as per the government guidelines and the average daily consumption of fruit and vegetables may all be used to describe different populations and make comparisons between them regarding relative health status. This information may be routinely collected, such as smoking prevalence in young people, or it may be obtained from commissioned surveys. For example, sun protection surveys are carried out annually in Victoria, Australia. These lifestyle measures are sometimes narrowed down to more specific behaviour in relation to the health services. For example, the percentage of children immunized against childhood illnesses, or the percentage of women screened for cervical and breast cancer, may be used to describe the health status of a population.

Socio-economic Indicators

SES, including educational attainment, occupational status and income, is related to health in developed countries, with higher SES being associated with better health. Other factors that are strongly associated with health include well-developed primary healthcare systems, more equal income distribution, high levels of female education and reduced racial conflict (Braveman and Gottlieb, 2014).

The socio-economic environment shapes resources, opportunities and exposures, and can directly and indirectly influence health. Characteristics of the socio-economic environment can be measured through specific data and provide a picture of health in a neighbourhood or population, for example,

- wealth and income: financial stress, older age provision
- housing: supply and affordability
- transport and infrastructure: travel time to work, access to public transport, internet access
- productivity and employment: innovation and new businesses, jobs available, rates of pay
- social support: voluntary groups.

The social environment may also be measured in terms of its 'healthiness'. One of the measures most commonly used to assess the social environment is wealth. The gross domestic product (GDP – the value of all goods and services produced within a nation in a given year) measures economic well-being, but this forms only part of social well-being (also called quality of life or social welfare). Happiness and life satisfaction are only weakly related to GDP in the developed Organisation for Economic Co-operation and Development (OECD) countries. The United Nations issues an annual report on levels of happiness in 156 countries. For the last decade, New Zealand and countries in Scandinavia have ranked in the top countries but the USA has not made the top 10. Norway has the highest GDP per capita, but ranks behind Finland in population happiness. Happiness is a different indicator of population health from those discussed earlier in this chapter. There is considerable discussion amongst statisticians and policymakers about the reliability of this measure. One of the debates is what factors are associated with population levels of happiness. Is it, for example, related to income level, life expectancy or employment opportunity? Consider this as you complete Learning Activity 3.8.

 Learning Activity 3.8   Measuring Happiness

What might account for the high scores for happiness in north-west European countries and the low score for the USA?

Environmental Indicators

The same method may be applied to physical environments. Measurements of the physical environment include air and water quality, and housing type and density. These measures are routinely collected by the environmental health departments of local authorities. The European Happy Planet Index is a global index of sustainable well-being, combining measures of carbon footprints, life expectancy and life satisfaction (happyplanetindex.org).

Many countries now have sustainability indicators that may measure a variety of factors pertaining to social capital, economic capital and natural capital. The United Nations' Sustainable Development Goals, as shown in Fig. 3.3, include many aspirations for a cleaner planet.

MEASURING DEPRIVATION

As we saw in Chapter 2, deprivation can have a significant negative impact on health and health outcomes. In the UK, deprivation has been calculated since the 1970s. Key to this is the Index of Multiple Deprivation (IMD) which defines deprivation in a range of domains including income; employment; health and disability; education, skills and training; access to services; barriers to housing and other services; living environment; and crime (Ministry of Housing, Communities and Local Government, 2019). Each domain includes several different indicators. For example, the income domain includes:

- adults and children in income support households
- adults and children in income-based job seeker's allowance households
- adults and children in working families' tax credit households whose equivalized income (excluding housing benefits) is below 60% of the median before housing costs
- adults and children in disabled person's tax credit households whose equivalized income (excluding housing benefits) is below 60% of the median before housing costs
- adults and children in pension credit (guarantee) families
- asylum seekers in England in receipt of subsistence or accommodation support, or both.

In addition, indices for income deprivation affecting children and older people have been developed. The indices of deprivation measure relative levels in small areas of England called super output areas (SOAs). Lower-layered SOAs include about 1500 people and enable smaller area analysis.

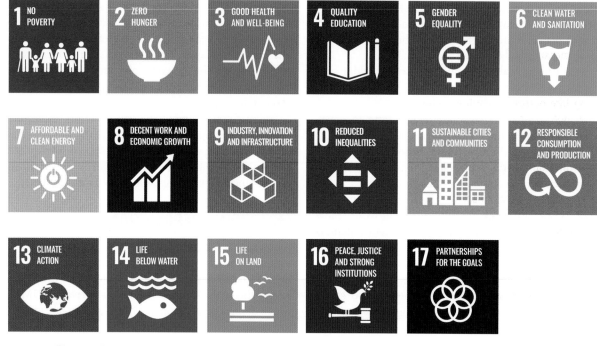

Fig. 3.3 The United Nations' Sustainable Development Goals (From https://www.un.org/sustainabledevelopment/. The content of this publication has not been approved by the United Nations and does not reflect the views of the United Nations or its officials or member states.)

Population health management is a new approach used by local health and care partnerships to proactively identify where there may be healthcare needs in the future and try to act immediately to prevent them. For example, adults and children who live in cold, damp housing may be more likely to develop respiratory problems over the next 20 years because their lungs are affected by the mould spores in their home. Improving housing now may mean they do not end up with various health conditions such as asthma in the future, which can result in poor quality of life.

SUBJECTIVE HEALTH MEASURES

The previous section outlined ways of measuring health as if it were an objective property of beings, societies or environments, capable of scientific scrutiny. However, it is apparent that health is not such a simple or uncontested attribute. Chapter 1 highlighted the importance of subjective interpretations of health and the multiple meanings health may have in different contexts. This has led some researchers to attempt to devise measurements of health which incorporate subjective meanings. Herzlich (1973) identified three different aspects of people's accounts of health:

1. Health as a vacuum (not being ill).
2. Health as a reserve (of strength and resilience).
3. Health as equilibrium (balance and well-being).

Bowling (2017) identifies five dimensions of subjective health:

1. Functional ability.
2. Health status.
3. Psychological well-being.
4. Social networks and social support.
5. Life satisfaction and positive morale.

There are numerous instruments that attempt to measure these dimensions but few composite measures. For example, the EuroQol measures five dimensions of mobility, self-care, usual activities, pain/discomfort and anxiety/depression. The ONS in the UK compiles a population well-being picture using a variety of measures in the National Well-being dashboard that include general life satisfaction.

PHYSICAL WELL-BEING, FUNCTIONAL ABILITY AND HEALTH STATUS

Most measures of functional ability use people's self-reports of physical activity, such as their degree of mobility and their ability to perform activities of daily living like personal care and domestic work. A widely used tool to measure health is the short-form 36-item (SF-36) health survey (Stewart et al., 1988). The SF-36 is a multi-item scale that assesses eight health dimensions.

1. Limitations in physical activities because of health problems.
2. Limitations in social activities because of physical or emotional problems.
3. Limitations in usual role activities because of physical health problems.
4. Bodily pain.
5. General mental health.
6. Limitations in usual role activities because of emotional problems.
7. Vitality.
8. General health perceptions.

A short version is the SF-12 health survey, which is published in both standard (4 weeks) and acute (1 week) recall versions for self-administration. Learning Activity 3.9 asks you to find a widely used health questionnaire (Short Form [SF-36]) and consider how useful it is to assess a patient or client's health and well-being.

 Learning Activity 3.9   Using the Short Form (SF-36) Health Survey

What are the advantages and disadvantages of the SF-36 health survey?

QUALITY OF LIFE

Because health is multidimensional and includes physical, social and mental domains, composite measures have been developed, known as health-related quality of life measures. The desire to include a measurement of health in evaluating healthcare outcomes has led to the development of quality-adjusted life years (QALYs). QALYs are an explicit attempt to include not just years of life saved but also the quality of life when making resource allocation decisions regarding different medical procedures. The quality of life includes things such as freedom from pain and discomfort and the ability to live independently. The assessment of quality of life is made by both health professionals and lay people. The QALY is the arithmetic product of life expectancy and an adjustment for the quality of the remaining life years gained. These two components are quite separate. QALYs are an important tool in making decisions about how to ration healthcare resources.

PSYCHOLOGICAL WELL-BEING

Several questionnaires have been developed to measure psychological well-being, including the general health questionnaire (GHQ) (Goldberg et al., 1997). The GHQ measures minor psychological distress and social dysfunction and includes factors such as:
- ability to concentrate
- enjoyment of normal activities
- capability to make decisions
- feeling unhappy and depressed
- losing much sleep.

Well-being, as discussed in Chapter 1, is a complex concept. It is commonly assessed using the Warwick–Edinburgh Mental Well-Being Scale (WEMWBS), which is a 14-item scale of subjective well-being covering psychological functioning and well-being in the past 2 weeks. In contrast to the other measures described, it is worded positively and addresses aspects of positive mental health. As WEMWBS scores show a roughly normal distribution, WEMWBS can be expected to capture the full spectrum of positive mental health without floor or ceiling effects, and is suitable for both monitoring trends over time and evaluating the effect of mental health promotion programmes or interventions.

MEASURING SOCIAL HEALTH

Health includes the dimension of social health, which may be defined as the degree to which people function adequately as members of their community. A key characteristic of social health as described in Chapter 1 is social support, incorporating both the extent of a person's social networks and their perceived adequacy. The Living Standards Framework of New Zealand measures social connections as part of its population well-being measures and includes experiences of discrimination, feelings of loneliness, connection to ancestry and weekly or more frequent face to face contact with friends who do not live with them (see https://lsfdashboard. treasury.govt.nz/wellbeing/). In the UK other domains that are measured in addition to social networks are personal relationships, civic engagement and trust and cooperative norms. Civic engagement and trust had declined in the UK but there are signs that the COVID 19 pandemic has reversed this, leading to greater engagement through collective responsibility, volunteering and social media connectivity.

The concept of 'social capital', widely used to describe the social networks and trust which link people together in a community (Wilkinson, 1996), is discussed further in Chapter 11. Higher levels of social capital are associated with better health, less violent crime, better schooling, more tolerance and more economic and civic equality (Putnam, 2001). It has been argued that a reduction or disinvestment in social capital, triggered by increased income inequality, leads to increased mortality (Kawachi et al., 1997). Related to social capital is the concept of social cohesion, which is commonly cited in policy debates. Social cohesion is often identified as 'solidarity' and 'togetherness', achieved through reductions in wealth disparities, and the existence of common values and a civic culture which create social solidarity, social networks and social capital. The peaceful co-existence and valuing of diverse groups is often seen as the heart of social cohesion. This section has discussed the concepts of social capital and cohesion. Learning Activity 3.10 asks you to consider when you might wish to assess or measure these items at an individual, family or community level.

 Learning Activity 3.10   Measuring Social Capital and Social Cohesion

Why and in what contexts might it be important to measure social capital, social cohesion or social connectedness?

There is much theoretical and methodological confusion in attempts to measure different aspects of positive health, and a lack of consensus in how this may best be achieved. It is an area which is currently being refined and researched.

RESEARCH EXAMPLE 3.1
The Framingham Heart Study

The Framingham Heart Study started in 1948, enrolling 5209 people in the town of Framingham in Massachusetts, USA. Their offspring cohort of 5124 started to be followed in the 1970s, and their offspring, a third generation of 4095 people, began to be followed in 2002. The original intention was to discover the risk factors for cardiovascular disease. For 20 years, from 1983 to 2003, the participants completed a happiness assessment. Clusters of happy and unhappy people are visible in the network of participants, and people's happiness extends up to three degrees of separation (e.g., to the friends of one's friends' friends). People who are surrounded by many happy people and those who are central in the network are more likely to be happy in the present and in the future. In other words, happiness is contagious. Interestingly the same researchers found that obesity also spreads through networks by influencing ideas about what appropriate behaviours are, or what an appropriate body image might be.

Based on Fowler, J., Christakis, N., 2008. Dynamic spread of happiness in a large social network: longitudinal analysis over 20 years in the Framingham Heart Study. BMJ 337, a2338.

CONCLUSION

Indicators used to describe health will depend on what they are being used for and the extent to which stakeholders such as local people are involved. But, as with all forms of measurement, indicators need to be:

- measurable
- understandable
- comparable
- available
- targetable
- geographic
- temporal.

Measuring health is an important activity for health promoters, and is integral to the planning and evaluation of health promotion programmes. Yet there is no consensus on the best means to measure health, and a wide variety of methods have been used. Some are opportunistic, relying on data already collected and available, such as the annual Health Survey for England and QALYs. The drawback of using these methods is that they use data which have been collected for specific reasons, often managerial or administrative, and which might therefore be restricted. Other methods, such as the SF-36, have arisen from research which has addressed the issue of how to measure health. The concept 'health' can have many different meanings, as outlined in Chapter 1, and this also contributes to the variety of methods used. Some methods focus on one dimension of health, whereas others try to span different dimensions. Different measures may suit different purposes. It is unlikely that any one method will ever prove to be a comprehensive measure of health, even if it combines different measurements within a weighted index. What is important is first to be specific about why you wish to measure health, and second to select the most appropriate means of measurement, bearing in mind constraints on the time and money you have at your disposal.

The final learning activity (Learning Activity 3.11) in this chapter is for healthcare practitioners to consider and discuss what information is available about a patient's health – in this case a mother and child.

 Learning Activity 3.11   Health Records

Susan is a 27-year-old mother of one child, 7-year-old Stephen. She collapses while out shopping with her son, and is taken by ambulance to her local accident and emergency department. The staff are keen to treat Susan as effectively as possible, which will entail checking her medical records to identify any pre-existing conditions or sensitivities to particular drugs. The staff are also anxious to keep an eye on Stephen and avoid any unnecessary distress to him. What information about Susan and Stephen will staff be able to access?

REFLECTIONS ON PRACTICE

- Thinking of your own or fellow workers' practice, how is health conceptualized and measured? Are you more likely to use positive (e.g., well-being) or negative (e.g., absence/presence of disease) indicators?
- The following information would be available for a needs assessment on stroke. What are the limitations of this information and what other information might you wish to include?
  - profile of the local population (e.g., age, sex, deprivation) prevalence of stroke
  - hospital admissions for stroke
  - mortality rates for stroke
  - risk factors for stroke (e.g., levels of obesity; smoking; hypertension)
  - capacity of local hospital(s) for managing stroke (including CT scan for diagnosis, thrombolytic facilities etc.)

SUMMARY

This chapter has examined the reasons for attempting to measure health, and demonstrated that the most commonly used measures of health are in fact measures of ill health, disease and premature death. Recently, there has been more activity directed towards trying to find ways of measuring health as an independent positive variable. Different approaches have been taken, including attempts to combine the measurement of health as an objective aspect of people or environments with the measurement of health as a subjective experience interpreted by people. These different approaches have been identified and described.

FURTHER READING AND RESOURCES

There are many accessible textbooks providing introductions to epidemiology. The following provide short overviews and examples of how health and social care professionals can use health information.

Carr, S., Unwin, N., Pless-Mulloli, T., 2007. An Introduction to Public Health and Epidemiology, second edn. Open University, Buckingham.
A basic introduction to epidemiology which explains core concepts in a simple and readable form.

Crichton, N., 2022. Epidemiology. In: Naidoo, J., Wills, J. (eds.), Health Studies: An Introduction, fourth edn. Springer, Singapore.
A concise and readable introduction to epidemiological theories and methods, including features designed to help readers reflect on the material and relate it to their own concerns.

Harvey, J., Taylor, V. (eds.), 2013. Measuring Health and Wellbeing. Sage Publications, London.
This very useful book provides an introduction to health surveillance practices for public health practitioners.

FEEDBACK TO LEARNING ACTIVITIES

3.1 It is likely that you included:
- information about the health status of the community (e.g., the number of deaths and the main causes of death; the number of episodes of illness and the main types of illness)
- information on the determinants of health (e.g., people's lifestyles; the quality of housing; levels of employment; the adequacy and accessibility of health services)
- information about the community itself (e.g., the age, gender, ethnic and socio-economic breakdown of the population).

3.2 Poor food hygiene in developed countries is likely to lead to illness but unlikely to lead to death. Mortality rates are therefore unlikely to flag up poor food hygiene as a priority. Poor food hygiene may be linked to ill health and loss of income, and may therefore be a priority for health promotion. In developing countries poor food hygiene may be linked with life-threatening illnesses (e.g., *Salmonella*, *Shigella*, *Campylobacter*), but mortality rates may be inappropriate when trying to gauge the extent and impact of poor food hygiene.

3.3 The use of medical conditions, illnesses and diseases in classifying causes of death tends to obscure the significance of lifestyle behaviours in causing ill health and premature death. This in turn impacts on the funding of health promotion, which is perceived as being of less importance than clinical medicine in reducing ill health and premature deaths. This has a knock-on effect on public awareness and knowledge of risk factors for ill health and premature death. The net result of the medicalization of classification of causes of death and ill health is less priority to, funding for, and awareness of, health promotion and the enormous benefits it could bring.

3.4 In the table, Zimbabwe had the lowest life expectancy for both sexes (47 years). The countries with the lowest life expectancy worldwide are the Central African Republic, Chad and Lesotho, with life expectancy of about 53 years. Hong Kong and Japan have the highest life expectancy for both sexes (85 years). Many factors contribute to life expectancy, for example economic factors; whether or not a country is at war; its infrastructure, for example, is clean water universally available; and the availability of medical help against disease and illness.

According to the table, Zimbabwe had the highest IMR. In the Central African Republic nearly 9% of all infants die. These very high rates are due to many factors including a lack of basic sanitation and clean water; lack of medical care and facilities; and lack of social stability.

Several countries have low IMR, for example, Finland, Iceland, Monaco and Japan all had an IMR of 2% in 2019. Again, this is due to several different factors, including economic infrastructure, stability of the country and the availability of medical help when required.

3.5 There are several reasons why mortality statistics may not be complete.
- In rural areas the infrastructure for recording may not exist.
- Particular causes of mortality may be easier to recognize or be less stigmatized than others.
- People in higher socio-economic groups are more likely to have sought medical care prior to death, and thus have a detailed cause of death recorded.

There were major differences in the recording of deaths due to COVID-19 in 2020, depending on whether or not it was assumed to have caused or contributed to the death.

3.6 HES is a secure data repository, established in 1987, that collects monthly data on all hospital admissions, outpatient appointments and accident and emergency attendances at NHS hospitals in England. The data enable hospitals to be paid for the services they provide, and are also used by providers, researchers and service users for a range of other purposes, including healthcare analysis, monitoring and regulation and research. HES enables activities such as monitoring of NHS hospital activity, supporting local service planning, enhancing patient choice and public accountability and revealing health trends.

HES will reveal local use of NHS hospital services, but does not provide details of the health status of local populations or their use of primary healthcare facilities, for example GPs or community nurses. The dataset is primarily administrative, and designed to enable NHS planning and payment for services provided.

3.7 A good indicator is one that accurately and reliably describes an aspect of the population's health. Most available indicators measure ill health or death rather than health. The SMR is the ratio of observed deaths in the study group to expected deaths in the general population. A ratio of 1.0 means the number of observed deaths is equal to that of expected deaths. If the SMR is greater than 1.0, there is a higher number of deaths than expected. IMRs and life expectancy are used to compare populations internationally, and were both used to set targets to reduce health inequalities in England. GCSE rates are used in the Marmot Review (Marmot et al., 2010) as an indicator of social disadvantage. Childhood obesity is measured through the National Child Measurement Programme. Smoking prevalence rates are estimates based on national surveys. Depression rates depend on the condition being identified as such and recorded by the clinician.

3.8 Happy life expectancy is calculated by multiplying life expectancy by a happiness index. Happiness is a subjective concept, but it is associated with various factors such as security and good health. Seventy percent of the statistical variance in happy life expectancy scores is explained by four characteristics: affluence, freedom, education and tolerance. The World Happiness report in 2020 ranked cities and found that, alongside reduced social inequalities, the social and natural environments are key to happiness.

3.9 The SF-36 measures people's subjective assessment of their physical, mental and social health. It does not measure physical health in an objective manner, for example screening for markers of disease. The main criticism of such measures is that people may become accustomed to limitations of bodily or social function and not perceive them as such.

3.10 Social capital is now measured as a contributor to health status. Higher levels of social capital are associated with better health, higher educational achievement, better employment outcomes and lower crime rates. There are a number of different aspects to social capital, which makes its measurement in communities complex. Generally, social capital focuses on:

- levels of trust – for example, whether individuals trust their neighbours and consider their neighbourhood to be a place where people help each other
- membership – for example, to how many clubs, societies or social groups do individuals belong

- networks and how much social contact individuals have in their lives – for example, how often individuals see family and friends.

3.11 Susan will have been monitored throughout her pregnancy, with the following information being routinely recorded:

- height and weight
- blood pressure
- whether or not she smokes, drinks alcohol (and if so, how much per week) and takes, or has ever taken, any illegal drugs
- results of tests for HIV, hepatitis B and C, syphilis, rubella, sickle cell, thalassaemia, foetal anomalies and blood glucose.
- Susan's records will also include demographic information about her SES:
- postcode, which gives an indication of her SES
- ethnicity
- employment status (of Susan and any partner)
- marital status.

Staff will be able to access a wealth of information about Stephen. All children are given an NHS number and registered in local child health and GP systems after they have been registered (civil registration) by their parent/s. Information on newborn babies includes medical conditions identified from a blood sample and recorded at birth (e.g., sickle cell disease, cystic fibrosis). Additional information recorded on the Child Health Information System (CHIS) includes whether or not Stephen was breastfed, measurements of his head circumference and body length, hearing and sight test results, and all his vaccinations. Any medical conditions will be recorded in Stephen's medical records. At school Stephen's weight will be recorded as part of the National Child Measurement Programme.

Everyone has their personal data held by different agencies, including health authorities. Linking up all the data held on someone by different agencies (health, education, housing, social services) can provide an overview of the person's health, living conditions and SES, but this is a time-consuming task. There is also concern about the levels of information held about individuals in relation to privacy.

REFERENCES

Australian Institute of Health and Welfare, 2020. Indigenous life expectancy and deaths. Available at: https://www.aihw.gov.au/reports/australias-health/indigenous-life-expectancy-and-deaths.

Bowling, A., 2017. Measuring Health: A Review of Quality of Life Measurement Scales, fourth edn. Open University Press, Buckinghamshire.

Braveman, P., Gottlieb, L., 2014. The social determinants of health: it's time to consider the causes of the causes. Public Health Rep. 129 (Suppl. 2), 19–31.

Floud, R., 1989. Measuring European inequality: the use of height data. In: Fox, J. (ed.), Health Inequalities in European Countries. Gower, Aldershot, pp. 231–249.

Goldberg, D.P., Gater, R., Sartorius, N., Ustun, T.B., Piccinelli, 1997. The validity of two versions of the GHQ in the WHO study of mental illness in general health care. Psychol. Med. 27 (1), 191–197.

Herzlich, C., 1973. Health and Illness. Academic Press, London.

Kawachi, I., Kennedy, B.P., Lochner, D., Prothrow-Stith, D., 1997. Social capital, income inequality and mortality. Am. J. Public Health 87, 1491–1498.

Marmot, M., Goldblatt, P., Allen, J., Boyce, T., McNeish, D., et al., 2010. Fair Society Healthy Lives: the Marmot Review. Report. Institute of Health Equity, London. Available at: http://www.instituteofhealthequity.org/resources-reports/fair-society-healthy-lives-the-marmot-review.

Ministry of Housing, Communities and Local Government, 2019. The English indices of deprivation 2019. Available at: https://assets.publishing.service.gov.uk/government/uploads/system/uploads/attachment_data/file/835115/IoD2019_Statistical_Release.pdf.

Putnam, R., 2001. Social capital: measurement and consequences. Isuma Can. J. Policy Res. 2, 41–51.

Rose, G., 1981. Strategy of prevention: lessons from cardiovascular disease. Br. Med. J. 282, 1847–1851.

Stewart, A.L., Hays, R.D., Ware Jr., J.E., 1988. The MOS short-form general health survey. Reliability and validity in a patient population. Med. Care 26 (7), 724–735.

Wilkinson, R.G., 1996. Unhealthy Societies: The Afflictions of Inequality. Routledge, London.

World Health Organisation, 2010. The International Classification of Disease, Injuries and Causes of Death. World Health Organization, Geneva.

Defining Health Promotion

LEARNING OUTCOMES

By the end of this chapter you will be able to:
- define health promotion, health education and public health and the differences between them
- describe the historical origins of health promotion and the importance of the Ottawa Charter
- critically evaluate the contribution of health promotion to the health of populations
- assess your own practice in relation to advocacy, mediation and enablement.

KEY CONCEPTS AND DEFINITIONS

Disease prevention Activities to prevent the onset of disease or to reduce or ameliorate its effects.

Health education Activities to facilitate health-related learning and behaviour change.

Health promotion A range of activities and interventions that enable people to take greater control over their health. Activities may be directed at individuals, families, communities or whole populations.

Public health Activities based on a biomedical understanding of health which focus on the identification of health-related needs and population-based actions such as immunization and screening.

IMPORTANCE OF THE TOPIC

Promoting health includes a range of interventions, for example:
- fostering and enabling healthy lifestyles
- encouraging access to services and involvement in health decisions
- encouraging the regulation and control of unhealthy products and seeking to promote an environment in which the healthy choice becomes the easier choice.

Until the 1980s most of these interventions were referred to as 'health education', and were almost exclusively located within preventive medicine or, to a lesser extent, education. In the last four decades the term 'health promotion' has become widely used. Many professions, including nursing, have embraced health promotion as part of an expanding job description. This development reflects the arguments presented in this book – that it

is health, not illness or disease, which should underpin healthcare work, and that understanding the conditions in which people live is key to understanding how their health can be improved. Yet what practitioners do in the name of health promotion varies enormously. This chapter outlines the historical development of health promotion and considers different views on the purpose, nature and scope of health promotion practice.

The term health promotion is recent and was used for the first time in the mid-1970s (Lalonde, 1974). The Alma Ata conference (World Health Organization, 1978) is cited as setting the agenda for health promotion. The foundations of health promotion are complex and differ between countries and regions, but in general arose from:
- a change in perceptions of the determinants of health and a shift away from the tendency to equate health with healthcare services

- the shift from communicable to chronic diseases attributable to people's lifestyles
- an awareness of the potential of primary healthcare as a first line for prevention.

Nutbeam (1998, pp. 1–2) defines health promotion as:

a comprehensive social and political process. It not only embraces actions directed at strengthening the skills and capabilities of individuals, but also actions directed towards changing social, environmental and economic conditions so as to alleviate their impact on public and individual health. Health promotion is the process of enabling people to take control over the determinants of their health and thereby improve their health.

Health promotion can thus be understood as:

- a discrete discipline that draws on other disciplines (e.g., psychology, education, sociology) to understand a particular problem
- a process or way of working that seeks to empower individuals and groups by valuing their experience and enabling them to address their own needs
- activity that includes supporting people to develop skills, fostering public participation, building partnerships and coordinating policy and strategy.

ORIGINS OF HEALTH PROMOTION IN THE UK

19th Century: The Social Hygiene Period

The first phase of health promotion development is known as the 'social hygiene period', and had roots in both public health and health education. These origins of health promotion date back to the 19th century, when epidemic disease eventually led to pressure for sanitary reform in overcrowded industrial towns. Alongside the public health movement emerged the idea of educating the public to improve their health. The medical officers of health appointed to each town under the public health legislation of 1848 frequently disseminated everyday health advice on safeguards against 'contagion'. Voluntary associations were also formed, including the London Statistical Society (1839), the Health of Towns Association (1842) and the Sanitary Institute (1876). The temperance movement held Band of Hope mass meetings, and lectured young people in schools

and churches on the virtue of abstinence from alcohol. By the 1920s health education had become associated with diarrhoea, dirt, spitting and venereal disease. The evidence that from 10% to 20% of soldiers in the First World War had contracted venereal disease led to propaganda, one-off lectures and the first 'shock-horror' techniques in which soldiers were shown lurid pictures of diseased genitals to dissuade them from having sex (Blythe, 1986; Welshman, 1997).

1920–80: Personal Services

The second phase of health promotion development is known as the 'personal services' period. Changing patterns of morbidity and mortality shifted attention away from disease to personal behaviour. The Central Council for Health Education was established in 1927, paid for by local authority public health departments, and public health doctors formed the majority of its members. An extract from some of the tasks it listed as important reflects an emphasis on information and education to bring about change in personal habits and behaviour:

- the provision of better and cheaper posters and leaflets
- the provision of exhibits for public exhibition
- the production of a readable monthly bulletin
- the provision of a panel of lecturers who could hold the attention of an audience.

The Central Council was principally concerned with propaganda and instruction. During the Second World War it delivered 3799 lectures on sex education and venereal disease, which were attended by 340,000 people (Amos, 1993).

England's Health Education Council (HEC), which was set up in 1968 as a quango – a quasi-autonomous non-governmental organization – reflected the Department of Health and Social Security's (as it then was) medical model of health. HEC members were drawn from public health and medical and dental professions, with the inclusion of advertising and consumer affairs representatives. Its brief was to create a 'climate of opinion generally favourable to health education, develop blanket programmes of education and selected priority subjects' (Cohen Committee, 1964). Similar health education agencies were set up in Wales, Scotland and Northern Ireland.

The HEC came to be associated with mass publicity campaigns such as 'Look After Yourself' (LAY), which was launched in 1978. LAY reflected the view that people could be encouraged to adopt lifestyles which would lead to better health. The HEC consistently promoted mass campaigns and short-term initiatives. Sutherland, the first director of education and training at the HEC, has vividly described the pressures and lobbying which removed the HEC from confrontation with vested interests, such as agriculture and tobacco, and kept it confined to mass-media campaigns, despite evidence of their limited effect (Sutherland, 1987).

By the 1970s there was an increasing recognition that health policy could not continue to be confined to clinical and medical services, which were expensive and not improving the health status of the population. Health education and the prevention of disease represented a means of cutting costs and an ideology which placed the onus of responsibility onto individuals. Learning Activity 4.1 presents part of a UK policy document from the 1970s and asks you to consider and discuss changing views about personal health responsibility.

Learning Activity 4.1   Changing Views on Disease Prevention

What does this extract from the government document Prevention and Health: Everybody's Business (Department of Health and Social Security, 1976) suggest about changing views on prevention, risk and individual behaviour?

To a large extent though, it is clear that the weight of responsibility for his own health lies on the shoulders of the individual himself. The smoking-related diseases, alcoholism and other drug dependencies, obesity and its consequences, and the sexually transmitted diseases are among the preventable problems of our time and, in relation to all of these, the individual must decide for himself.

1990 Onwards: Social Determinants of Health

From 1990 grew an awareness that poor health is linked to poverty. In 1980 the Black Report, commissioned by the UK government, showed how those in lower socio-economic groups had a far higher risk of dying prematurely than more advantaged groups (Townsend and Davidson, 1982). The last four decades have seen a recognition of the need to address the social, economic and environmental determinants of health (see Chapter 2). In all countries, making the connection between the social determinants of health and health

promotion policy and action is a major task, as discussed by the International Commission on the Social Determinants of Health (http://apps.who.int/iris/bitstream/10665/43943/1/9789241563703_eng.pdf).   Yet the view that improving health depends on individuals changing the way they live in order to avoid 'lifestyle' diseases still permeates the strategies of most nations. Many strategies include targets to promote healthy lifestyles across the life course, for example, reducing the numbers of people who smoke, are obese or who have unprotected sex (e.g., the Kenya Health Policy 2014–2030 http://publications.universalhealth2030.org/uploads/kenya_health_policy_2014_to_2030.pdf).

In many countries health promotion remains 'downstream', focusing on the behaviours associated with ill health, such as smoking, rather than going upstream and challenging the material factors and socio-structural conditions that determine health outlined in Chapter 2. In addition, most governments are reluctant to challenge or curtail the industries that produce ill health, such as tobacco, alcohol and armaments. Learning Activity 4.2 presents the concept of 'upstream' and 'downstream' interventions through a well-known public health parable. Fig. 4.1 illustrates the implications for interventions using the upstream–downstream analogy.

Learning Activity 4.2   Refocusing Upstream

McKinlay (1979) trying to persuade us of the need to refocus upstream on the factors that contribute to health problems, tells a story:

There I am standing by the shore of a swiftly flowing river and I hear the cry of a drowning man. So I jump into the river, put my arms around him, pull him to shore and apply artificial respiration. Just when he begins to breathe, there is another cry for help. So I jump into the river, reach him, pull him to shore, apply artificial respiration, and then just as he begins to breathe, another cry for help. So back in the river again, without end, goes the sequence. You know I am so busy jumping in, pulling them to shore, applying artificial respiration, that I have no time to see who the hell is upstream pushing them all in.

- What examples of short-term problem-specific activity can you identify in your own work?
- What would a reorientation upstream involve?
- Who or what do you think is pushing people in?

From the late 1990s, some countries began to adopt alternative terms for health promotion. For example, in England the term 'health development' came and went and now the term 'health improvement' is used. In the USA, health promotion as a term was used (e.g., American Journal of Health Promotion), but in practice it never replaced the dominant terminology of public and school health education. Health promotion is sometimes defined as one of the processes used to secure public health. In many countries there is a clear distinction between public health and public health medicine, which emphasizes the prevention and control of disease, referred to in the UK as health protection, and described in Chapter 8. Fig. 4.2 shows the relationship between health promotion, health protection and actions related to service improvement.

 Learning Activity 4.3   Critical Health Promotion

Green et al. (2019, p. 40) refer to health promotion as the critical conscience of public health. What do you think they mean? Do you agree?

THE WORLD HEALTH ORGANIZATION AND HEALTH PROMOTION

The World Health Organization (WHO) has played a key part in proposing a broader agenda for health promotion. In 1977 the World Health Assembly at Alma Ata committed all member countries to the principles of Health for All 2000 (World Health Organization, 1977) that there 'should be the attainment by all the people of the world

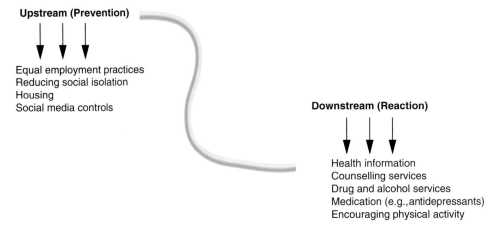

Fig. 4.1 Upstream and downstream interventions to improve mental health

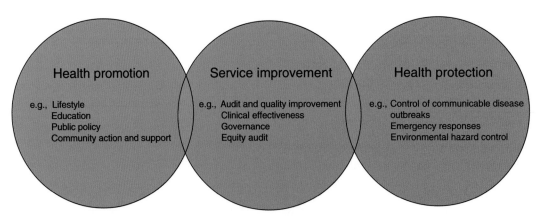

Fig. 4.2 Domains of public health, health protection and health promotion

by the year 2000 of a level of health that will permit them to lead a socially and economically productive life'. The WHO identified five key principles for health promotion in a discussion paper (World Health Organization, 1984) commonly referred to as the Copenhagen document as shown in Research Example 4.1.

The context for the development of broad-based health strategies thus needs to be based on equity, community participation and intersectoral collaboration. The WHO also noted that improvements in lifestyles, environmental conditions and healthcare will have little effect if certain fundamental conditions are not met. These include:

- peace and freedom from the fear of war
- equal opportunity for all and social justice
- satisfaction of basic needs, including food and income, safe water and sanitation, housing, secure work and a satisfying role in society
- political commitment and public support (World Health Organization, 1985).

RESEARCH EXAMPLE 4.1
The Principles of Health Promotion

1. **Holistic:** It involves the population as a whole in the context of their everyday lives, rather than focusing on people at risk of specific diseases.
2. **Equitable:** It is directed towards action on the causes or determinants of health to ensure that the total environment which is beyond the control of individuals is conducive to health.
3. **Multi-strategy:** It combines diverse, but complementary, methods or approaches, including communication, education, legislation, fiscal measures, organizational change, community development and spontaneous local activities against health hazards.
4. **Participatory:** It aims particularly at effective public participation supporting the principle of self-help movements and encouraging people to find their own ways of managing the health of their community.
5. **Multisectoral:** Although health promotion is basically an activity in the health and social fields and not a medical service, health professionals – particularly in primary healthcare – have an important role in nurturing and enabling health promotion.

Based on Rootman, I., Goodstadt, M., Hyndman, B., McQueen, D., Potvin, L., et al. (eds.), 2001. Evaluation in Health Promotion. WHO Regional Publications, European Series, No. 92. WHO Regional Office for Europe, Copenhagen. Available at: https://www.euro.who.int/en/publications/abstracts/evaluation-in-health-promotion-principles-and-perspectives.

The WHO launched a programme for health promotion in 1984, and conferences in Ottawa (1986), Adelaide (1988), Sundsvall (1991), Jakarta (1997), Mexico (2000), Bangkok (2003), Nairobi (2009), Helsinki (2013) and Shanghai (2016) have outlined further areas for action. The practice and principles of health promotion developed in the Ottawa Charter (World Health Organization, 1986) are still widely used to provide a framework for practice, as shown in Fig. 4.3. In this figure the outer circle represents the goal or action area of 'building healthy public policy' and the need for policies to hold the other action areas together. The small circle stands for the three central strategies of 'enabling, mediating and advocacy'. The four wings are the other action areas:

1. Creating supportive environments.
2. Developing personal skills, including information and coping strategies.
3. Strengthening community action, including social support and networks.
4. Reorienting health services away from treatment and care, and improving access to health services.

Each of these health promotion actions is the subject of a chapter in Part II of this book. Table 4.1 shows examples of dietary and nutrition interventions related to these action areas.

THE METHODS AND PROCESSES OF HEALTH PROMOTION

The Ottawa Charter referred to three key processes needed to achieve positive results in the action areas.

Advocacy

Advocacy in health promotion is the process of defending or promoting a cause. It may mean representing the interests of disadvantaged groups and speaking on their behalf, or lobbying to influence policy. It may also mean action to gain political commitment, policy support, social acceptance and support systems for a particular goal or cause. For example, health promotion networks in Australia, New Zealand, the USA and Canada have long advocated for a focus on the health of indigenous people.

Enablement

Enablement means working in partnership with others to enable everyone to achieve their fullest health potential. This involves identifying needs and developing networks and resources in the community; assisting people

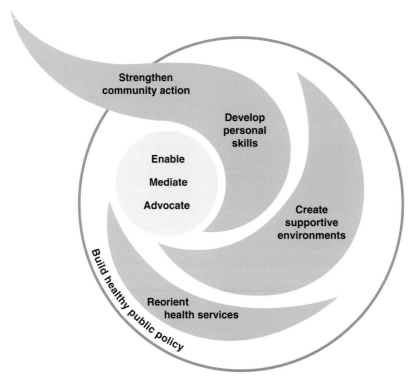

Fig. 4.3 Key action areas and strategies of the Ottawa Charter for Health Promotion (Adapted from World Health Organization, 1986. Ottawa Charter for health promotion. World Health Organization, Geneva. Available at: http://www.who.int/healthpromotion/conferences/previous/ottawa/en.)

TABLE 4.1	Improving Diet and Nutrition
Ottawa Charter Action Area	**Example of Intervention**
Building a healthy public policy	Restricting the online advertising to children of high fat, high sugar and high salt foods
	Levying a tax on sugary drinks
	Food labelling of calories
Create supportive environments	Workplace canteens that have food labelling and subsidized healthy options
	Nutritional school meals
	Licensing control of take away outlets
Develop personal skills	Cookery classes
Strengthening community action	Community allotments to grow food
Reorienting health services	Weight management as part of primary care

to develop knowledge and skills; and helping people to identify and address the determinants of their own health. Enablement is an essential core skill for health promoters which requires them to act as a catalyst and then stand aside, giving control to the community (see Chapter 11 for further discussion of working with communities).

Mediation

Health promotion requires coordinated action from many sectors including governments, health, social and economic sectors, local government, non-governmental organizations (NGOs), industries and the media. Health promoters mediate between these different sectors by providing evidence and advice, and influence local and national policy through lobbying, media campaigns and participation in working groups.

HEALTH PROMOTION – WHAT IT IS AND WHAT IT IS NOT

Is Health Promotion the Same as Health Education?

Health education may be defined as planned opportunities for people to learn about health and change their behaviour. It includes:

- raising awareness of health issues and factors contributing to ill health
- providing information
- motivating and persuading people to seek changes in their lifestyle to promote their health
- equipping people with the skills and confidence to make lifestyle changes.

The awareness that individuals' health choices contribute to the development of disease led to the view that it was possible to influence these health choices through providing information about the prevention of disease, motivating people to change their behaviour through the use of persuasion and mass-communication techniques and educating people in the skills for a healthy lifestyle. The development of 'personal skills', an action area of the Ottawa Charter, is the subject of Chapter 10. Traditional health education has often been criticized for having a narrow focus on information provision, based on the mistaken assumption that knowledge leads to behaviour change. Chapter 10 discusses the complexities of health decision-making in which people may adopt behaviours that they know are harmful, for example, smoking. This poses challenges for a healthcare practitioner; Learning Activity 4.4 asks you to reflect and discuss an interaction in primary care with a heavy drinker.

 Learning Activity 4.4   Health Education Approaches

Consider the following case of a middle-aged manual worker and appropriate health education approaches.

John is a labourer on the roads. He is 47 and single, and his social life revolves around the pub. He drinks a few pints with his sandwiches at lunchtime and usually drinks another four pints on his way home. John visits his GP complaining of backache. The GP takes his blood pressure and finds it is dangerously high.

Which of the following do you do?

1. Tell him that the recommended drinking limit for adult males is 28 units per week. Stress the damage alcohol does to his heart and liver, and that he risks a heart attack if he continues drinking at his current level.
2. Discuss the reasons for his drinking behaviour, and whether he sees it as causing problems.
3. Prescribe medicine to lower his blood pressure, and tell him to visit the practice nurse in 2 weeks to see if his blood pressure has come down.

The assumption that individuals can take control of their health simply through having information leads to a further assumption that individuals are therefore responsible for their own health. If people do not act in accordance with health information messages they can be viewed as ignorant or foolish or reckless. Victim blaming makes individuals feel guilty, and exonerates policy makers of any duty of care, although it may be factors beyond people's control (e.g., poverty, social and environmental factors) that prevent them from making health changes. The idea that individuals are responsible for their health is widely accepted but a conditional access to healthcare based on personal lifestyle is very controversial. Learning Activity 4.5 asks you to reflect on your own position in relation to individual responsibility for health.

 Learning Activity 4.5   Is Health an Individual Responsibility?

Is your health in your own hands?

Is Health Promotion About Empowerment?

Power is one of the most important determinants of people's health, whether this be through knowledge or money or skills. Empowerment is the process of people acquiring more power or control over their lives through the provision of information, the development of self-efficacy and skills to put knowledge into practice and the opportunity to take control over one's life. When we look at the practice of health education, we might be led to believe that it is the *giving* of information, and that success is when the client follows advice. This approach may be criticized as a way of achieving compliance with predetermined objectives. By contrast, education for empowerment means client-led learning, where people define their own needs and objectives and the most appropriate methods to achieve their goals. An essential element is 'critical consciousness-raising' to increase people's awareness of the fundamental causes of ill health – a notion first espoused by the Brazilian priest Paolo Freire. This process can identify the structural influences on health that need be addressed through policy change (see Chapter 5 for a discussion of Tones' model of health promotion). Learning Activity 4.6 asks you to consider and discuss the concept of empowerment, what this means at an individual level and how healthcare practitioners can enable people to take greater control over their health.

 Learning Activity 4.6   Individual Empowerment

How can individuals be empowered to take more control over their health?

The concept of empowerment applies not only to individuals but also to communities, societies and nations. Community engagement and involvement in decision-making is discussed in Chapter 11. Recent concern about environmental sustainability is a good example of how whole nations, societies and generations can be mobilized in an attempt to take control of global phenomena such as climate warming. The concept of glocalization – think globally, act locally – has evolved to describe initiatives that seek to develop and protect the local environment while simultaneously reducing the need for global trading, and hence protecting the global environment.

For practitioners, there is often a tension between persuading people to adopt a recommended behaviour, or giving them fuller information which enables the exercise of free choice. Some practitioners might argue that the long-term benefits of behavioural changes justify the use of coercive measures to bring about such changes. They might also argue that such tactics are necessary to counter-persuasive advertising and marketing of unhealthy products and lifestyles. Others might argue that respecting people's autonomy is paramount, even if this leads to unhealthy choices. Chapter 6 discusses the ethical dilemmas of creating and respecting people's autonomy, and the tension between individual choice and the social good.

The principle of public involvement and engagement is integral to health promotion and underpins health and social care programmes in the UK. This is reflected in:

- User participation in decisions about treatment and care.
- User involvement and co-production of service development.
- User evaluation of service provision and a shift to public accountability.
- User involvement and co-production of research.

Learning Activity 4.7 asks you to consider and discuss why patient and public involvement and engagement (PPIE) is desirable.

 Learning Activity 4.7   Involvement and Engagement

Why is involving the public or patients seen as a 'good thing'?

Is Health Promotion Part of Healthcare?

Whilst the health sector is crucial to promoting population health, it is only through multi or intersectoral policy and action that the determinants of health and threats to health can be addressed. Much of the disease burden and health-related suffering in the world is avoidable and arises from the choices we make as societies and as individuals. Avoiding disease is largely determined by policies beyond medical care. Many of the behavioural and environmental risk factors discussed in Chapter 2 (e.g., tobacco and alcohol use, air pollution, unsafe sexual behaviour) are strongly influenced by complex existing and emerging social factors. These social factors include rapid urbanization, climate change, pandemic threats, the proliferation of unhealthy commodities, extreme poverty and inequities and multimorbidity. Addressing the causes of these causes will require action in multiple sectors including central fiscal measures such as taxes and subsidies, laws and regulations, planning and changes in the built environment and information, education and communication in numerous settings (see Part III). Teachers, workplace managers and social and welfare workers alongside healthcare professionals are therefore all involved in promoting health.

There are, as we saw in Chapter 2, a range of factors which influence people's health including material–structural and behavioural factors. These factors need to be addressed by policy changes as well as by education. Health promotion thus involves public policy change and community action to enable people to make changes in their lives (see Chapter 12). A phrase first coined by Milio (1986) 'making the healthy choice the easier choice' has come to encapsulate health promotion. It is easy for practitioners to confine their health promotion role to offering information and advice on how to adopt a healthier lifestyle. However, for people to make such changes, the factors and situations which led them to adopt 'unhealthy' behaviours need to be addressed. People may smoke because of stress, even though they know it is bad for their health. Others may use an illegal drug because it is widely used by their peer group and is part of their social life. Equally, some people find it easier than others to make healthy choices, for example, it is easier for people with reasonable incomes who have easy access to supermarkets or high-street shopping to eat a healthy diet including fresh fruit and vegetables. Many factors affecting individual health are beyond individual control, for example, inadequate housing, busy roads or lack of childcare.

Changing health behaviours without regulation will always be difficult. Yet regulation of individual behaviour lays government open to the charge of being a nanny state. Chapter 6 discusses the nature and scope of intervention strategies, whether they include a 'nudge', which aims to change the 'choice architecture' in which individuals make decisions by, for example, removing confectionery counters from supermarket checkout areas, or the use of stronger triggers for action, for example, taxing sugary drinks.

Is Health Promotion About Preventing Disease?

The WHO has shifted the definition of health promotion away from the prevention of specific diseases or detection of risk groups and towards the health and well-being of whole populations. Instead of experts and professionals diagnosing problems, people themselves define health issues of relevance to them in their local community. Instead of health being seen solely as the responsibility of individuals, the social factors determining health are taken into account, and health is viewed as a collective responsibility of society which needs to be prioritized by organizations and governments.

The variety of approaches to health promotion are outlined and discussed in Chapter 5 and range from the medical model, focusing on health surveillance and achieving behaviour change, to the educational model, which relies on the provision of knowledge to inform. Other approaches include community development, which emphasizes the need to take collective action for health, and a social model which focuses on the need to influence decision-makers at local and national levels.

Whilst health promotion is part of national efforts to improve health, its rejection of a disease-oriented pathogenic model of health differentiates it from medical approaches. Its goals derive from a positive, salutogenic concept of health and well-being (as discussed in Chapter 1). Its methods are empowering, enabling individuals and groups to have a say in how their health is promoted, valuing their perspective and supporting people to acquire the skills and confidence to take greater control over their health.

In practice, health promotion encompasses different political orientations which can be characterized as the individual versus structural approaches. The individual approach views health promotion as a narrow field of activity which explains health status by reference to individual lifestyles. Health promotion is largely determined by experts who advise on beneficial lifestyle changes. In its emphasis on personal responsibility the individual approach advocates a minimal role for the state, and has thus come to be associated with a conservative viewpoint (see Chapter 7). For others, including the WHO, health promotion recognizes that health and wealth are inextricably linked, and seeks to address the root causes of ill health and problems of inequity using radical approaches that challenge the status quo (www.who.int/social_determinants/en/). It is not helpful to debate whether one form of activity is better or worse than the other: both are necessary. Health promotion may involve lobbying and political advocacy, but it may just as easily involve working with individuals and groups to enhance their knowledge and understanding of the factors affecting their health.

Many practitioners believe that their role in achieving the social changes necessary to eliminate health inequalities, or the community change necessary to provide social support, is limited. Yet there are ways in which individual practitioners can promote health over and beyond merely informing, advising or listening.

Skills and Competences for Health Promotion

A range of practitioners see themselves as promoting health and the term specialist health promoters is used to identify these practitioners and to differentiate them from mainstream health promotion, which can be embedded into the work of many health promoters both inside and outside the health sector, for example, in schools, sport and fitness settings, workplaces and prisons. This raises the question of identifying the recommended skills required to practice health promotion, and how to develop a health promotion workforce. In the UK, standards for public health specialists and practitioners have been developed that relate to the key functions and competences that need to be achieved in order to be able to register to practise. The International Union of Health Promotion and Education (IUHPE) has identified core competencies and professional standards for health promotion (http://www.ukphr.org/wp-content/uploads/2017/02/Core_Competencies_Standards_linkE.pdf). Health promotion is, as we have seen in this chapter, a field of activity with its own ideology and knowledge base. Its values relate to a holistic view of health that includes equity, self-determination, social justice, participation and empowerment. Despite the articulation in the Ottawa Charter, numerous NGOs such as the Thai Health Promotion Foundation and the IUHPE and specialized journals such as *Health Promotion International*, health promotion is constantly needing to assert itself as a moral and political value-based project (Wills and Douglas, 2008) that makes a distinctive contribution to the improvement of population health.

Although many professions include health promotion as part of their role, this can be limited, primarily because of workload constraints, inadequate educational training in health promotion and a traditional focus on biomedical models of health and disease treatment. Whitehead (2018), who has written extensively on health promotion in nursing practice, claims that much of nursing-related health promotion practice is 'out of step' with the wider health promotion described in this chapter, and that nurses are most likely to be engaged in health education. Research Example 4.2 illustrates how many healthcare professions include health promotion as part of their expected competences or standards and how that health promotion role is described.

Following these descriptors of health promotion roles, Learning Activity 4.8 asks you to reflect on how this would be demonstrated through an example of a nurse–stroke patient interaction.

RESEARCH EXAMPLE 4.2
Health Promotion Roles

1. Nursing

At the point of registration, the registered nurse will be able to:

Understand and apply the aims and principles of health promotion, protection and improvement and the prevention of ill health when engaging with people.

(https://www.nmc.org.uk/globalassets/sitedocuments/education-standards/print-friendly-future-nurse-proficiencies.pdf; Section 2.1.)

2. Midwifery

At the point of registration the midwife will be able to:

Demonstrate the ability to share information on public health, health promotion and health protection with women, enabling them to make evidence-informed decisions, and providing support for access to resources and services.

(https://www.nmc.org.uk/globalassets/sitedocuments/standards/standards-of-proficiency-for-midwives.pdf; Section 3.3.)

3. Allied Health Professionals

Allied Health Professionals make an enormous contribution to tackling public health challenges.... Examples of support could come in the form of brief advice on healthy behaviours, detecting signs of more serious ill-health or helping people to live independent, fulfilling lives. For instance, a physiotherapist might offer advice on healthy eating while a dietitian might signpost a smoker to local stop smoking support. Many AHPs, such as podiatrists, also play an important role in spotting symptoms of serious conditions like cardiovascular disease, by detecting irregular pulse through routine checks. AHPs play a critical role in supporting people to re-build their lives following a serious physical or mental illness for example, developing confidence and coping skills to return to work.

(https://publichealthmatters.blog.gov.uk/2019/05/09/allied-health-professionals-have-a-major-role-to-play-in-prevention.)

Learning Activity 4.8   Health Promotion Role of a Nurse

Mr C is 58 and has had a stroke which has caused right-sided weakness. Mr C can walk a few steps with sticks and can transfer from the bed to the chair with assistance. He has no swallowing problems though his appetite is poor. He is uncommunicative and repeats certain phrases such as 'what is the time?'

What is the health promotion role of the nurse?

CONCLUSION

Many health workers are strongly committed to health education and the promotion of health. However, this has often been manifested in one-to-one programmes limited to providing information. Many may be daunted by the broad definition of health promotion, and feel that this broad approach is beyond their professional remit. Indeed, it would not be possible for any one worker or group to bring about the changes needed for a health promoting society. It is important that we remind ourselves of the WHO's view, which describes the process of promoting health as not only involving political change and interagency collaboration, but also enabling people to take more control over their own health and equipping them with the means for well-being. Health promotion thus includes increasing individual knowledge about the functions of the body and ways of preventing illness, raising competence in using the healthcare system and raising awareness of, and strengthening community action on, the political and environmental factors that influence health.

REFLECTIONS ON PRACTICE

- What term do you use to describe your work in improving people's health – health promotion, health education, health improvement, public health or another term? Why do you use this term?
- How do you explain the current emphasis on health promotion in healthcare job remits?
- To what extent do you work 'on behalf of' clients or the public? Is advocacy a part of your health promotion role?
- To what extent, and how, do you encourage participation and enable your clients to take more control over their health?

SUMMARY

This chapter has looked at the origins of health promotion, and shown how different interpretations of health promotion arise from different origins. This chapter has shown that health promotion is a broad term encompassing interventions which differ in aims and in the role accorded to the practitioner. Health promotion may be seen as a set of activities intended to prevent disease and ill health, to educate people to adopt a healthier lifestyle or to address the wider social and environmental factors which influence people's health. Health promotion may also be seen as a set of principles to orient health work towards addressing inequality and promoting collaboration and participation. Health promoters thus need to be clear in their understanding of what health is, what aspect of health is being promoted and the ways in which health is affected by influences other than individual behaviour. Health promoters must also be able to argue the value or worth of health promotion, whether through the economics of prevention, or as an ethical approach to practice or both.

FURTHER READING AND RESOURCES

Green, J., Cross, R., Woodall, J., Tones, K., 2019. Health Promotion Planning and Strategies, fourth edn. Sage Publications, London.
A useful textbook which includes thoughtful and provocative discussion on health promotion goals and methods.
Keleher, H., MacDougall, C., 2015. Understanding Health, fourth edn. Oxford University Press, Melbourne.
An interesting Australian textbook that applies equity approaches to health promotion.
Nutbeam, D., 1998. A Health Promotion Glossary. Available at: https://www.who.int/healthpromotion/about/HPR%20 Glossary%201998.pdf?ua=1.
Nutbeam, D., Harris, E., Wise, W., 2010. Theory in a Nutshell: A Practical Guide to Health Promotion Theories, third edn. McGraw-Hill, Sydney.
This short text explains different relevant theories of change in individuals, communities and organizations. It provides concise reviews of established theories, such as social cognitive theory and health belief model.
National health promotion agencies or associations can provide useful insights into health promotion work. See, for example, the following.
Australia: Australian Health Promotion Association at www.healthpromotion.org.au and Victorian Health Promotion Foundation at www.vichealth.vic.gov.au.

Canada: Public Health Agency of Canada at http://www.phac-aspc.gc.ca/index-eng.php.

New Zealand: Health Promotion Agency at http://www.hpa.org.nz.

Northern Ireland: Public Health Agency for Northern Ireland at www.publichealth.hscni.net. See health and social well-being improvement.

Scotland: Public Health Scotland at https://www.publichealthscotland.scot/.

Thai Health and Information at https://en.thaihealth.or.th/.

USA: Office of Disease Prevention and Health Promotion at https://health.gov.

Wales: https://phw.nhs.wales/.

Journals can also be helpful. For example, see the following.

American Journal of Health Promotion
Critical Public Health
Health Education Research
Health Promotion International
Health Promotion Journal of Australia
Scandinavian Journal of Health Promotion

The Ottawa Charter can be downloaded from the WHO website. Available at: www.who.int/healthpromotion/conferences/previous/ottawa/en/.

FEEDBACK TO LEARNING ACTIVITIES

4.1. Ill health is often viewed as a consequence of the way that people live and as a matter of individual choice. Nowadays there is much greater recognition of the many pressures put on individuals to adopt unhealthy behaviours, and health promotion is directed at changing these pressures as well as encouraging individual change.

4.2. The concept of refocusing upstream is a powerful and persuasive argument for health promotion. It can help us to reorient our thinking away from a belief that medical care can, or will, solve most health problems, and towards prevention.

4.3. Critical conscience or consciousness is a concept developed by Freire which focuses on understanding the social and political contradictions that exist in the world, and on taking action against the oppressive forces in one's life. Health promotion as being the critical conscience of public health implies that health promotion takes a broader view of health as a socio-economic concept rather than a medical concept. Health promotion seeks correspondingly broader actions to promote health, such as building a healthier environment, rather than medical interventions such as immunization against diseases.

4.4. The first approach is health education, telling the patient what health risks he faces as a result of his drinking habits. The second approach is health education and promotion – more enabling and patient-oriented and seeking to understand his perspective. The third approach is medically oriented and seeks a result (lower blood pressure), with little active involvement from the patient.

4.5. The underlying principle of health education is to enable people to make their own informed choices about health behaviour. For those who believe the roots of ill health lie in social structures, this emphasis on choice is merely illusory. In Chapter 6 we explore further the limits to freedom of choice and how far an ethical principle such as the promotion of autonomy can govern our practice as health educators. As we saw in Chapter 2, many factors that impact on health are not in our control (although our actions may have a limited effect), for example, air pollution. Other factors are more directly controllable, for example, exposure to sexually transmitted infections and maintaining a healthy weight.

4.6. Empowerment is seen as a cornerstone of health promotion philosophy and practice. At an individual level, empowerment may mean developing health literacy, self-efficacy, self-esteem and coping skills. At a wider level, as discussed in Chapter 11, empowerment means enabling those without power to understand how structural processes (e.g., patriarchy and gender inequality or moneylending) impact on them and mobilizing the community to take action.

4.7. Involving the public or patients:
- Enables organizations to get a clear idea of what is important to local communities.
- Identifies unmet needs.
- Enables resources to be targeted effectively and to prioritize future spending.
- Ensures that services will be used and are relevant for the local context, and improves quality through measuring satisfaction.
- Encourages people to feel a greater ownership and commitment to services and interventions that they have been involved in designing and may help to restore confidence in public services.
- Contributes to greater openness and accountability.

4.8. The patient's priorities are likely to be to resume daily activities and be able to go home quickly. The nurse's health promotion role might include:

- Listening to the patient's and families' concerns and identifying needs in his daily activities such as returning to work and driving.
- Involving the patient in their healthcare plan including, for example, how to use a dosette box so he can remember to take his medication.
- Offering a short, focused intervention to Mr C and his family and skills to decrease risk factors based on safe drinking levels and the importance of weight control.

- Providing information to Mr C and his family about home modifications and rehabilitation services.
- Referring to community programmes, for example, cooking or hobby groups and to support programmes for stroke survivors.

More upstream interventions for the individual nurse might be to raise awareness of the demographic and socio-economic risk inequities for stroke and the need for cultural awareness given the high numbers of Black and Asian people who experience stroke.

REFERENCES

Amos, A., 1993. In her own best interests: women and health education – a review of the last 50 years. Health Educ. J. 52 (3), 141–150.

Blythe, M., 1986. A century of health education. Health Hygiene 7, 105–115.

Cohen Committee, 1964. Health Education. Report of a Joint Committee of the Central and Scottish Health Services Councils. HMSO, London.

Department of Health and Social Security, 1976. Prevention and Health: Everybody's Business. HMSO, London.

Green, J., Cross, R., Woodall, J., Tones, K., 2019. Health Promotion Planning and Strategies, fourth edn. Sage Publications, London.

Lalonde, M., 1974. A New Perspective on the Health of Canadians. Government of Canada, Ottawa.

McKinlay, J.B., 1979. A case for refocussing upstream: the political economy of health. In: Jaco, E.G. (ed.), Patients, Physicians and Illness. Macmillan, Basingstoke, pp. 234–248.

Milio, N., 1986. Promoting Health through Public Policy. Canadian Public Health Association, Ottawa.

Nutbeam, D., 1998. Health Promotion Glossary. World Health Organization, Geneva. Available at: http://heapro.oxfordjournals.org/content/13/4/349.full.pdf.

Sutherland, I., 1987. Health Education: Half a Policy. National Extension College, Cambridge.

Townsend, P., Davidson, N., 1982. Inequalities in Health: The Black Report. Penguin, Harmondsworth.

Welshman, J., 1997. Bringing beauty and brightness to the back streets: health education and public health in England and Wales, 1890–1940. Health Educ. J. 56, 199–209.

Whitehead, D., 2018. Exploring health promotion and health education in nursing. Nurs. Stand. 33, 38–44.

Wills, J., Douglas, J., 2008. Health promotion still going strong? Crit. Public Health 18 (4), 431–434.

World Health Organization, 1977. Health for All by the Year 2000. World Health Organization, Geneva.

World Health Organization, 1978. Declaration of Alma Ata, International Conference on Primary Health Care, Alma Ata. World Health Organization, Geneva, September 6–12. Available at: http://www.who.int/publications/almaata_declaration_en.pdf.

World Health Organization, 1984. Health Promotion: A Discussion Document on Concepts and Principles. World Health Organization, Geneva. Available at: http://apps.who.int/iris/bitstream/10665/107835/1/E90607.pdf.

World Health Organization, 1985. Targets for Health for All. World Health Organization, Geneva.

World Health Organization, 1986. Ottawa Charter for Health Promotion. World Health Organization, Geneva. Available at: http://www.who.int/healthpromotion/conferences/previous/ottawa/en/.

5

Models and Approaches to Health Promotion

LEARNING OUTCOMES

By the end of this chapter you will be able to:
- analyse different approaches to health promotion
- understand different conceptual and analytical models of health promotion and how they might be applied in practice
- appreciate the importance of theory-based approaches to planning health promotion.

KEY CONCEPTS AND DEFINITIONS

Medical model This model uses medical concepts of health and sickness rooted in physical or psychological changes that can be measured and quantified.

Model A simplified description or graphic representation of reality (processes, organizations, beings). Models are often used to hypothesize the outcomes of specific inputs or processes.

Social model This model uses sociological concepts to theorize about health and illness. Health is normal social functioning, whereas illness is any impairment (physical or psychological) of social functioning.

Theory An idea or proposition, often using general principles, used to explain a specific thing.

IMPORTANCE OF THE TOPIC

The diversity in concepts of health, influences on health and ways of measuring health leads, not surprisingly, to a number of different approaches to health promotion. If health is seen as the absence of disease, clinical interventions will be seen as appropriate. If the prevention of physiological risk factors is deemed most important, then changing people's behaviour will be the main goal. If health is viewed as the product of interaction and interdependence between the individual and the environment, then legislative or regulatory interventions will be seen as relevant. In Chapter 1 we examined how different views of health have been described in different models or representations. The medical model, sometimes called the biomedical model, has dominated thinking. The medical model defines and

measures health as the absence of disease and having a high level of function as described in Chapter 3. In the holistic model of health outlined in the World Health Organization Constitution, mental and social well-being and physical health are viewed as of equal importance. The term 'parity of esteem' is used in England to refer to a whole-person response in which physical and mental health needs are treated equally (HM Government, 2011). The biopsychosocial model acknowledges that health and well-being cannot be understood without reference to the social and cultural context. Socio-ecological models also emphasize the interrelationships between individual, interpersonal, community or institutional and wider social and economic factors.

Ischaemic heart disease is a major cause of mortality and morbidity across the world. What you consider to be the cause of heart disease will influence how you think it should best be addressed. If your perspective is predominantly biomedical, you will be more likely to expect treatment with statins and/or surgery. If your perspective is that individual lifestyles are a major risk factor, you would be more likely to recommend the use of information or community-based support such as a cooking skills programme. If you believe that behaviours are a response to the social context in which people live, you would be more likely to direct your efforts to changing the socio-economic environment through advocacy, for example, restrictions on the advertising and marketing of unhealthy foods.

In this chapter, five different approaches will be discussed:

- medical or preventive
- behaviour change
- educational
- empowerment
- social change.

These approaches are examined in terms of their different aims, methods and means of evaluation. The approaches have different objectives:

- to prevent disease
- to encourage people to adopt healthy behaviours
- to ensure that people are well informed and able to make health choices
- to help people to acquire the skills and confidence to take greater control over their health
- to change policies and environments in order to facilitate healthy choices.

All the approaches reflect different ways of working. The framework is descriptive – it does not indicate which approach is best, nor why a practitioner might adopt one approach rather than another. There are also a number of theoretical frameworks or models of health promotion which are outlined, discussed and assessed in relation to practice in the latter part of this chapter.

It is common for a practitioner to think that theory has no place in health promotion, and that action is determined by work role and organizational objectives rather than by values or ideology. However, all approaches to health promotion embody values which determine how the world is seen, which activities and priorities are selected and how strategies are implemented.

Models of health promotion are not guides to action but attempts to delineate a contested field of activity, and to show how different priorities and strategies reflect different underlying values. They are useful in helping practitioners think through:

- aims
- implications of different strategies
- what would count as success
- one's own role as a practitioner.

THE MEDICAL APPROACH

Aims

This approach focuses on medical interventions which aim to reduce morbidity and premature mortality. Activity is targeted towards whole populations or high-risk groups.

The medical approach to health promotion is popular for several reasons.

- It has high status because it uses scientific methods such as epidemiology (the study of the pattern of diseases in society).
- In the short term, prevention and the early detection of disease are much cheaper than treatment of people who have become ill. Of course, in the long term this may not be the case, as people live longer, experience degenerative conditions and draw pensions for a longer period.
- It is an expert-led, or top-down, type of intervention. This kind of activity reinforces the authority of medical and health professionals, who are recognized as having the expert knowledge needed to achieve the desired results.
- There have been spectacular successes in public health as a result of using this approach, for example, the worldwide eradication of smallpox as a result of the vaccination programme.

As we saw in Chapter 1, the medical approach is conceptualized around the absence of disease. It does not seek to promote positive health, and can be criticized for ignoring the social and environmental dimensions of health. In addition, the medical approach may encourage dependency on medical knowledge and remove people's ability to make their own health decisions. Healthcare workers may persuade patients to cooperate and comply with prescribed treatment.

Public health medicine specializes in prevention, and most day-to-day preventive work is carried out by the community health services, which include community health workers, specialist community public health nurses and district nurses.

Methods

The principle of preventive services such as immunization and screening, which are described in Chapter 8, is that they are targeted to groups at risk of particular conditions. While immunization requires a certain level of take-up for it to be effective, screening is offered to specific groups. For example, cervical screening every 3 to 5 years is offered to all women aged 25–64 in the UK.

Preventive procedures need to be based on a sound rationale derived from epidemiological evidence. The medical approach also relies on having the infrastructure capable of delivering screening or an immunization programme. This includes trained personnel, equipment and laboratory facilities, information systems which determine who is eligible for the procedure and record uptake rates and, in the case of immunization, a vaccine which is effective and safe. Having screening or immunization facilities available is effective only if people can be persuaded to use them. The medical approach to health promotion is therefore a complex process which may depend on the establishment of national programmes or guidelines.

Outbreaks of vaccine-preventable diseases (e.g., polio in the Russian Federation and measles in Wales), and the development of vaccination against COVID-19, reflect the challenges to public health authorities in obtaining optimum levels of vaccination. A key factor is gaining public trust through media campaigns, face-to-face communication and support materials to address the population's perception on the necessity, safety and efficacy of a vaccine.

Evaluation

Evaluation of preventive procedures is based ultimately on a reduction in disease rates and associated mortality. This is a long-term process, and an example of a more popular measure capable of short-term evaluation is an increase in the percentage of the target population being screened or immunized. This chapter outlines several different approaches to promote health without indicating that one is better than another, nor may only one approach be used. This section has reviewed the medical approach which holds that health is the absence of disease and thus focuses on identifying risk factors. Learning Activity 5.1 asks you to consider and discuss the medical approach.

 RESEARCH EXAMPLE 5.1

Screening for Hypertension in the Community

Hypertension is a problem among Black men who are less likely to have this condition controlled by pharmacists or family doctors. The use of alternative settings such as hairdressers and barbershops for health promotion has been advocated for some time (see, e.g., Linnan and Ferguson, 2007). In a trial in California, barbers measured blood pressure and arranged in shop meetings with pharmacists who prescribed blood pressure medication. In the control group, barbers measured blood pressure and promoted follow-up with primary care providers and lifestyle modification. At 12 months, the average systolic blood pressure fell by 28.6 mm of mercury (mmHg) to 123.8 mmHg in the intervention group and by 7.2 mmHg (to 147.4 mmHg) in the control group.

There are many reasons for the success of this intervention.

- Pharmacists made drug therapy convenient by bringing it to the barbershop.
- The intervention was tailored to Black men and endorsed by the involved barbers as trusted community members.
- Patrons of barbershops are consistent in their visits, usually every 2 weeks, which facilitates hypertension management.

Learning Activity 5.1   The Medical Approach to Health Promotion

What might be some of the critiques of the medical approach?

BEHAVIOUR CHANGE

Aims

This approach aims to encourage individuals to adopt healthy behaviours, which are seen as the key to improved health. Chapter 10 shows how making health-related decisions is a complex process and, unless a person is ready to take action, encouraging behaviour change is unlikely to be effective. As we saw in the previous chapter, seeking to influence or change health behaviour has long been part of health education.

The approach is popular because it views health as a property of individuals. It is then possible to assume that people can make real improvements to their health by choosing to change their lifestyle. It also assumes that if people do not take responsible action to look after themselves, then they are to blame for the consequences.

 Learning Activity 5.2   Barriers to Behaviour Change

What are the reasons why people may not be able to put a healthy diet into practice?

It is clear that there is a complex relationship between individual behaviour and social and environmental factors. Behaviour may be a response to the conditions in which people live, and the causes of these conditions (e.g., unemployment, poverty) are outside individual control.

Methods

Behaviour change approaches aim to affect a range of behavioural outcomes, for example:

- preventing and stopping people from engaging in harmful or risky behaviours (e.g., smoking)
- promoting health protective behaviours (e.g., exercising or vaccination programmes)
- switching from more harmful to less harmful forms of a behaviour (e.g., reducing the amount of sugar or salt added to drinks or food)
- promoting effective self-management of diseases (e.g., blood pressure monitoring).

The behaviour change approach has been the bedrock of activity undertaken by the lead agencies for health promotion. Campaigns persuade people to desist from smoking, adopt a healthy diet and undertake regular exercise. This approach is targeted towards individuals, although mass means of communication may be used to reach them. It is most commonly an expert-led, top-down approach, which reinforces the divide between the expert who knows how to improve health and the general public who need education and advice. However, there are exceptions. Interventions may be directed according to a client's stated needs when these have been identified. For example, social marketing techniques (see Chapter 13) focus on finding out what consumers want and need, and then providing it. The national archive for public information films (http://www.nationalarchives.gov.uk/films) provides examples of some of the ways the public have been encouraged to change their health behaviour over the years.

Many healthcare workers educate their clients about health by providing information and one-to-one counselling. Patient education about a condition or medication may be undertaken to seek compliance – in other words, a behaviour change – or it may be more client-directed.

Evaluation

Evaluating a health promotion intervention designed to change behaviour would appear to be a simple exercise: has the health behaviour changed after the intervention? But there are two main problems: change may only become apparent over a long period of time, and it may be difficult to attribute any change to a health promotion intervention (as discussed in Chapter 21). There are also a host of influences that could intervene and mediate the link between behaviour and outcome.

Behaviour change approaches, while popular with politicians and policymakers, are often unsuccessful, and may be victim blaming. Population-based behaviour change approaches, such as mass-media campaigns, assume a homogeneity which may not exist amongst the receivers of the health promotion messages. The National Institute of Health and Care Excellence (NICE) issues guidance on behaviour change and the principles for selecting interventions and programmes aimed at individuals. These are outlined in Research Example 5.2.

RESEARCH EXAMPLE 5.2
Guidelines for Individual Behaviour Change

NICE guidelines PH49 cover changing adults' unhealthy behaviours through one-to-one advice, group teaching and media campaigns, and NG 183 covers the development and use of digital and mobile interventions.

The guidance advises that effective interventions include working with individuals to:

- agree goals for behaviour and resulting outcomes
- develop action plans and prioritize actions
- develop coping plans to prevent and manage relapses
- consider achievement of outcomes and further goals and plans
- encourage and support the self-monitoring of behaviour and its outcomes
- provide feedback on behaviour and its outcomes.

Additionally, behaviour change interventions are more effective if there is social support and if appropriate, the healthcare worker may advise on, and arrange for, friends, relatives, colleagues or 'buddies' to provide practical help, emotional support, praise or rewards.

THE EDUCATIONAL APPROACH

Aims

The purpose of this approach is to provide knowledge and information, and to develop the necessary skills so that people can make informed choices about their health behaviour. The educational approach should be distinguished from a behaviour change approach in that it does not set out to persuade or motivate change in a particular direction. However, education is intended to have an outcome. This will be the client's voluntary choice, which may not be the one preferred by the health promoter.

The educational approach is based on a set of assumptions about the relationship between knowledge and behaviour, for example, increasing knowledge will change attitudes which in turn may lead to changes in behaviour. The goal of a client being able to make an informed choice may seem unambiguous and consensual. However, this ignores the very real constraints that social and economic factors place on voluntary behaviour change, and also the complexities of health-related decision-making (see Chapter 10).

Methods

Psychological theories state that learning involves three aspects:
1. cognitive (information and understanding)
2. affective (attitudes and feelings)
3. behavioural (skills).

An educational approach to health promotion will provide information to help clients make informed choices about their health behaviour. Information may be provided via leaflets and booklets, visual displays or one-to-one advice. This approach may also provide opportunities for clients to share and explore attitudes to their health through, for example, group discussion or one-to-one counselling. Educational programmes may develop clients' decision-making skills through role play and activities designed to help explore options. Clients may take on roles or practise responses in simulated 'real-life' situations, for example, clients taking part in an alcohol programme may role-play situations where they refuse the offer of a drink. Educational programmes are usually led by a teacher or facilitator, although the issues for discussion may be decided by the clients. Educational interventions require the practitioner to understand the principles of adult learning and the factors which help or

> ### RESEARCH EXAMPLE 5.3
> #### Antenatal Education
>
> Antenatal education is offered to pregnant women in most high-income countries and sometimes includes expecting fathers. It has the overall aim of providing expecting parents with strategies for dealing with pregnancy, childbirth and parenthood, and providing information about labour, pain relief and breastfeeding. Brixval et al. (2015) highlight how antenatal education differs in its focus, which may be on maternal exercise and relaxation techniques or information; and in its delivery, which may be in small classes with group discussions emphasizing the support that comes from others in the same situation, or in lectures in large auditoriums providing information on childbirth and breastfeeding. Group-based models have been successfully implemented in a number of countries worldwide, including Australia, Sweden and the USA. In England, a group-based approach in 'pregnancy circles' aims to empower women, giving them more of 'a voice', enhancing informed decision-making and enabling them to tailor antenatal care to their own needs (Wiggins et al., 2018). The expected outcome is that if women feel they have more autonomy and choice, this will increase their sense of control around childbirth. Yet despite considerable research the effect of antenatal education on childbirth or parenthood remains largely unknown (Gagnon and Sandall, 2007).

hinder learning. This is illustrated through the example of antenatal education in Research Example 5.3.

Evaluation

Increases in knowledge are relatively easy to measure. Health education programmes using mass-media campaigns, one-to-one education and classroom-based work have all shown success in increasing information about health issues, or the awareness of risk factors for a disease. Information alone is, however, insufficient to change behaviour and, as we shall see in Chapter 10, even the desire and ability to change behaviour are no guarantee that the individual will do so.

EMPOWERMENT

Aims

The World Health Organization (1986) defined health promotion as enabling people to gain control over their lives. This approach helps people to identify their own concerns and gain the skills and confidence to act upon them. It is unique in being based on a 'bottom-up' strategy, and calls for different skills from the health promoter. The health promoter needs to become a facilitator whose role is to act as a catalyst, getting things going and freeing up resources, and then to withdraw from the situation. The Ottawa Charter refers to 'enabling' as a core process, although latterly the term 'empowerment' is more commonly used. Essentially this means that individuals and communities directly participate in the planning and implementation of health promotion activities determining not only what they want and need in relation to health but also how they wish to get it. This is particularly important in communities that have suffered historical social injustices and have been 'disempowered'. Learning Activity 5.3 asks you to reflect on what an empowering approach would mean for your practice.

? Learning Activity 5.3   Defining Empowerment

- What do you understand by the term 'empowerment'?
- Can a practitioner empower a client?
- Are there health promotion actions which can disempower someone?

There is a difference between self-empowerment and community empowerment. Self-empowerment refers to approaches to promoting health based on counselling which use non-directive, client-centred methods aimed at increasing people's control over their own lives. For people to be empowered they need to:

- recognize and understand their powerlessness
- feel strongly enough about their situation to want to change it
- feel capable of changing the situation by getting information, support and life skills.

Empowerment also refers to increasing people's power to change their circumstances and 'social reality'. Chapter 11 includes a discussion of community development as a way of working which seeks to create active, participating communities which are empowered and able to challenge and change the world about them. This may or may not include political consciousness raising, such as that advocated by the radical educationist Paulo Freire (1972).

Methods

Many health, education and social care practitioners use empowerment strategies, which may be referred to as client-centred approaches, advocacy or self-care. Laverack (2005) states that the challenge for practitioners is to use their own power (power over) to help clients to gain power (power from within).

Community development is a similar strategy to empower groups of people to identify their concerns, and then work with them to plan a programme of action to address these concerns. Some health promoters have a specific remit to undertake community development work; most do not. Community development work is time-consuming, and most health promoters have clearly defined priorities which take up all of their time. Funding for this kind of work is invariably insecure and short term; and the communication, planning and organizational skills necessary for this approach may not be included in professional training. For many health promoters, relinquishing their expert role to fully embrace community development work may be difficult and uncomfortable. Ways of working with communities are discussed more fully in Chapter 11.

There are numerous examples of social movements in health promotion and of health activists using

---

📋 CASE STUDY 5.1
Empowering Through Reminiscence

Reminiscence is an example of a communication strategy which encourages older people to tell their story and recall past events. This provides opportunities for them to say what kind of care they want. It shifts the power balance of the relationship towards the client or patient, and helps build trust and understanding. In dementia care, older people can be encouraged to retrieve their past experience and maintain their personality. Some ethnic groups with strong oral traditions use reminiscence to preserve their cultural identity (Coleman and O'Hanlon, 2004). Football memories is a collaboration between Alzheimer Scotland and the Scottish Football Museum. It trains volunteers to spend time with people with dementia, and to encourage them to remember and discuss their football memories.

empowerment approaches. Laverack (2013) gives examples of activists seeking to:

- develop healthy public policy (e.g., sex worker collectives)
- tackle the social determinants of health (e.g., members of the community visiting elderly neighbours)
- use the media (e.g., the BUGA UP campaign – Billboard Utilizing Graffitists Against Unhealthy Promotions)
- use coalitions and networks (e.g., for the homeless).

Evaluation

Evaluating empowering activity is problematic, partly because the process of empowerment and networking is typically long term. This makes it difficult to be certain that any changes detected are due to the intervention and not some other factor. In addition, positive results of such an approach may appear to be vague and hard to specify, especially when compared to outcomes used by other approaches, such as changes in behaviour which are quantifiable, for example, reducing drink driving offences. Evaluation includes the extent to which specific aims have been met (outcome evaluation) and the degree to which the group has gelled, or been empowered, as a result of the intervention (process evaluation). Evaluation therefore needs to include qualitative methods that reveal people's perceptions and beliefs as well as quantitative methods that demonstrate outcomes such as behaviour change.

SOCIAL CHANGE

Aims

This approach, which is sometimes referred to as radical health promotion, acknowledges the importance of the socio-economic environment in determining health. Its focus is at the policy or environmental level, and the aim is to bring about changes in the physical, social and economic environment which will have the effect of promoting health. This may be summed up in the phrase 'to make the healthy choice the easier choice'. For example, a healthy food choice of fresh fruit exists, but to make it a realistic option for most people requires changes in its cost, availability or accessibility. Chapter 12 discusses the processes involved in creating healthy public policies. This section has discussed a social change approach, and Learning Activity 5.4 asks you to consider how this might be demonstrated through the example of healthy eating interventions.

Learning Activity 5.4   Social Change Approaches and Healthy Eating

Several studies have shown that a healthy diet which includes fruit and vegetables costs more than the typical diet of a low-income family. What should be the focus of health promotion interventions on healthy eating?

Methods

The social change or radical approach is targeted towards groups and populations, and involves a top-down method of working. Change may be in organizations (e.g., nutritional standards for school meals), communities (e.g., age-friendly cities) or policies and laws (e.g., smoke-free legislation). Although there may be widespread consultation, the changes being sought require commitment at the highest levels. Chapter 12 discusses healthy public policy and how legislation has had an enormous impact on the nation's health. The successful implementation of policy and legislation requires the support of the public, which is achieved through education, lobbying and social marketing. Chapter 13 discusses social marketing in greater detail.

For most health promotion workers, the scope for this type of activity will be more limited than for the traditional medical or behaviour change approaches. The necessary skills for working in this way, such as advocacy, lobbying, policy planning, negotiating and implementation, may not be included in professional training. Working in such a way may be interpreted as being beyond the brief of the job, too political or someone else's remit. There is, however, scope for professional organizations to become involved as stakeholders in social change processes. For example, health practitioners' professional bodies were involved in lobbying for a total smoking ban in public places, alongside pressure groups such as ASH (Action on Smoking and Health). Individuals may also campaign on specific issues, for example, recently nurses in the USA have highlighted the environmental threats from healthcare and used their nursing skillset for activism (Terry et al., 2019).

Evaluation

Evaluation of the social change approach includes outcomes such as legislative, organizational or regulatory changes which promote health, for example, regulations governing food labelling, a ban on tobacco sponsorship and advertising and a ban on smoking in public places.

The extent of partnership working and the profile of health issues on common agendas may also be used to demonstrate a greater degree of commitment to social change for health. These social change outcomes are typically long-term, complex processes, making it difficult to prove a link to particular health promotion interventions.

 Learning Activity 5.5   Social Change Approaches in Practice

Are there parts of your work which are aimed at social change? Have you sought to influence policies and practices which affect health?

Table 5.1 uses the example of physical activity to show how different approaches to health promotion will have different aims and use different methods.

 Learning Activity 5.6   Approaches to Healthy Eating

Choose one of the current public health priorities (reducing obesity, encouraging sensible drinking or improving mental health and well-being). Consider how health promotion interventions in this area will be affected by working with the five identified approaches to health promotion: medical, behaviour change, educational, empowerment and social change.

- In each case what would working within this approach entail in terms of:
  - aims or focus,
  - methods,
  - worker–client relationship?
- How would you evaluate your success using each approach?
- With which approach would you feel most comfortable?

MODELS OF HEALTH PROMOTION

The outline of different approaches to health promotion in Table 5.1 is primarily descriptive. Table 5.1 illustrates what health promoters do, and it is possible to move into and out of different approaches depending on the situation. A more analytic means of identifying types of health promotion is to develop models of practice. All models, be they building models, diagrammatic maps or theoretical models, seek to represent reality and show how different things connect. Implicit in the use

TABLE 5.1	Approaches to Health Promotion: the Example of Physical Activity		
Approach	**Aim**	**Method**	**Worker/Client Relationship**
Medical	To identify those at risk from disease	Screening, individual risk assessment, e.g., measurement of body mass index, cardiovascular function	Expert led, passive, conforming client
Behaviour change	To encourage individuals to take responsibility for their own health and choose healthier lifestyles	Persuasion through one-to-one advice and information; mass-media campaigns, e.g., get moving messages	Expert led, dependent client; possible victim-blaming ideology
Educational	To increase knowledge and skills about healthy lifestyles	Information and exploration of attitudes through individual or small-group work; development of skills, e.g., stretching	May be expert led; may also involve client in negotiation of issue for discussion
Empowerment	To work with clients or communities to meet their perceived needs	Advocacy; negotiation; networking; facilitation, e.g., walking projects	Health promoter is facilitator; client becomes empowered
Social change	To address inequalities in health based on class, race, gender or geography, adopting a population perspective	Development of organizational policy, e.g., transport to work policies; public health legislation, e.g., cycle routes; fiscal controls	Entails social regulation and is top down

of models is a theoretical framework that explains how and why the elements are connected. Themes, conceptual maps and models structure our thinking and action about a problem, and provide a rationale for acting or developing an approach. Models of health promotion may help to:

- conceptualize or map the field
- interrogate and analyse existing practice
- plan and chart possible interventions.

Using a model can be helpful because it encourages you to think theoretically and come up with new strategies and ways of working. It can also help you to prioritize options and locate more or less desirable types of interventions.

There has been a proliferation of models in health promotion literature, with large areas of overlap but little consensus on terminology or underlying criteria. Thus we find that Beattie (1991) uses criteria of 'mode of intervention' (authoritative–negotiated) and 'focus of intervention' (individual–collective) to generate four paradigms (see Fig. 5.1). The terminology for models also varies. For example, French (1990) calls a social change approach 'politics of health', while Caplan and Holland (1990) distinguish between a radical model and a Marxist model. This can be extremely confusing for the reader.

Beattie's (1991) Analytic Model

Beattie offers a structural analysis of the repertoire of health promotion approaches. He suggests that there are four paradigms for health promotion (see Fig. 5.1). These are generated from the mode of intervention, which ranges from authoritative (top down and expert led) to negotiated (bottom up and valuing individual autonomy). Much health promotion work involving advice and information is determined and led by practitioners. Equally, policy work may also be expert led,

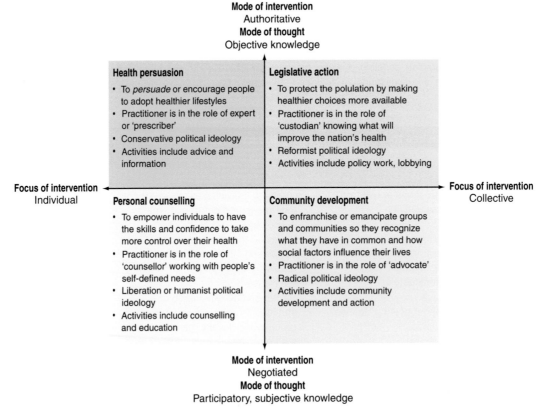

Fig. 5.1 Using Beattie's model to analyse practice (Based on Beattie, A., 1993. The changing boundaries of health. In: Beattie, A., Gott, M., Jones, L., Sidell, M. (eds.), Health and Wellbeing: A Reader. Macmillan/Open University, Basingstoke.)

with the priorities determined by epidemiological data. These approaches use objective explanations for health as opposed to approaches which prioritize subjective accounts of what health means. The other dimension relates to the focus of the intervention, which ranges from individuals who are responsible for their own health to collective bodies and the roots of ill health.

Beattie's typology generates four strategies for health promotion.

1. Health persuasion. These are interventions directed at individuals and led by professionals. An example is a primary healthcare worker encouraging a pregnant woman to stop smoking. This approach is based on the premise that the expert knows best. Health persuasion may range from straightforward signposting to brief interventions that seek to motivate a person to change.
2. Legislative actions. These are interventions led by professionals which are intended to protect communities. Examples are lobbying for tighter controls on food labelling, and limiting the number of licenced premises that serve alcohol in a neighbourhood.
3. Personal counselling. These interventions are client led and focus on personal development. The health promoter is a facilitator rather than an expert. An example is a youth worker working with young people, either individually or in groups, to increase their confidence and skills. Another example is motivational interviewing (see Chapter 10), which is widely used in primary care settings.
4. Community development. These interventions seek to empower or enhance the skills of a group or local community, for example, a community worker working with a local tenants' group to increase opportunities for further education and active leisure pursuits. The community development process is based on principles of social justice, and can therefore be viewed as a radical approach to health promotion.

Fig. 5.1 shows how Beattie's model can identify the following aspects of community development:
- goals and activities
- client–practitioner relationship
- political ideologies.

Each of the four strategies is linked to a different political perspective. Thus conservative reformist perspectives see health promotion as attempting to correct or repair a deficit (e.g., lack of information) or an aspect of deprivation (e.g., difficulties of access). These perspectives give rise to authoritative and prescriptive approaches.

Libertarian and radical perspectives see health promotion as seeking to empower or enfranchise individuals. The radical perspective seeks to mobilize and emancipate communities. Each of these perspectives also casts the practitioner in a different role in relation to clients.

Beattie's model is useful for health promoters because it identifies a clear framework for deciding a strategy, and reminds them that the choice of intervention is influenced by social and political perspectives. Learning Activity 5.7 asks you to apply Beattie's model and interrogate the current interventions to address a specific issue or priority.

Learning Activity 5.7 Applying Beattie's Model of Health Promotion

Choose one of the following programme objectives, and use Beattie's model to plot the different strategies which might be employed to reduce:
- smoking among pregnant women
- drinking among young people
- accidents among older people
- mental ill health.

Which interventions are directed towards the individual level, for example, counselling and which at population level? Which interventions are 'top down' and which are negotiated and aimed at empowering individuals or groups?

Tannahill's Descriptive Model

This model (Downie et al., 1996) was developed to illustrate the scope of health promotion activity which includes three overlapping spheres of activity: health education, health protection and prevention of ill health.

Health education – communication to enhance well-being and prevent ill health through influencing knowledge and attitudes.

Prevention – reducing or avoiding the risk of diseases and ill health primarily through medical interventions.

Health protection – safeguarding population health through legislative, fiscal or social measures. This is not how the term 'health protection' is currently used, which is to control infections (see Chapter 8).

Tannahill's diagrammatic representation (Fig. 5.2) shows how these different approaches relate to each other in an all-inclusive process termed 'health promotion'. Within the three overlapping circles are seven different domains, each of which refers to a different type of activity, all of which are part of health promotion.

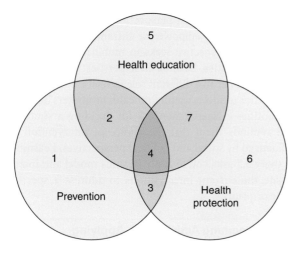

Fig. 5.2 Tannahill's model of health promotion; *1* stands for prevention service, *2* preventive health education, *3* preventive health protection, *4* health education for preventive health protection, *5* health education, *6* positive health protection, *7* health education for positive health protection (Adapted from Downie, R.S., Tannahill, C., Tannahill, A. 1996. Health Promotion: Models and Values, second edn. Oxford Medical Publications, Oxford.)

Tannahill's model can seem confusingly complex. Table 5.2 shows how this model can be applied and what is encompassed in the different domains.

Tannahill's model is primarily descriptive of health promotion practice. It is useful for health promoters to see the potential in other areas of activity and the scope of health promotion. The model does not however give any insight into why a practitioner might choose one approach over another. The model suggests that all approaches are interrelated despite reflecting distinctive ways of looking at health issues.

Tones' Empowerment Model

This model (Tones and Tilford, 2001) claims to be an empowerment model which has as its cardinal principle the goal of enabling people to gain control over their own health. It prioritizes empowerment, which is seen as both the core value and core strategy underpinning and defining the practice of health promotion. Tones makes a simple equation that health promotion is an overall process of healthy public policy × health education (see Fig. 5.3). These twin approaches underpin health promotion practice.

TABLE 5.2 Tannahill's Model and Domains of Health Promotion Activity		
Domains	**Characteristics**	**Example of Typical Interventions**
1. Prevention service	Programmes and services designed to prevent disease and ill health	Immunization screening programmes Nicotine replacement therapy
2. Preventive health education	Education to influence lifestyles to prevent ill health combined with encouragement to use prevention services	Smoking cessation advice conjunction with the provision of nicotine replacement therapy
3. Preventive health protection	Policies and regulation to prevent disease and ill health	Fluoridation of water supplies to prevent dental health problems
4. Health education for preventive health protection	Educating policymakers for the need for preventive regulations while educating a community to seek or accept changes	Lobbying for policies on seat belts
5. Health education	Influencing behaviour on positive health grounds to encourage the development of healthy attributes including self-esteem and communication	Life skills and relationship training
6. Positive health protection	Regulations and policies that promote positive health and well-being	Workplace smoking policies
7. Health education for positive health protection	Educating policymakers on the need for positive health regulations while educating a community to accept or seek change	Lobbying for a smoking public places

Numbers in the column 'Domains' refer to the areas of activity as shown in Fig. 5.2.
Based on Sykes, S., 2014. Fundamentals of approaches to promoting health. In: Wills, J. (ed.), Health Promotion for Nurses. Wiley Blackwell, West Sussex, p. 52.

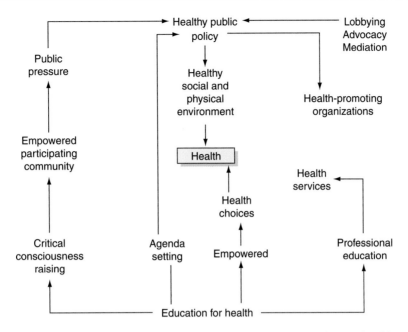

Fig. 5.3 Tones' empowerment model for the contribution of education to health promotion (Adapted from Tones, K., Tilford, S., 2001. Health Education: Effectiveness, Efficiency, Equity, third edn. Nelson Thornes, Cheltenham.)

Tones considers education to be the key to empowering both lay and professional people by raising consciousness of health issues. People are then more able to make choices and create pressure for healthy public policies. An example of this is the media attention generated by Jamie Oliver on school dinners. This created public pressure, which in turn led to the introduction of school meal standards in 2013 and universal free school meals for infants in England. We have seen how there is a distinction between self-empowerment and community empowerment. Tones argues that there is a reciprocal relationship between the two. Changes in the social environment achieved through healthy public policies will facilitate the development of self-empowered individuals. People who have the skills to participate effectively in decision-making are better able to access resources and shape policy to meet their needs. The support of individuals is also necessary for implementing change. Empowerment, as opposed to prevention or a radical political approach, is the main aim of health promotion in Tones' model (Tones and Tilford, 2001). Working for empowerment enhances individual autonomy and enables individuals, groups and communities to take more control over their lives.

THEORIES IN HEALTH PROMOTION

So far in this chapter we have looked at models of health promotion, which are visual representations seeking to explain this emerging area of thinking and practice. The terms theory and model are often used interchangeably. Theories are organized sets of knowledge applicable in a variety of circumstances. In most disciplines the building of theory and progress towards understanding a phenomenon are an accepted part of research. Theories seek to analyse, explain or predict a particular phenomenon or why something happens, and the ways in which change takes place in individuals, communities, organizations or societies. Theories underpin the processes used to plan, implement and evaluate health promotion interventions, reminding us of our goals, of how activities are supposed to work and what needs to be in place for them to work. Health promotion draws on a number of disciplines for its theory:

- Teaching and learning theory, for example, social learning theory assists in the development of health education campaigns.
- Communication theory, for example, social marketing theory is used to maximize communication with targeted audiences.

TABLE 5.3   Health Promotion Action Areas and Associated Theories

Level of Activity	Key Area for Change	Theory or Model	Chapter in This Book
Individual	How can we motivate individuals to change?	Health belief model Stages of change/model	10
	How do individuals learn?	Social learning theory	
	What is the influence of social norms?	Theory of planned behaviour	
	Why do individuals relapse or not comply?	Theory of reasoned action	
Community	Why do some people adopt new ideas readily, while others are more conservative?	Diffusion of innovation theory Community mobilization	11
Organizational change	Why do some organizations resist change?	Theories of organizational change	14–19
	What factors in settings create health?	Settings' theories: socio-ecological, salutogenesis	
Population	How do we market or design effective communication to the general public?	Social marketing theory	13

- Sociological theory, for example, to assist the targeting of specific groups defined by gender, ethnicity or social divisions.
- Psychological theory, for example, to assist in understanding individual constructs like self-esteem, self-efficacy, locus of control and the different stages of the life cycle. These ideas are valuable in understanding the attitudes and needs of clients.

CASE STUDY 5.2
Using Theory in Health Promotion Planning

Consider the example of partner notification as a priority in sexual health promotion. It is known that there is a reluctance to notify partners if a person has an STI (sexually transmitted infection) for fear of introducing conflict into a relationship, although people are more likely to inform 'steady' partners than casual ones. Studies show there is anxiety about raising the issue of STI and persuading a partner to go for testing and possible treatment. It is also known from case audits that partner notification is frequently not discussed by medical staff and patients (National AIDS Trust, 2012).

A psychosocial/behavioural theory may predict that:
- a greater intention to notify would be associated with higher levels of self-efficacy and a greater likelihood of notifying all partners.

Organizational theory may predict that:
- the lack of case notes on partner notification may reflect organizational structures and processes rather than actual activities.

- Theories of organizational change, for example, to assist in explaining the development and implementation of public policy.

As health promotion is essentially about enabling change at different levels, a theory-driven approach provides a direction and justification for activities. Table 5.3, adapted from Nutbeam et al. (2010), matches the focus of interventions to theories or models that seek to explain change processes at the appropriate level. This facilitates action informed by theory (rather than by tradition or knee-jerk response).

CONCLUSION

A number of different activities are subsumed under the label 'health promotion'. For example, there are a number of different approaches to tackling an issue such as teenage pregnancy:
- medical approach: providing contraception
- behavioural approach: contraceptive advice
- educational approach: sex education
- empowerment approach: life skills, including negotiation, assertiveness and communication
- social change approach: review of services and benefits (education and training, medical, financial, housing) available to young women.

Attempts to organize these activities into different categories have generated a plethora of models and typologies. The most obvious starting point is to describe the variety of current practices, and this is the approach taken at the beginning of this chapter.

However, there are limitations to this method, and it may be criticized as being insufficiently analytical. Theorists who have taken this one step further have identified key criteria which serve to locate different forms of practice, both existing and potential. Adopting a more analytical approach enables judgements to be made about more and less desirable forms of practice, and opens up these judgements for debate. If health promotion is to progress as a discipline and an activity in its own right, a strong theoretical framework is necessary.

The search to clarify models and typologies of practice may appear to be academic and unrelated to the 'here and now' of your activities to promote health. However, we would argue that for practice to develop beyond a reactive response to demands made by others, practitioners need to have an idea of all available options and reflect on which approaches are most effective and most congruent with their own beliefs and values. It is only when we can contemplate different ways of promoting health that we can make judgements as to what is possible and what is preferable. Recognizing that the two are not always synonymous may be frustrating in the short term, but must in the long term contribute towards the effectiveness and efficiency of health promotion.

Learning Activity 5.8 in this chapter asks you to synthesize your learning and understanding of different approaches to health promotion.

? Learning Activity 5.8 Using Health Promotion Models to Plan Strategy

The smoking rate among women on low incomes increases with:
- greater disadvantage
- more children to care for
- children in poorer health
- caring alone
- carrying extra responsibility for family members.

Using one of the models discussed earlier, map those health promotion interventions which you would regard as:
- most appropriate for women smokers on a low income
- most likely to be adopted
- ones you would use.

If the answers to these three criteria are different, what might account for this?

▌SUMMARY

This chapter has examined five different approaches to health promotion: the medical or preventive approach, the behaviour change or lifestyle approach, the educational approach, the empowerment and community development approach, and the social change or radical approach. In practice, the edges between them may be blurred. However, they do differ in significant ways. They encompass different assumptions concerning the nature of health, society and change. The preferred methods of intervention, necessary skills and means of evaluation all differ. Many health promoters will find that the approach they adopt is dictated, in part at least, by their job role and functions. This chapter stresses the importance of examining your approach to health promotion and identifying any changes you may wish to make.

FURTHER READING AND RESOURCES

Cragg, L., Davies, M., Macdowall, W., 2013. Health Promotion Theory. McGraw Hill, London.
A useful synthesis of theory and its application.

Laverack, G., 2005. Public Health: Power, Empowerment and Professional Practice. Palgrave Macmillan, Hampshire.
This book explores the concept of power and discusses the potential and dilemmas for professional practitioners seeking to empower their clients, in both individual and community settings.

Nutbeam, D., Harris, E., Wise, M., 2010. Theory in a Nutshell, third edn. McGraw Hill, Sydney.
A useful short guide to theories across the disciplines that health promotion draws on.

Wills, J., 2012. Understanding and using theory and models. In: Jones, L., Douglas, J. (eds.), Public Health: Building Innovative Practice. Open University, Buckingham.
A brief summary of health promotion models and theories.

FEEDBACK TO LEARNING ACTIVITIES

5.1. Critiques of a medical approach to an issue might include:
- does not seek to understand or address the underlying cause, which is probably related to social determinants of health
- does not seek to promote positive health
- may encourage a dependence on medical solutions, including technology and medication
- probably removes decision-making from lay people.

5.2. Barriers to changing behaviour such as a healthy diet include:
- cost, for example, of fruit and vegetables, lean meat and fish
- negative perceptions, for example, healthy food is not tasty
- beliefs, for example, that their current diet is already healthy
- lack of knowledge, for example,. about portion sizes or the different food groups in their diet
- lack of cooking skills
- lack of availability of healthy foods
- family or peer pressure, for example, to eat the same (unhealthy) diet as friends and family.

5.3. Empowerment is a complex, albeit popular, concept. Empowerment is the giving of power or control, and may occur at individual, organizational or community levels. Empowerment is both a process and an outcome. Practitioners can empower clients by providing information and skills. Health promotion actions, even if they lead to better health, can be disempowering if decisions are taken with no consultation. See Woodall et al. (2010) for a review of the evidence on empowerment and well-being.

You may have included some of the following:
- changes in pricing structures, such as reducing the price of wholemeal bread compared to white bread
- working with food manufacturers and distributors to promote food labelling, making it easier for customers to identify low-fat, low-sugar foods
- farming subsidies which encourage the production of lean meat
- the provision of healthy food in workplaces and hospitals
- ensuring that the existing nutritional standards for school meals, which promote healthy food including fruit and vegetables, are maintained.

5.4. The focus of health promotion interventions towards healthy eating might include organizational development, environmental health measures, economic or legislative activities and public policies on housing, education or the provision of services are all examples of health promotion aimed at social change.

Partnership working with other agencies enables the socio-economic and environmental determinants of health to be targeted, for example, health, education and environment practitioners may work together to lobby for the provision of safe outdoor recreation areas.

Practitioners may seek to address the root causes of ill health by developing health profiles, conducting health equity audits, working in partnerships with other agencies, social commentary and research.

5.5. For many health workers whose work is predominantly with individuals on your caseload, it may be difficult to work towards social change. Most of your work may include education (e.g., about the calories in different foods) and advice on behaviour change (e.g., avoiding calorific snacks, exercising more). There is, however, a lot you can do to document and record the social determinants and factors that are affecting your patient's health. For others, advocacy and lobbying for change may be part of your work where an issue affects your setting, for example, those working with children may seek to reduce pollution in urban areas or those working in clinical settings may seek to address environmental waste.

5.7. What you may find is that there is a preponderance of strategies in one quadrant. The approach which used to be most popular was health persuasion, but currently there are increasing numbers of state-led legislative interventions.

5.8. It is likely that there may be a discrepancy between the model you as a health professional would adopt and the model that might be most effective or acceptable to the woman living on a low income. As a health professional you might feel most comfortable with the health education or prevention models, providing information or Nicorette to the young mother. Such an approach vindicates your authority and expertise. However, the young mother might feel more comfortable with a health protection model, which introduces restrictions on smoking in public places but does not target her behaviour at home. Health professionals are constrained by their workload and budget, and their primary role is to provide care for individual patients rather than to lobby for societal changes regarding health behaviours (such as smoking bans in public places).

REFERENCES

Beattie, A., 1991. Knowledge and control in health promotion: a test case for social policy and social theory. In: Gabe, J., Calnan, M., Bury, M. (eds.), The Sociology of the Health Service. Routledge, London, pp. 162–202.

Brixval, C.S., Axelsen, S.F., Lauemøller, S.G., Andersen, S.K., Due, P., et al., 2015. The effect of antenatal education in small classes on obstetric and psycho-social outcomes: a systematic review. Syst. Rev. 4, 20. Available at: https://doi.org/10.1186/s13643-015-0010-x.

Caplan, R., Holland, R., 1990. Rethinking health education theory. Health Educ. J. 49, 10–12.

Coleman, P.G., O'Hanlon, A., 2004. Ageing and Development. Arnold, London.

Freire, P., 1972. Pedagogy of the Oppressed. Penguin, Harmondsworth.

French, J., 1990. Boundaries and horizons: the role of health education within health promotion. Health Educ. J. 49 (1), 7–10.

Gagnon, A.J., Sandall, J., 2007. Individual or group antenatal education for childbirth or parenthood, or both. Cochrane Database Syst. Rev. 3, CD002869.

HM Government, 2011. No health without mental health. Available at: https://assets.publishing.service.gov.uk/government/uploads/system/uploads/attachment_data/file/213761/dh_124058.pdf.

Laverack, G., 2005. Public Health: Power, Empowerment and Professional Practice. Palgrave Macmillan, Hampshire.

Laverack, G., 2013. Health Activism: Foundations and Strategies. Sage Publications, London.

Linnan, L.A., Ferguson, Y.O., 2007. Beauty salons: a promising health promotion setting for reaching and promoting health among African American women. Health Educ. Behav. 34 (3), 517–530.

Nutbeam, D., Harris, E., Wise, M., 2010. Theory in a Nutshell. McGraw Hill, Sydney.

Terry, L., Bowman, K., West, R., 2019. Becoming and being an environmentally 'woke' nurse: a phenomenological study. Nurs. Outlook 67, 725–733. Available at: https://doi.org/10.1016/j.outlook.2019.04.011.

Wiggins, M., Sawtell, M., Wiseman, O., McCourt, C., Greenberg, L., et al., 2018. Testing the effectiveness of REACH Pregnancy Circles group antenatal care: protocol for a randomised controlled pilot trial. Pilot Feasibility Stud. 4, 169.

Woodall, J., Raine, G., South, J., Warwick-Booth, L., 2010. Empowerment and Health and Wellbeing: Evidence Review. Available at: http://eprints.leedsbeckett.ac.uk/id/eprint/2172/.

World Health Organization, 1986. Ottawa Charter for Health Promotion. World Health Organization, Geneva. Available at: http://www.who.int/healthpromotion/conferences/previous/ottawa/en/.

6

Ethical Issues in Health Promotion

LEARNING OUTCOMES

By the end of this chapter you will be able to:

- critically analyse the ethical values and principles underpinning health promotion
- discuss various ethical issues that arise in promoting health

- reflect upon your personal ethics and practice
- defend health promotion as an ethically sound activity.

KEY CONCEPTS AND DEFINITIONS

Autonomy A person's ability to be independent and free, and make their own decisions.

Beneficence (doing good) Actions taken to benefit and help other people.

Ethics A branch of philosophy that focuses on defining moral principles and what concepts and behaviours are morally right or wrong.

Morality Principles and beliefs about what is right and wrong, or good and bad, behaviour.

Non-maleficence (doing no harm) Actions that are not intended to harm other people.

Social justice Justice or fairness regarding the opportunities, privileges and distribution of wealth and power within a society.

IMPORTANCE OF THE TOPIC

Health promotion involves working to improve people's health. This requires making judgements about what better health means for the individual and society, and about whether, when and how to make a health promotion intervention. The understanding of ethics helps us to clarify, prioritize and justify courses of action based on principles, values and beliefs. Many courses of action will have competing claims and pose challenging problems, and the values underpinning actions may not be equally shared, for example, people may disagree as to:

- whether it is justified to implement health promotion interventions which have not been sufficiently evaluated,
- the extent to which health promotion should influence the public to choose what is deemed to be the

healthy (and, by implication, correct and good) choice,

- the legitimacy of the state to influence the environment to encourage healthy behaviour.

This chapter explores how to establish a just, transparent process for decision-making based on a commitment to:

- respect for the rights, dignity, confidentiality and worth of individuals and groups:
  - prioritizing the needs of those experiencing poverty and social marginalization
  - ensuring that health promotion action is beneficial and causes no harm
  - being honest about what health promotion is, and what it can and cannot achieve
  - building autonomy and self-respect as the basis for health promotion action
  - being accountable for the quality of one's own practice and taking responsibility for maintaining

and improving one's knowledge and skills (Abbasi et al., 2018; Dempsey et al., 2011).

THE NEED FOR A PHILOSOPHY OF HEALTH PROMOTION

Debate in health promotion has centred on discussion of practice and some attempts to develop a theoretical base. However, there has been relatively little discussion concerning the philosophy of health although this is integral to how we understand the world. Health promotion involves decisions and choices that affect other people and requires judgements to be made about whether particular courses of action are right or wrong. There are no definite ways to behave. Health promotion is, according to Seedhouse (2009), 'a moral endeavour'. Philosophical debate helps to clarify what it is that one believes in most and how one wants to live. It helps practitioners reflect on the principles of practice, which then inform practical judgements about whether to intervene and which strategies to adopt.

Philosophy has three main branches:
1. logic – the development of reasoned argument,
2. epistemology – enquiry into the nature and origins of knowledge and meanings,
3. ethics – enquiry into the principles underpinning practice and how we ought to act and conduct ourselves.

Morals refers to beliefs about how people 'ought' to behave. These debates about right and wrong, good and bad and duty are part of everyday discourse. Is it wrong to tell a lie? Is it ever justified to kill another person? Is it our duty to look after ageing parents? Judgements about the morality of people's actions derive from our personal values and moral beliefs, which in turn derive from religion, culture, ideology, professional codes of practice or social etiquette, the law and our life experience. The function of ethical theory is not to provide answers, but to inform these judgements and help people work out whether certain courses of action are right or wrong.

Western philosophy has been shaped by two theories of ethics – deontology and consequentialism. Deontology comes from the Greek word deonto, meaning duty. Deontologists believe that we have a duty to act in accordance with certain universal moral rules. Consequential ethics are based on the premise that whether an action is right or wrong depends on its end result.

DUTY AND CODES OF PRACTICE

Deontologists believe that there are universal moral rules that it is our duty to follow. Many of the philosophical discussions about the nature of duty are based on the theories of Immanuel Kant. The essence of Kant's thinking is encapsulated in the categorical imperative which can help us to discover, through reason, if a rule or moral principle exists (Kant, 1909).

The major features of Kant's theory are as follows:
1. Act as if your action in each circumstance were to become law for everyone, yourself included, in the future. In other words, if everyone always behaved this way, would the overall effect be good? If the answer is yes, then this action may be applied in all similar situations. The biblical 'Do unto others as you would they do unto you' becomes a universal moral imperative.
2. Always treat human beings as 'ends in themselves' and never merely as a 'means' to achieve other goals. A moral rule respects all people.

Deontological theories make decision-making apparently easy, because as long as we obey the rules then we must be doing the right thing, regardless of the consequences.

Screening can identify individuals at increased risk of or in the early stages of a disease (see Chapter 8) but it raises many ethical issues and is widely debated. Examples include consent and the extent to which it is informed and the utility of the actual tests performed. Learning Activity 6.1 asks you to consider and discuss as many issues as possible that pertain to the ethics of antenatal screening.

 Learning Activity 6.1   The Ethics of Antenatal Screening
How ethical is antenatal screening?

Many healthcare workers have codes of practice which set out guidelines for the fulfilment of duties. For example, doctors take the Hippocratic Oath, which requires them as a first principle to avoid doing harm. The Nursing and Midwifery Council (www.nmc-uk.org) states that nurses have a duty to respect life, to care for patients and to do no harm. Kant (1909) would have added 'the duty to be truthful in all declarations is a sacred, unconditional command of reason, and not to be limited by any expediency'.

Sindall (2002) argues that health promotion has not engaged in the kind of debate necessary to establish the principles, duties and obligations which health promoters would need to agree to before working in the field. Codes of conduct are simply devices offering a framework in which to practice; they do not help practitioners involved in the messy and complex everyday world of healthcare (Duncan, 2021). For example, Article 3 of the nursing code declares that the registered nurse, midwife or specialist community public health nurse must obtain consent before any treatment or care, but the concept of informed consent is complex. Learning Activity 6.2 asks you to focus on this issue of consent and to consider and discuss what is actually meant by consent being 'informed'.

 Learning Activity 6.2   Defining Informed Consent

What do you understand by the concept of informed consent? What difficulties might there be in complying with this aspect of the code of practice?

CONSEQUENTIALISM AND UTILITARIANISM: THE INDIVIDUAL AND THE COMMON GOOD

The other classical school of ethics is consequentialism, and utilitarianism is its best-known branch. Consequentialism differs from deontological theories because it is concerned with ends and not only means. The utilitarian principle is that a person should always act in such a way that will produce more good or benefits than harms. Utilitarians such as John Stuart Mill and Jeremy Bentham aimed for the greatest good or pleasure for the greatest number of people. Utilitarians can thus respond to all moral dilemmas by reviewing the facts and weighing up the consequences of alternative courses of action. This can, of course, prove difficult. What exactly is a good end? How does one predict whether an outcome will be favourable? One of the main problems with utilitarianism is that if the aim of all actions is to achieve the greatest good, does this justify harm or injustice to a few if the majority benefits?

There are many questions over health promotion's ends and means.

- Good health is a relative concept, so whose definition should take precedence? Is it ethical for a practitioner to persuade someone to adopt their perception of a healthier lifestyle?
- What means are justifiable to promote good health in the population? Should the interests of the majority always prevail?
- Since most ill health is avoidable, should those who knowingly adopt unhealthy behaviours be refused treatment?

In Chapter 12 concern over 'social engineering' in health promotion is discussed in relation to public policy used to promote health, and whether government intervention risks becoming government intrusion. Many interventions are justified as being in the interests of a 'healthy society', yet they may not have been requested or desired by the lay population. Learning Activity 6.3 identifies several examples of state intervention and public policies, some of which may be in place in your country and some may not. Consider and discuss whether you would support each of these and whether there are ethical issues involved.

 Learning Activity 6.3   The Ethics of Healthy Public Policy

Consider these examples of healthy public policies and whether, in your view, they are ethical:

- fluoridation of tap water,
- subsidy of lead-free petrol,
- ban on smoking in green areas run by local government, for example, parks, sports grounds, beaches,
- complete ban on drinking and driving (requiring a 0 mg blood alcohol level for drivers),
- compulsory testing of all visitors to the UK for human immunodeficiency virus (HIV) infection,
- government subsidy of child-minding,
- compulsory immunization for all children entering educational institutions.

ETHICAL PRINCIPLES

Ethical principles can help clarify the decisions that have to be taken at work. Sometimes decisions may be guided by trying to do the best for the greatest number of people; at other times they may be guided by an overriding concern for people's right to determine their own lives; and sometimes decisions may be guided by other ethical principles or a professional code of conduct.

There are four widely accepted ethical principles (Beauchamp and Childress, 2019):

1. Respect for autonomy (a respect for the rights of individuals and their right to determine their lives).
2. Beneficence (the commitment to do actions that are of benefit).
3. Non-maleficence (the obligation not to harm other people; if there is doubt, precaution should prevail).
4. Justice (the obligation to act fairly when dealing with competing claims for resources or rights).

These principles provide a framework for consistent moral decision-making. However, in practice increasingly complex and sometimes conflicting choices between these principles must be made. The World Health Organisation (2015) highlights the ways that ethical principles can be called into question in public health and health promotion practice:

Harm prevention, public good and individual liberty

If infectious disease threatens the health and welfare of others, is it legitimate to restrict people's privacy and liberty in order to protect others in the community?

Treatment and prevention

Prevention is better than waiting for harm to develop and then focusing on treatment. However, when resources are limited, devoting greater attention to prevention may take away needed resources from treatment. How should priorities be identified?

Health promotion and equity

Ill health related to chronic disease is rising across the world. Ill health and chronic disease are often linked to lifestyle choices, such as smoking tobacco, drinking alcohol, overeating and not exercising enough. Those in lower socio-economic groups have fewer opportunities to change these aspects of their lives, which may also help them to cope with stress. How can health promotion actions avoid widening inequalities?

States have long intervened to reduce the impact of epidemics through, for example, quarantine and the forcible detention of the sick during plagues. Other examples of state intervention include actions to tackle pollution or the tobacco industry, which are discussed in Chapter 12. The COVID-19 pandemic has raised several ethical and policy dilemmas. Collins and Garlington (2020) proposed two new principles – compassion and solidarity – with an extra emphasis on justice in recognizing that the burden of pandemics falls on the most marginalized in society. The ethical issues

RESEARCH EXAMPLE 6.1

Consequentialist Ethics: Trading Off Health Impacts Versus Societal Impacts

A study in the Netherlands (Chorus et al., 2020) during the COVID-19 pandemic asked a sample of citizens to choose between various lockdown and policy measures according to their effects on health, the economy, education and personal income. They found that:

…the average citizen, in order to avoid one fatality directly or indirectly related to COVID-19, is willing to accept a lasting lag in the educational performance of 18 children, or a lasting (>3 years) and substantial (>15%) reduction in net income of 77 households…

…the elderly, known to be at relatively high risk of being affected by the virus, are relatively reluctant to sacrifice economic gain and educational disadvantages for the younger generation, to avoid fatalities.

posed by COVID-19 in relation to individual and social actions are discussed in Research Example 6.1.

Seedhouse (2009) has developed the principles into an ethical grid which provides health promoters with an easy-to-follow guide on which to ground their work on moral principles (Fig. 6.1).

The Ethical Grid

The grid provides a tool for practitioners, helping them to question basic principles and values, and be clear about what they intend to do. It suggests ways in which practitioners can work through proposed actions. In any situation we should be asking ourselves certain questions:

1. Central conditions in working for health
   a. Am I creating autonomy in my clients, enabling them to direct their own lives?
   b. Am I respecting the autonomy of my clients, whether or not I approve of their chosen direction?
   c. Am I respecting all people as equal?
   d. Do I work with people on the basis of needs first?
2. Key principles in working for health
   a. Am I doing good and avoiding harm?
   b. Am I telling the truth and keeping promises?
3. Consequences of ways of working for health
   a. Will my action increase the individual good?
   b. Will it increase the good of a particular group?
   c. Will it increase the good of society?
   d. Will I be acting for the good of myself?

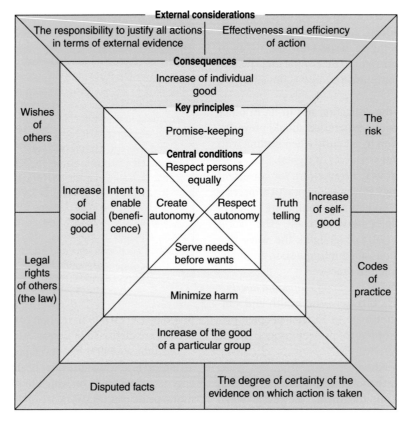

Fig. 6.1 The ethical grid (From Seedhouse, D., 1988. Ethics: The Heart of Health Care. Wiley, Chichester.)

4. External considerations in working for health
   a. Are there any legal implications?
   b. Is there a risk attached to the intervention?
   c. Is the intervention the most effective and efficient action to take?
   d. How strong is the evidence on which this intervention is based?
   e. What are the views and wishes of those involved?
   f. Can I justify my actions in terms of all this evidence?

Health promotion involves working to improve people's health. This requires a series of value judgements about what health means for the individual and society, and about whether, when and how to intervene.

Learning Activity 6.4 considers an example of incentives and their ethical basis which you are asked to assess by using Seedhouse's framework. In Learning Activity 6.5 you will continue to identify ethical issues posed through different scenarios and again try to justify the actions you would take in each case.

 Learning Activity 6.4   The Ethics of Incentivizing Change

In the USA a charity has offered young women addicted to heroin or crack cocaine, and who have frequent pregnancies resulting in abortions, stillbirths or addicted babies, a sum of money to be sterilized. Use Seedhouse's ethical grid illustrated in Fig. 6.1 to consider whether or not such action is morally justified.

 Learning Activity 6.5   Ethical Decision-Making

In the following scenarios, decide what ethical issues are involved, and what action you would take, and why.

1. You are nursing a 50-year-old who has chronic obstructive pulmonary disease. The patient has smoked 40 cigarettes a day since he was 17. He has become very distressed by advice to stop smoking.
2. A child has recently died from glue-sniffing at a local secondary school. The community police officer is keen to visit all local schools to show a video depicting a group of children who sniff glue and get into all kinds of trouble.
3. As part of a local mental health strategy, a general practice has introduced questionnaires to detect early indicators of mental health problems at all its clinics. A middle-aged, single, unemployed man regularly attends the diabetic clinic. His questionnaire indicates that he has sleep disturbance and high levels of anxiety.

Autonomy

Autonomy derives from the Greek word autonomous, meaning self-rule. It refers to people's capacity to choose freely for themselves and ability to direct their own lives. Since people do not exist in isolation from each other, there will be restrictions on individual autonomy and autonomous people have a sense of responsibility: they cannot do entirely as they like. Thus, people do not have complete freedom of choice. The limits to an individual's autonomy are when that individual's action affects others in a negative way. Apart from this restriction, traditional notions of liberal individualism see autonomy as essential to all human beings. It is only constrained by:

- reason and the ability to make rational choices
- the ability to understand one's environment
- the ability to act on one's environment.

In addition, a person needs to be free from pressures such as fear and hunger, and have the personal and social circumstances to make any chosen action possible.

Autonomy must, therefore, be thought of not as an absolute but as attainable to a greater or lesser extent. Not everyone has autonomy. When people's capacity for rationality is affected in some way, decisions are often taken on their behalf on the basis that 'they do not know what's best for them'. Thus people with a learning disability or mental illness, young children and older people with mental confusion are often assumed to be unable to make a rational choice. It was not until the 20th century that women were deemed able to make a rational choice in a democratic election. The Children

Act of 1989 first recognized the rights and capacity of children to have a say in their care. Equality, rights and ethics all come into play when considering the sexual relationships of people with learning disabilities. Sexual expression and experiences are a human right but it can be difficult to assess if a person with learning disabilities can give informed consent to partnered sexual activities. Learning Activity 6.6 asks you to consider and discuss this contested issue.

Learning Activity 6.6   Ethical Issues: The Sexual Rights of People with Learning Disabilities

The rights of young people with profound learning disabilities to determine their sexual health is a contested area.

- Should young people with a severe learning disability have sexual relationships?
- Should they decide whether or not to use contraception?
- Should they decide if they wish to have children?

What do we mean by autonomy? In part, we must mean respecting those we work with as people and helping them to cope with the consequences of their choices. Seedhouse (2009) makes a distinction between creating and respecting autonomy, which he regards as central conditions when working for health.

Creating autonomy is trying to enhance what a person is able to do. In health promotion work this is often called empowerment. It may involve giving information to enable clients to make choices, or developing clients' skills in analysing situations and making decisions by increasing self-awareness and assertiveness. As stated elsewhere in this book, it is of prime importance in health promotion practice to recognize the limits to individual autonomy, and that social and economic circumstances can constrain individual health choices. Health promoters may claim they are creating autonomy by explaining the health hazards of smoking and thereby enabling individuals to make an informed choice to quit. Yet the autonomy of smokers may be compromised by addiction, social circumstances in which cigarettes may serve as a 'drug of solace' or a means of belonging, advertising and peer pressure.

Respecting autonomy is respecting a person's choices, whether or not they are approved by others – for example, respecting a pregnant woman's autonomy to smoke or to have a termination of pregnancy. Creating and respecting autonomy are closely related. People cannot express a free wish if they are not aware of the possibilities open to them, and thus it may, in some circumstances, be ethically justifiable not to respond to a client's expressed wishes, but to attempt to open up to them other options. The implications of this for professional practice are raised in Learning Activity 6.7.

 Learning Activity 6.7   Creating Autonomy

Think of some examples from your work when you have attempted to create autonomy in your clients so they are able to express their wishes and wants.
    How did you go about trying to create autonomy?
    At what point did you decide that the client is autonomous and to respect their wishes?

Chapter 11 explores the community development way of working which aims to empower people with regard to their own health agenda. This chapter explores the dilemma of control and autonomy, and to what extent community development workers impose, their own agenda, or genuinely facilitate local or community health needs. Chapter 10 looks at how practitioners support individuals to change, and whether such approaches empower individuals or merely get them to make the desired changes.

Perhaps the starkest example of the ethical problems associated with respecting autonomy is what confronts the health worker when a patient or client chooses not to follow advice or treatment which is known to be beneficial. It would seem straightforward that this is the client's right, and that the health worker should respect the client's autonomy and choices if the client is properly informed and understands any risks involved. However, the health worker is committed to 'doing good' and may feel it is their duty to persuade the client, especially if the client's decision has implications for other people. Such action is paternalistic, and places the health worker's need to do good above the client's wish for autonomy. Yet by not seeking to persuade or motivate the client, the practitioner may, by omission, be doing harm.

Respecting autonomy involves respecting another person's rights and dignity so that the person reaches a maximum level of fulfilment as a human being. In the context of health promotion and healthcare this means that the relationship with patients or clients is based on a respect for them as people with individual rights. It follows that we must then see them as 'whole people', with physical, social, emotional and spiritual needs, as equal and unique individuals. Learning Activity 6.8 raises another contested issue which is whether treatment should ever be conditional.

 Learning Activity 6.8   Ethical Issue: Refusing Treatment

A patient who has undergone heart bypass surgery continues to smoke after the operation.
- Is it justifiable to refuse further treatment?
- What factors do you take into account in making your judgement?

Rights in relation to healthcare are usually taken to include:
- the right to information
- the right to privacy and confidentiality
- the right to appropriate care and treatment.

Health workers are often placed in the position of deciding whether to inform patients or relatives of an adverse prognosis. Although the patient's right to information is usually considered paramount, there are occasions when the health worker's duty of beneficence – to do good and avoid harm – may outweigh this right.

Beneficence (Doing Good) and Non-maleficence (Not Doing Harm)

Beneficence means doing or promoting good as well as preventing, removing and avoiding evil or harm. The common good is often put before individual good. Wearing a seat-belt may halve the risk of death to the driver, but the odds that a particular individual will ever benefit are not great, as few people are killed while driving. Rose (1981) termed this the 'prevention paradox', according to which a measure that brings large benefits to the community offers little to each participating individual. The alternative to a mass approach is to focus on risk groups, but this may stigmatize certain groups. Learning Activity 6.9 considers the issue of vaccination which is also discussed in Chapter 8. The ethics of compulsory vaccination became a hugely contested issue during the COVID-19 pandemic.

Learning Activity 6.9 Ethical Issue: Vaccination

- Is getting vaccinated an individual choice?
- Is it right to require individuals to participate in an immunization programme for the sake of the communal benefit of herd immunity?
- Should people be able to refuse a vaccination if they believe it to be dangerous?
- Should the state be able to make immunization compulsory?

Informing individuals and ensuring that they understand the information and implications of any actions can be said to be beneficial. By so doing, the health worker can be said to be avoiding harm and fulfilling their duty of care. However, simply providing a choice for the individual may potentially harm others, as in the case of vaccination uptake.

In the field of drug education, harm reduction has been adopted as a way of working. This is perhaps more realistic than the encompassing principle of doing no harm. The healthcare worker recognizes that clients may not wish to change their behaviour, and therefore seeks to encourage a safer way of life and to reduce harm. Drug workers may give clients clean needles and condoms, and provide information about emergency first aid to reduce the risks of HIV infection and accidents. The harm-reduction approach to smoking is outlined in Case Study 6.1.

📋 CASE STUDY 6.1

Tobacco and Harm Reduction

NICE (National Institute for Health and Clinical Excellence) public health guidance (PH45, 2013) recommends a harm-reduction approach for people who are highly dependent on nicotine and who may not be able to stop smoking in one step. Nicotine is highly addictive, but it is the toxins and carcinogens in tobacco smoke that are most harmful. A harm-reduction approach to tobacco control encourages smokers who cannot, or are unwilling to, stop smoking to switch to using nicotine in a less harmful form which would include:

- using a licensed nicotine product
- smokeless tobacco (snus)
- cutting down on tobacco use
- using electronic cigarettes
- temporary abstinence.

 Learning Activity 6.10 Ethical Issue: Condoms in Prisons

Should condoms be provided in prisons?

The example of screening which is discussed in Chapter 8 illustrates the complexities of ethical decision-making, and how attempting to follow the key ethical principles of doing good and avoiding harm is not a simple process. Most preventive services are offered with an explicit promise that they will do some good and an implicit understanding that they will do no harm. Yet what is the nature of that good? Screening, for example, only tells people that they are healthy at the present time. A negative result does not mean that illness will not develop the following year. Screening cannot promise a good outcome. Early detection can mean more effective or less radical treatment in some cases, but there may be no medical benefit and no treatment available. This latter outcome used to be the case with HIV infection. However, anti-retroviral drug therapies may prevent or delay illness in some people with HIV. Ethically, screening represents the tension between beneficence and non-maleficence. Poorly conducted screening can cause psychological harm by, for example, giving false-positive results. Pressure to ensure adequate take-up and to demonstrate the success of a service means screening is often 'sold' to the public and consent is often presumed, making refusal difficult.

Justice

Philosophers suggest three versions of justice:

1. The fair distribution of scarce resources.
2. Respect for individual and group rights.
3. Following morally acceptable laws.

Thus justice requires that people are treated equally. But what is meant by equal? Does it mean according to equal need? Or according to merit? Or according to equal contribution? Or ensuring non-discriminatory practices?

The equal distribution of resources can mean different things. It could mean that resources should be distributed equally in mathematical terms. Or it could mean resources should be distributed according to how much was contributed so that those who have put in the most get the most out. Or the Marxist adage 'From each according to his ability, to each according to his needs' could be applied. See Chapter 7 for further discussion of the politics of health promotion.

The National Health Service in the UK was established on the basis of free medical care to all who need it.

In an era of scarce resources, demand far exceeds supply. Need is an obvious criterion for distributing care, but it is not sufficient. Tudor Hart (1971), whose inverse-care law was described in Chapter 2, observed that those who most needed healthcare received the least. As we shall see in Chapter 19, although we may use some objective measurements to assess individual health needs, for example, the ability to self-care or perform certain tasks, this does not override the subjective value judgement involved in making these decisions. In recent years health economists have tried to establish objective and measurable criteria to compare competing claims. These criteria include, for example, the relative financial costs of treatment, or an assessment made on quality-adjusted life years, which are described in Chapter 3.

Issues of social justice are glaringly evident in health promotion. We noted earlier the evidence of wide differences in health status between different groups in society. Whilst health promoters may be unable to alter society's inequities, they may nevertheless be able to work on programmes which acknowledge that people's abilities to achieve health differ, to avoid victim blaming and to tackle discriminatory practices.

Being fair to everyone might seem to suggest adopting public health measures which iron out differences in resources, healthcare or environmental quality. Yet any kind of state intervention means addressing the issue of individual rights versus the common good. For instance, would it be just for top wage earners to pay 50% income tax to finance public spending on health and welfare? Chapter 7 examines different political perspectives on health promotion, and the fundamental differences between the right and left wings of the political spectrum towards health and welfare. Learning Activity 6.11 raises the difficult question of whether universalism is ethical or whether it is more ethical or fair to direct health interventions for the most disadvantaged. The concept of proportionate universalism is discussed in Chapter 2.

 Learning Activity 6.11   Ethical Issue: Universal or Targeted Programmes
Are universal health programmes ethical?

Telling the Truth

The process of health education and giving information in health promotion also involves complex ethical decisions. Seedhouse (2009) identifies telling the truth and keeping promises as principles which the health promoter should hold on to when deliberating a course of action. As we saw earlier the individual's right to information and the health promoter's duty to tell the truth may conflict with the duty of beneficence.

Practitioners want people to make healthy choices. When convinced of the 'good' of an action, practitioners may seek to persuade people to adopt the action, perhaps through raising clients' anxiety, or selecting which information or evidence to give people. Yet ethical health promotion also includes a commitment to enhancing autonomy. As we saw in Chapter 4, the essential nature of health promotion is that it is based on the principle of voluntarism. Health promotion should not seek to coerce or persuade, but rather to facilitate an informed choice.

 Learning Activity 6.12   Ethical Issue: Opportunistic Health Promotion
Is it ethical to carry out opportunistic health education in primary healthcare? For example, a patient goes to their GP with back pain. The doctor uses the opportunity to deliver some health education and take the patient's blood pressure and family history.

All education may involve some persuasion, and it is too simplistic to suggest that a desire to empower and create autonomy rules out persuasion. However, the role of persuasion should be minimal compared to the role of empowerment. This means that the health promoter must be sure that clients seek advice and help, and are not persuaded against their will. Yet many health promoters would argue that the only way to balance this need to empower people and facilitate healthier choices is to make this easier through policy decisions and frameworks (see Chapter 12). This takes us back to the argument that developing healthy public policy prioritizes the public good over individual freedom of choice, and may not even be mandated by public opinion.

There may also be debate about the point at which enough information has been collected to justify legislative or coercive means of health promotion. The UK government's ban on unpasteurized green-top milk and France's ban on tomato ketchup are examples where government action could be criticized for removing choice and leading to negative effects on employment and economic activity. Yet government inaction in the field of regulation and labelling of food could also be criticized for removing people's right to make decisions based on information. In Chapter 7 we explore how information about what is deemed 'healthy' is often influenced by political decisions and vested interests.

Because the knowledge base of health promotion is constantly changing, there are few areas where recommendations can be made on a factual basis. It is possible to think of numerous examples in recent years where information on the risks or benefits of certain behaviours has changed, for example, the contribution of saturated fat to a healthy diet and recommended levels of safe drinking of alcohol. Learning Activity 6.13 asks you to reflect on how you might present a public health message when evidence changes.

 Learning Activity 6.13   Ethical Issue: How Important Is Evidence?

Should the public be made aware of debates over the evidence for health promotion advice?

Should interventions be employed when the evidence for their effectiveness is in doubt?

CONCLUSION

Health promotion can involve complex layers of decision-making generating many ethical dilemmas. Screening, for example, a frequently unchallenged lynchpin of preventive health promotion, raises key issues about its benefits for an individual versus the social good, as well as questions about the extent to which screening is honestly presented. Before we can make any sort of ethical judgement, we need to be clear about the values and principles which underpin our actions. If we return to the questions asked earlier in this chapter, what do we mean by doing good and avoiding harm? At what point should we switch from creating autonomy to respecting autonomy? What do justice and equity mean in health promotion practice?

Tools to enable clear thinking around ethical issues, such as codes of practice or the Seedhouse (2009) ethical grid, provide a way to clarify decision-making and make the process more transparent. But dilemmas remain, and following different principles (each of which is sound and desirable) may lead to contradictory courses of action. While there may never be absolute answers in ethical decision-making, a way forward is to be clear about which principles and duties you value

most, and to encourage an open debate about ethical principles and how these translate into health promotion practice.

Many professions have codes of practice which provide guidelines on how practitioners should and should not act. The Public Health Knowledge and Skills Framework includes a section on public health ethics and the dilemmas posed by reducing childhood obesity and fluoridating the water supply (https://assets.publishing.service.gov.uk/government/uploads/system/uploads/attachment_data/file/609620/PHSKF_public_health_ethics_in_practice.pdf).

REFLECTIONS ON PRACTICE

- Reflect on how you communicate health messages and the extent to which you seek to persuade or cajole. Are you satisfied that your behaviour is ethical? Why?
- The Good Public Health Practice Framework (https://www.fph.org.uk/professional-development/good-public-health-practice/) states that 'You must respect the right of people to decline to take part in interventions, initiatives, teaching or research even if it may be of benefit to them'. Do you agree and what tensions does this pose for actions to try to control the COVID-19?

SUMMARY

Health promoters need to be clear that what they do involves certain values and principles about what is 'good' health and health promotion. Beneficence, justice and respect for people and their autonomy are fundamental ethical principles in health promotion. Their application in practice, however, is often problematic. Every situation or potential intervention involves a judgement not only of its possible effectiveness but also of its morality – whether it is 'right' or 'wrong'. In this chapter we have defined these key ethical principles and considered how they are manifested in common dilemmas for health promotion practitioners. An understanding of ethics is thus a key competency for health promoters. At times, it is necessary to deliberate and evaluate ethical issues, and be able to identify and assess the ethical components of a health problem and the ethical implications of responding to it in different ways.

FURTHER READING AND RESOURCES

Coggon, J., Viens, A.M., 2017. Public Health Ethics in Practice. Available at: https://assets.publishing.service.gov.uk/government/uploads/system/uploads/attachment_data/file/609620/PHSKF_public_health_ethics_in_practice.pdf.
A background paper to support the UK Public Health Skills and Knowledge Framework.

Cribb, A., Duncan, P., 2002. Health Promotion and Professional Ethics. Blackwell, Oxford.
An exploration of ethical issues and their impact on practice. Case studies explore value conflicts and issues such as codes of practice.

Duncan, P., 2022. Ethics and law. In: Naidoo, J., Wills, J. (eds.), Health Studies: An Introduction, fourth edn. Palgrave Macmillan, Basingstoke, pp. 401–431.
An introduction to the key principles of ethics and law as applied to health. The chapter includes a detailed analysis of the ethics of banning junk-food advertising.

Holland, S., 2014. Public Health Ethics, second edn. Polity, Cambridge.
An interesting and useful introduction to the ethical dilemmas involved in protecting and promoting public health. The book introduces aspects of moral and political philosophies, and debates key issues such as screening and immunization.

➤ FEEDBACK TO LEARNING ACTIVITIES

6.1. Antenatal screening programmes are in place to reduce the birth prevalence of a chromosomal disorder. The assumption underlying screening for conditions such as Down's syndrome is that parents with a positive result will decide to terminate the pregnancy. Some positive-testing parents who do not choose termination may indirectly benefit from the test because they will be better able to adjust to the condition of their baby. The Kantian objection is that the screened population becomes a mere means to achieve the public health goal of reducing chromosomal disorders in the population. Some might argue that there is a contradiction in offering termination for a foetal abnormality while maintaining a positive societal attitude towards disability.

6.2. Patients have different capacities to understand the nature of treatment or intervention. Patients may feel they will be judged, or other interventions will be withheld, if they refuse. Consent is so obviously presumed in many cases, for example, in the 'invitation' to screen or test, that refusal can seem impossible. Practitioners may also not communicate risk clearly, so patients may not be fully informed when they consent to a procedure. Practitioners may believe they are acting in the best interests of the individual and society because the action they are advocating is beneficial for health.

6.3. Some of these actions are intended to protect the population from possible harm. For example, fluoridation of water is a public health strategy. The loss of individual choice is overridden by the proven benefits for all of such an action. Others are promoting evidence-based health interventions, although their universal application can restrict the actions of some

people. Smoking bans restrict individual choice but benefit the whole population.

6.4. You probably concluded that offering money as an inducement for sterilization is a coercive measure that does not respect the autonomy of the individual. Although it may give women greater control over their reproduction, having more money may result in increased drug use. Sterilization is an irreversible procedure about which women need to be fully and freely informed. This action is not, then, one which increases morality. It is a quick-fix solution which fails to deal with the root causes of drug addiction.

6.5. Each of these three scenarios involves ethical decisions:

1. Although your patient is distressed by advice to quit smoking, your duty to tell the truth and do good would suggest that such advice needs to be given. Addressing the reasons why he is so distressed, and providing support, are ethically sound actions. Bear in mind however, that cigarettes serve a purpose for this man by enabling him to cope with stress.

2. You need to balance the possible negative effect of showing the video with its possible positive outcomes. The negative impact might be to dramatize drug-taking (and make it more appealing) and to blame the student who died for their actions. The positive impact may be to deter children from drug-taking. It might be more effective and ethically sound to integrate education about drug-taking into the normal curriculum, rather than have an outsider deliver the messages.

3. Your duty to do good would suggest you to intervene and try to help this patient with his anxiety

and sleep disturbance. As long as this is done in a respectful way that acknowledges his autonomy, such an intervention will be ethically sound.

6.6. In recent years the courts have ruled that a young woman with a learning disability should be sterilized to avoid the possible trauma of pregnancy and childbirth or abortion, for which it was considered she would not be prepared. This decision was also deemed to be in the best interests of a possible child, who would not be able to be brought up by the young woman. The rights of people with learning disabilities to determine whether, how and with whom to have sex and intimate relationships is a long-running campaign. According to Section 1 of the Mental Capacity Act, a person must be assumed to have capacity until it is established that they do not, and a person is not to be treated as unable to make a decision.

6.7. Respecting clients' autonomy can be difficult for health promoters. There is often a tendency to give advice, exert pressure on them to make the 'right' decision or persuade clients to change their behaviour. The challenge for health promoters is to accept a role of partner and enabler rather than expert and controller. This means the following:

- not imposing their own solutions to the clients' problems;
- not instructing clients on what to do because they take too long to work it out for themselves;
- not dismissing clients' ideas without providing an adequate explanation or the opportunity to try them out.

Children and young people may be encouraged to express their wishes as part of growing up. People with mental health problems may also be encouraged to express their wishes. Autonomy is usually deemed appropriate for fully functioning adults – those aged 18 and over who have capacity.

6.8. A healthcare professional following a code of conduct ought to treat the patient if that is what the patient wants and if some treatment is available which will provide net benefit to the patient. The healthcare professional may also fulfil their duty by advising that the most effective way of regaining and maintaining health is to alter one's lifestyle. But coercion will generally be contraindicated by the requirement to respect people's autonomy, and withdrawal of care from those who reject one's advice will generally be contraindicated by a doctor's personally and professionally undertaken duty of care, or obligation of beneficence.

6.9. Although it could be argued that people have a duty not to infect others, and not simply to reap the benefits of herd immunity, the risks of vaccination are contested. Coercion therefore seems unjustified.

6.10. In England and Wales condoms can be prescribed by the prison medical officer where there is risk of HIV transmission. Condoms are not available in the prisons of Northern Ireland.

The argument in favour of condoms being made available in prisons is based on reducing risk: prisoners are disproportionately affected by HIV and other blood-borne viruses such as hepatitis C. Condoms are tools for prevention and risk reduction. Needle exchanges and the provision of clean needles are available in some European prisons but not in UK prisons.

6.11. Universal health promotion programmes target the whole population, but raise two concerns: First, they may not be taken up by the individuals most at risk and will therefore widen the inequality gap. Second, universal health promotion programs might actually lead to a 'flattening up' of inequalities – if they are taken up uniformly across a population, they could improve overall population health, but without necessarily reducing the gap. Hence, a just approach might be proportionate universalism, i.e. targeting those most in need.

6.12. The patient had not sought a health check, nor was she made aware beforehand of the implications if her blood pressure was found to be raised. The patient had not freely chosen to have her blood pressure checked in this way. Although she gave her consent, it might not be regarded as fully informed.

6.13. There is no definitive answer to this question. Evidence does change – in 2015, for example, considerable press time was devoted to challenging public health advice to reduce saturated fat based on a research study suggesting that this advice was premature (http://openheart.bmj.com/content/2/1/e000196.full). The evidence supporting some public health measures, for example, mandatory vaccination of healthcare workers, is not strong, and if an argument is made for a compulsory policy or key message that hinges on controversial evidence, the reputation of public health becomes damaged. The media has a role to play in providing responsible and knowledgeable reporting of risk that enables the public to make informed decisions.

REFERENCES

Abbasi, M., Majdzadeh, R., Zali, A., Karimi, A., Akrami, F., 2018. The evolution of public health ethics frameworks: systematic review of moral values and norms in public health policy. Med. Health Care Philos. 21 (Sept. (3)), 387–402.

Beauchamp, T.L., Childress, J.F., 2019. Principles of Biomedical Ethics, eighth edn. Oxford University Press, Oxford.

Chorus, C., Sandorf, E.D., Mouter, N., 2020. Diabolical dilemmas of COVID-19: An empirical study into Dutch society's trade-offs between health impacts and other effects of the lockdown. PLoS One 15 (9), e0238683.

Collins, M., Garlington, E., 2020. Three Moral Virtues Necessary for a Pandemic Response and Reopening. Available at: https://medicalxpress.com/news/2020-06-moral-virtuesethical-pandemic-response.htm.

Dempsey, C., Battel-Kirk, B., Barry, M., 2011. The CompHP Core Competencies Framework for Health Promotion Handbook. Available at: https://www.iuhpe.org/images/PROJECTS/ACCREDITATION/CompHP_Competencies_Handbook.pdf.

Duncan, P., 2021. Ethics and law. In: Naidoo, J., Wills, J. (eds.), Health Studies: An Introduction, fourth edn. Palgrave Macmillan, Basingstoke, pp. 401–431.

Kant, I., 1909. On the supposed right to tell lies from benevolent motives. Cited in: Rumbold, G. (1991), Ethics in Nursing and Midwifery Practice. Distance Learning Centre, South Bank University, London.

National Institute for Health and Care Excellence, 2013. Smoking: harm reduction, Public health guideline (PH45). Available at: https://www.nice.org.uk/guidance/ph45.

Rose, G., 1981. Strategy of prevention: lessons from cardiovascular disease. Br. Med. J. 282, 1847–1851.

Seedhouse, D., 2009. Ethics: The Heart of Health Care, third edn. Wiley, Chichester.

Sindall, C., 2002. Does health promotion need a code of ethics? Health Promot. Int. 17 (3), 201–203.

Tudor Hart, J., 1971. The inverse care law. The Lancet 1, 405.

World Health Organization, 2015. Global Health Ethics: Key Issues. World Health Organization, Luxembourg. Available at: https://www.who.int/ethics/publications/global-health-ethics/en/.

7

The Politics of Health Promotion

LEARNING OUTCOMES

By the end of this chapter you will be able to:
- critically analyse issues of power and politics in health promotion policy and practice
- understand different ideological positions in relation to health promotion.

KEY CONCEPTS AND DEFINITIONS

Government The group of people with the authority to govern a state or country.

Ideology A set of ideas or beliefs which underlies and justifies the actions of governments, corporations or religious groups, or conversely attempts to undermine these bodies.

Neoliberal An economic or political approach that favours the free market and deregulation.

Politics The achievement and exercise of control over human communities, for example, states.

Power The ability or right to control people or things.

Social policy Planned government activities to regulate society.

IMPORTANCE OF THE TOPIC

Politics and health promotion are usually thought of as separate activities although different approaches to health promotion reflect different political positions. This chapter outlines the diversity of social and political philosophies, which helps us to understand how health promotion has developed in the social and political context of the late 20th and 21st centuries. Understanding our own values helps us to see the logical consequences for health promotion. The political dimensions of health promotion in relation to its organization, methods and activities are then explored.

WHAT IS POLITICS?

Heywood (2015) identifies a fourfold classification of politics.
1. Politics as government – party politics and state activities.

2. Politics as public life – the management of community affairs.
3. Politics as conflict resolution – negotiation, compromise and conciliation strategies.
4. Politics as power – the production, distribution and use of scarce resources.

Although these are separate concepts, they are arguably united by the fourth definition – politics as power – which is the main focus of this chapter. In democratic countries people use their vote to give power to the political party of their choice. The elected party then governs public life and thus wields power on behalf of the populace. Power includes not only material or physical resources but also psychological and cultural aspects, which may be equally effective in limiting or channelling people.

Power is distributed unequally worldwide, and globalization has contributed to increasing the divide between high-income regions, for example, Europe, the USA and Canada, and low-income regions such as sub-Saharan Africa. For example, 15,000 children under the age of 5 years die each day, almost all in poor countries or poor areas of middle-income countries, and half of these deaths are caused by diarrhoeal disease (https://ourworldindata.org/what-are-children-dying-from-and-what-can-we-do-about-it).

 Learning Activity 7.1   A Question Posed by Aristotle

If
A made the flute
B plays it best
C will die if s/he can't have it,
who should have the flute?

POLITICAL IDEOLOGIES

One of the areas in which power relationships are manifest is social policy, defined as planned government activities designed to maintain, integrate and regulate society. This includes both welfare and economic policies, and ranges from national legislation to local policy developments within local authorities. (See Chapter 12 for a discussion of developing healthy public policy.)

Government policies are determined according to its beliefs and ideas – its ideological position. Different political positions give rise to certain types of policy interventions. Analysts have identified many different frameworks and pointed to the shift in ideologies since the 1960s (Bambra et al., 2021). A mid-20th century spectrum of political beliefs, from the hard-line left (Marxism) via socialism and liberalism to the right wing (conservatism), no longer describes accurately the political beliefs and ideologies of nations and parties. Globalization, the demise of Soviet rule over Eastern Europe, and the permeation of national boundaries through international trade have instigated new political beliefs, in particular neoliberalism and neoconservatism. The relationship between ideology and welfare provision is summarized in Table 7.1.

Views on health and health promotion reflect a complex mix of values and beliefs, which in turn reflect different political ideologies. The central proposition of this chapter is that health, and therefore health promotion, is political. Health promotion takes place in the policy area and embodies ideological values. Bambra et al. (2005) describe ideology as a system of inter-related ideas and concepts that reflect and promote the

political, economic and cultural values and interests of a particular societal group. Thus in the 1970s and 1980s feminist, Black and development perspectives were prominent ways of thinking. In the 1990s faith and disability perspectives became prominent. In the last decade there has been strong attention to environmental issues and planetary health (Haines et al., 2012). The ideological viewpoints of different political parties vary widely. People differ in their beliefs in relation to promoting health, for example:

- the extent of personal responsibility
- the role of government legislation and intervention
- the role of the economy, and whether or not it should be regulated by government
- legitimate means to encourage choices and decisions
- the nature of society and the extent to which people are connected to each other
- the extent to which inequalities should be reduced.

On the right of the political spectrum there is a belief in individual self-determination and an antipathy to government intervention, which not only restricts

---

 CASE STUDY 7.1
Planetary Health and Health Promotion

In the 21st century, climate change poses a profound threat to human health and well-being. The World Health Organization (WHO) estimates that climate changes over the past 30 years have led to the loss of over 150,000 lives and 5 million disability adjusted life years (DALYs) per year throughout the world (World Health Organization, 2002). All population groups are vulnerable to climatic variability and the consequences of policies to mitigate against climate change, for example, carbon levies. The Ottawa Charter (World Health Organization, 1986) proposed a socio-ecological approach to health that recognizes the interdependent relationship between people and the environment. Some have argued that health promotion has largely ignored environmental and ecological issues due to its focus on equity (Patrick et al., 2012). Planetary health is a different concept that, at its simplest, is concerned with the state of the natural systems on which we all depend. Indigenous peoples' view is that planetary health concerns the health and well-being of Mother Earth, and of human beings as an inextricable part of natural ecosystems. Jones (2019) argues that these 'place based conceptualizations of agency' should act as an alternative to anthropocentric conceptions of empowerment.

TABLE 7.1 A Typology of Health and Welfare Ideologies

Political Party	Political Ideology	Role of State	View of Economy	View of Society	View of Healthcare	Core Values
Marxist/socialist	Socialism	Collectivist, state control	Regulated	Equality of opportunity and economic and political freedom are safeguarded by the state; the state should enable individual self-fulfilment and social justice through redistribution	Universal and free state provision to promote social cohesion and redistribution, plus individual provision if desired	Equality; collective responsibility; humanitarianism; social harmony
New Left	Social democracy	Collectivist	Mixed economy	The state should provide a safety net, although people should be encouraged to fend for themselves	State provision to safeguard the vulnerable alongside individual choice and private provision	Individualism; social justice; collectivism
New Right	Neoliberalism	Anticollectivist	Market deregulation and state decentralization	The individual is central; state intervention in economic affairs should be reduced and market economics resurrected	Paternalistic state should provide a safety net of healthcare provision alongside individual responsibility	Individualism; social justice; freedom; responsibility; authority
Conservatives	Neoconservatism	Anticollectivist	Free market	Society is made up of self-interested individuals; inequalities in wealth are inevitable and desirable because they stimulate innovation and success; market forces ensure people's needs are met in a satisfactory manner; state intervention should be minimal	Individual responsibility and freedom of choice; needs are best met through free-market consumerism	Tradition; individualism; freedom; self-discipline; choice; competition

freedom but can also inhibit enterprise. Conservatism sees differences as potentially beneficial in that they act as a stimulus for people to succeed, resulting in innovation and productivity. Neoconservatism stresses the need to restore traditional values and a shared culture.

Neoliberalism has evolved since the 1960s as an attempt to combine the twin goals of social justice and economic growth. Neoliberalism is committed to reducing state intervention in the economy, and advocates market deregulation as the means to economic growth and social welfare. Such views are associated with the rugged individualism of Margaret Thatcher, who famously asserted, 'there is no such thing as society, only individuals and their families'.

Socialism is based on a belief in equality, fellowship and community, and a sense of responsibility for others. The government has a key role to play in ensuring everyone's basic needs are met, redistributing material resources and promoting a sense of social stability and cohesion. Social democracy, whilst embodying the same core beliefs, also embraces the notion of individual choice within a free market.

GLOBALIZATION

Globalization, defined primarily as the economic processes of free trade supporting a global marketplace, is another reason for the shifting positions of political parties. No political party can ignore the immense power of global capitalism, which reaches across the world, ignoring national or regional boundaries. McDonald's, Microsoft and Philip Morris are known worldwide for promoting junk food, internet communication and tobacco, respectively. Proponents of globalization argue it is more efficient and allows poorer countries to benefit from the technological advances of more developed countries. Critics argue that globalization destabilizes national economies, reduces everything to a market value and increases inequalities of wealth and health. It has been argued that the socio-economic determinants of health have become globalized, leading to increased inequalities between rich and poor countries as well as within countries (Labonte and Schrecker, 2007). Whatever the stance adopted, health promotion needs to develop and function within an increasingly global economy and world. Learning Activity 7.2 asks you to consider whether free trade between nations contributes to population health improvement.

 Learning Activity 7.2   The Politics of Free Trade

Globalization is based on free trade. Is free trade good for health?

Globalization in politics is mirrored by globalization in health. Health risks are now increasingly global in their scope and spread, fuelled by the displacement of people (through war and natural disasters), global trade and movement of people and products. For example, the spread of human immunodeficiency virus/acquired immunodeficiency syndrome (HIV/AIDS), severe acute respiratory syndrome (SARS), the Ebola virus and COVID-19 requires continued vigilance and concerted action by nations and international agencies. Chapter 12 discusses some of the challenges of developing a global public health policy on issues such as environmental degradation and the fragmentation of labour markets that contribute to lower standards of occupational health and safety, and also to a loss of workers, in poorer countries. The political challenge for health promotion is to foreground health as a valued goal and a key component of the global public good.

This century has seen a considerable investment in global public health, for example, the Sustainable Development Goals promulgated by the United Nations and the WHO Commission on the Social Determinants of Health (CSDH). The CSDH, launched in 2005 and headed by Michael Marmot, was a group of policymakers, researchers and civil society organizations whose aim was to support the tackling of social causes of poor health and avoidable health inequalities (health inequities). The dominant theme in global health initiatives is the reduction of risk factors. Health is often reduced to the prevention of a threat to the population, as in the Ebola outbreak of 2014, when the main concern in Western countries was to prevent immigrants bringing Ebola into their territories, followed by a focus on finding an effective treatment for the disease. The COVID-19 pandemic led to the closure of borders even within the Schengen Treaty area of Europe, and international collaboration was frequently supplanted by insular nation-state interests. The promotion of positive health and the prevention of poverty and disease do not rank highly in political terms. However, there are exceptions to the rule, and the Framework Convention on Tobacco Control, first ratified in 2005, is an example of positive global public health (see Chapter 12).

HEALTH AS POLITICAL

In the WHO Alma Ata declaration (World Health Organization, 1978) health was seen as both a human right and a global social issue. The Universal Declaration of Human Rights, adopted by the United Nations (1948), proclaimed that 'everyone has the right to a standard of living adequate for the health and well-being of oneself and one's family, including food, clothing, housing, and medical care'. The right to healthcare, including reproductive choices, is asserted in the constitution of South Africa, which includes a Bill of Rights. Economic globalization has threatened these views of health as a human right. The People's Health Movement (www.phmovement.org) is a group of political activists opposed to globalization. This group argues that it is health, not the economy, that should be prioritized.

Within nation-states, the political context affects all areas of government policy that have an impact on health, both directly and indirectly. Bambra et al. (2021) argue that health is political because power is exercised over health and its correlates (such as citizenship and organization). The American national health promotion and disease prevention programme, Healthy People 2030 (https://health.gov/healthypeople) identifies the following as some of the social determinants of health:

- availability of resources to meet daily needs
- access to healthcare
- education and job training
- transport options
- public safety
- incidence of crime, violence and disorder
- socio-economic conditions
- language/literacy
- access to emerging technologies.

Evidence suggests that these social determinants are the best predictors of individual and population health, that they structure lifestyle choices and that they interact to produce health. This, in turn, leads to the notion of health as political and the outcome of national and international policy decisions. A strong welfare state that provides people with access to the social determinants of health is arguably the best means to promote health.

 Learning Activity 7.3   Politics and Health

Can you take politics out of health? Why might people say this?

THE POLITICS OF HEALTH PROMOTION STRUCTURES AND ORGANIZATION

Internationally and nationally, health promotion has enjoyed varying levels of support throughout the 20th and 21st centuries. The first International Conference on Health Promotion in 1986 led to the adoption of the Ottawa Charter for Health Promotion (World Health Organization, 1986), whose five action areas – building a healthy public policy, creating supportive environments, developing personal skills, strengthening communities and reorienting health services – are still widely used. The subsequent WHO global conferences focused on developing or consolidating an approach to make health promotion centre stage in international policy making (Table 7.2).

The following brief chronology of the development of health promotion in England highlights the changing views and dominant discourses that emerge at different times.

Around the world health promotion has struggled to have a visible presence, challenged by more dominant public health disciplines and professions (e.g., Rootman et al., 2017; Scott-Samuel and Springett, 2007;

TABLE 7.2 WHO Global Conferences	
Location and Date	**Concepts and Approaches to Influence International Decision-Making**
Adelaide, 1988	Concept of healthy public policy
Sundsvall, 1991	Supportive environments and settings approach
Jakarta, 1997	Globalization and engaging developing countries
Mexico, 2000	Sustainable health promotion through capacity building
Bangkok, 2005	Health Promotion as a core responsibility of government and key component of corporate practice
Nairobi, 2009	Closing the implementation gap in health and development through health promotion
Helsinki, 2013	Consolidation of Health in All Policies (HiAP)
Shanghai, 2016	Health as essential to achieving sustainable development

Based on World Health Organization, 1986. Ottawa Charter for Health Promotion. World Health Organization, Geneva. Available at: https://www.euro.who.int/__data/assets/pdf_file/0004/129532/Ottawa_Charter.pdf.

Smith et al., 2016). In the UK, health promotion is now termed 'health improvement' and is just one part of the remit of a range of other agencies and staff, including public health practitioners. In many other countries the ascendance of neoliberalism combined with traditional biomedical approaches inhibits the wholesale adoption of the Ottawa Charter principles for health promotion (Raphael, 2008). The term 'health promotion' is, however, still used worldwide.

Health promotion activities are structured by the prevailing policy framework, which has the effect of legitimizing certain approaches and excluding others. In the UK a combination of free-market economics and authoritarianism favoured medical preventive approaches and those which focus on individual lifestyles (see Case Study 7.2). Health promotion was seen as a means to prevent morbidity and mortality from specified diseases. Education and advice were the key strategies to encourage healthier lifestyles.

Neoliberal ideology advocates a more interventionist role for government, although the free-market economy is also emphasized as the means to meet needs. There is an emphasis on partnership working and consumer choice, attempting to transfer free-market economic relationships into the service sector. However, there is also recognition that state support and intervention are required to mitigate the inequalities in health that are driven by socio-economic inequalities (Bambra and Scott-Samuel, 2005). This runs parallel to a pervasive life-course discourse which states that health lies in the hands of the individual. (See Chapter 2 for more discussion of socio-economic inequalities in health.)

 CASE STUDY 7.2
The Politics of Health Promotion in England

1800–1900: Public Health Movement
- The movement arose out of a conservative tradition of reluctant collectivism: that the state had to intervene to ensure national efficiency, economic advantage and social stability.

1900–40s: Health Education
- A liberal, laissez-faire agenda which allowed voluntary organizations to provide preventive health education.

1940–70s: Rise of Prevention
- A broadly conservative ideology with the emphasis on individual responsibility for health, with information and advice being provided by health professionals; this was coupled with state intervention to provide a safety net for the most vulnerable.

1980s: The Rise of the Individual
- Despite calls for a coherent national programme to tackle widespread inequalities in health and the WHO Ottawa Charter, New Right ideology dominates the health service and individual freedom is emphasized.

1990s: The Rise of the Market
- Emphasis is on public accountability to the consumer in services, and the need to consult lay views.
- Collaboration is advocated as a means to achieve efficiency and reduce demands on the health service.
- Despite environmental consciousness this is not seen as an agenda for government action.

1997–2011: Community, Responsibility and Equality
- Acknowledgement of the role of socio-economic factors in health.
- Emphasis on public participation in care and services.
- Promotion of community cohesion.
- Emphasis on the free market, individual choice and the commodification of health as a means to satisfy needs.

2011–15: Citizens, Responsibility and Choices
- The public health function shifts to local government, acknowledging wider influences on health.
- Localism leads to areas deciding their own priorities.
- 'Ambitions' rather than performance targets are set for key priorities such as tobacco control, obesity and alcohol.
- 'Nudging' rather than state intervention is used to encourage healthy practices.
- Focus on well-being.

2015–Now: Austerity and Social Intervention
- Cuts in public spending and focus on delivery of acute healthcare.
- COVID-19 focused attention on mental health and isolation and issues of overcrowding.
- Rapid interventions in the furlough scheme lead to the provision of a universal basic income and the delivery of services online.

THE POLITICS OF HEALTH PROMOTION METHODS

The methods used in health promotion are often viewed as a technical choice. Health promotion specialists are seen as possessing the expertise to decide which methods will prove most effective given the circumstances. However, methods imply political perspectives, and the choice of which methods to use is not a politically neutral decision.

Health promotion has at its disposal a large repertoire of methods, which are discussed in greater detail in Part II of this book. Fig. 7.1 illustrates how different political philosophies privilege different methods and approaches, and have differing views about the role of the state and responsibility of the individual.

 Learning Activity 7.4   Political Philosophies

The following statements reflect particular political philosophies. Can you identify these political philosophies? Which statements do you agree with?

- There should be a safety net of economic and social support for the needy.
- Energy and enterprise should be rewarded, not stifled by high taxation.
- All people in a society have a commitment and a responsibility to others.
- Inequality is inevitable, and necessary for development and growth.
- High levels of benefits make people dependent on state support.
- Certain public services are essential and should be run by the state.

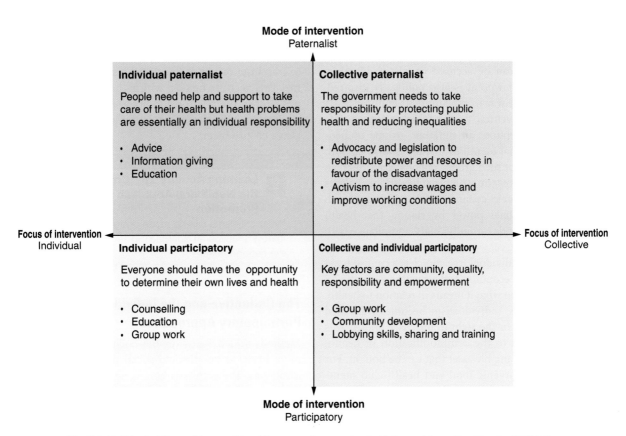

Fig. 7.1 Political philosophies and health promotion methods (Adapted from Beattie, A., 1993. The changing boundaries of health. In: Beattie, A., Gott, M., Jones, L., Sidell, M., (eds.), Health and Wellbeing: A Reader. Macmillan/Open University, Basingstoke.)

- Macropolitics is of less significance than issues, particularly those affecting local communities.
- People cannot be equal, but everyone should have the same chances.
- Shared values and a common culture are vital to the maintenance of social cohesion.
- A person's lot in life is determined by luck.

The Individual Paternalist Approach

This approach is likely to come from a conservative perspective that questions the extent of legitimate state intervention, the value accorded to public services, and the degree to which the economy should be managed or controlled. It has a long history, remaining perennially popular. Methods focused on the individual send a clear message about personal responsibility for health. Such methods rely on the belief that individuals can make significant changes in their lifestyle or environment. The focus on the individual also implies that everyone has equal resources and ability to comply with health promotion messages. This view may be seen as ineffective or incorrect, and can be accused of 'victim blaming'. However, such a viewpoint is also politically inspired, which may go some way to explaining its endurance.

By ignoring structural factors which affect the life chances and perceptions of different groups of people, people's personal identities that are bound up with their membership of such groups are obscured. Such an approach also ignores the structured health inequalities that are linked to socio-economic status. This approach reinforces professional power by stating that health improvement depends on individuals' compliance with expert advice.

The notion of individual free choice is a central tenet of the free-market economy and Learning Activity 7.5 asks you to reflect on what it means in relation to health. In economic terms, individualism becomes translated into consumerism, or the right to purchase goods. This approach is linked to the commodification of health, which is seen as a tangible asset that can be bought. For example, sales of organic food and health-club memberships have risen sharply in the UK, due in large part to their promotion as routes to health and well-being. This process in turn further exacerbates inequalities in health, as only the richest people can afford these healthier lifestyle choices.

 Learning Activity 7.5   Is There a Healthy Choice?

Do you think there is such a thing as a 'healthy choice'? Is it your role to inform patients and clients about healthy choices?

The Individual Participatory Approach

The individual participatory approach differs from the paternalistic individual approach by being premised on a different, and more equal, relationship between the health promoter and the client. This approach includes negotiated methods such as counselling, education and group work which take into account people's beliefs, attitudes and knowledge. The client is an active partner in the process, and the end goal is enhanced client autonomy. Many professional groups in recent years have tried to become more person-centred and develop approaches and services through collaboration with clients. Many health promoters feel more comfortable using these methods. Patient and public involvement and engagement (PPIE) has as its overarching principle 'no decisions about me without me'. This needs to be seen within the context of a political shift in the relationship between the state and the citizen, whereby the citizen is not just a consumer but also a co-producer.

 Learning Activity 7.6   Critique of the Neoliberal Approach to Health Promotion

What criticisms can be made of the individual participatory (neoliberal) approach in terms of promoting the nation's health?

The Collective and the Individual Participatory Approaches

Methods which focus on the collective approach are more likely to be allied to social democratic political ideologies. The emphasis here is on understanding the processes which shape health outcomes, and assisting people to develop the skills to challenge and reshape these processes. All collective approaches stress participation and active involvement, whether of communities or individual consumers. Being well integrated into a community (sometimes called communitarianism) is increasingly recognized as an independent source of health as well as of self-esteem.

Governments have sought to encourage social inclusion and collective participation through neighbourhood and community initiatives. Place-based approaches are increasingly advocated to address systemic and structural inequalities

The Collective Paternalist Approach

Collective paternalist methods of working are associated with left-wing beliefs. These beliefs include the primacy of socio-economic status in predicting culture, social status and life chances. Socialism views individual identity as shaped by social interaction and membership of social groups. The owners of the means of production (the middle class) and those who have only their labour power to sell (the working class) have conflicting economic goals (to maximize profits or maximize wages, accordingly). Class conflict is seen as inevitable according to this perspective.

Karl Marx's (1875) famous phrase, 'from each according to his ability, to each according to his need', sums up the socialist goal of equality and social solidarity. Actions can be top down (e.g., advocacy on behalf of lower socio-economic groups, or equity audits to expose inequalities) or bottom up (e.g., activism to increase wages and improve working conditions). Other methods may include promoting social cohesion through community development (see Chapter 11). Wilkinson and Pickett (2009) present a strong case for arguing that more egalitarian societies have healthier populations, even if they are poorer than wealthy capitalist societies.

The methods adopted by practitioners in response to particular issues reflect their political values about:
- humanity – the rights of people
- responsibility – whether health is in the hands of the individual, or a result of particular social patterns which are reproduced and maintained by social policies
- the role of the practitioner – whether practitioners should hold power in the form of professional expertise, or should corroborate knowledge defined and shared by lay people
- the role of the citizen – whether citizens have the autonomy and resources to exercise free choices, or

whether they are constrained by social and national norms and the exercise of professional power
- the role of the community – whether as active sources of solidarity, or as sources of disadvantage, vulnerability or marginalization
- the role of government – whether the state should take an active role in protecting and promoting its citizens' health, or whether responsibility for health should lie with the individual
- the role of the economy – whether there is a free market and competition, or a regulated economy overseen by the government.

 Learning Activity 7.7   The Political Values Underpinning an HIV Prevention Programme

Consider the following methods which might be adopted in an HIV and sexually transmitted infection (STI) prevention programme with vulnerable young people.
- Enhancing self-esteem.
- Peer education.
- Educational media campaigns.
- Young people's sexual health clinic run by nurses.
- Funding for a telephone helpline run by a voluntary self-help group.
- Easier access to condoms.
- More opportunities for young people to gain work experience and skills.
- Creation of hostels and sheltered housing for homeless young people.

What political values are being reflected in each approach?

This discussion has presented the view that the methods chosen to promote health are not politically neutral. Certain methods fit into, maintain and reproduce the ideological assumptions of certain political perspectives. However, it is important not to overstate this view. Methods and ideology are not deterministically linked in a cause-and-effect manner. A variety of methods across all four ideological perspectives shown in Fig. 7.1 may be used by health workers who espouse a particular political viewpoint. There may be convincing reasons for adopting an eclectic methodology to promote health. However, it is a fallacy to assume that methods are a technical, and politically neutral, aspect of a health promoter's activity.

The Politics of Health Promotion Content

The previous sections have examined the view that the structure, organization and methods used in health promotion have a political dimension. It is sometimes stated that although the process of promoting health is a political activity, the content of health promotion is neutral. However, it can be argued that health promotion content is inevitably political. The framing of suitable agendas and the construction of relevant information are not value-neutral activities; on the contrary, they imply certain political values.

> ### Learning Activity 7.8   Health Promotion for the 21st Century
> The Royal Society of Public Health have listed achievements of the 21st century. What do you think these are?

Perhaps the clearest example of the political nature of health promotion is the debate surrounding the social determinants of health. As outlined in Chapter 2, a wealth of research evidence from the 1980s linked poverty and disadvantage with ill health, but governments reacted differently according to their political allegiances. For almost two decades (1979–97) the Conservative UK government refused to recognize the evidence on social inequalities and health, referring instead to 'variations in health status between different socio-economic groups within the population' (Department of Health, 1992, p. 121). By denying the evidence, a non-interventionist policy could be adopted, which argued that the free market is the best means of meeting health needs. The Labour government elected in 1997 acknowledged the link between social inequalities and health, and adopted targets to reduce health inequalities (Department of Health, 2003). The Marmot Review, Fair Society, Healthy Lives (Marmot, 2010) marked a clear agenda shift, reframing the narrative around determinants of health and clearly signalling its political stance that reducing health inequalities is a matter of fairness and justice and economic growth is not the most important measure of a country's success (see www.instituteofhealthequity.org).

Practitioners are called upon to base their work on evidence. Yet it has been argued that political interest can drive the use of evidence and override its scientific basis (Parkhurst, 2017). For example, in 2013 it was

> ### CASE STUDY 7.3
> **The Political Discourse of Obesity**
>
> The discourse of obesity frames concerns as a societal panic and obesity as a consequence of immoral behaviour. If obesity is framed as a lifestyle choice, as is most common in public health discourse, then it becomes a matter of individual responsibility: people eat too much of the wrong kind of food and exercise too little. This may fuel the stigmatization of ethnic minorities and people living in poverty, who are more likely to be obese. Foucault describes how governments dictate how people act in certain ways through the construction of knowledge (Coveney, 1998). Thus, obesity is referred to as an individual threat or risk, and citizens are expected to be responsible and active consumers, whilst the actions of food companies goes unchallenged.
>
> The Lancet Commission on obesity, undernutrition, and climate change (Swinburn et al., 2019) describes a global syndemic of biological and social factors and the importance of understanding the role of politics. The authors emphasize that we should understand how food industries contribute to the availability and accessibility of foods for consumption, and propel an insatiable appetite for sugar that motivates its exploitative production.

claimed that President Obama was politically motivated in a decision to impose a minimum age restriction of 15 years for access to emergency contraception (the so-called morning after pill), even though the US Food and Drug Administration (FDA) stated the pill was safe and effective for girls of all ages. Appeals to evidence may also shift debates to focus on particular questions, and marginalize political and social issues that are too complex to address using an evidence-based model of decision-making. The process of research is also not immune to political considerations: what evidence filters through to the general public as the scientific consensus on health topics is also the result of political processes. The COVID-19 pandemic exposed many conflicts between scientific evidence and politics where concerns about, for example, the effectiveness of rapid diagnostic tests were bypassed to support mass screening in Liverpool. An editorial in November 2020 in the respected *British Medical Journal* was actually titled 'Covid-19: politicisation, 'corruption,' and suppression of science' (Abbasi, 2020).

BEING POLITICAL

We have seen how health promotion arises from, and reinforces, political values and beliefs, and takes place in a political context. Health promoters hold values and beliefs which are underpinned by established sets of ideas or ideologies. Many health promoters are engaged in practice which accords (more or less) with their personal values. The medical model of health provides a clear role for practitioners because it recognizes their expertise. It also gives a clear role for individuals to act to protect their own health. Health promoters may find that their professional role sometimes conflicts with their political beliefs and values. For example, a belief in collective health goals and the need to empower people to be involved and take control over factors influencing their health may be at odds with a health promotion role bound by corporate contracts and the need to meet limited and predetermined targets.

 Learning Activity 7.9 Radical Health Promotion

Adapted from Adams and Slavin (1985); O'Neill (1989).

The following are suggestions for developing radical health promotion practice. How many do you think are feasible for you? Be clear and honest about your own political standpoint.

- Develop an equal relationship with clients, where beliefs and values are respected and information is shared.
- Try to ensure real community involvement in policies and decision-making.
- Try to address health as a collective issue, making explicit the facts about health inequalities and supporting collective action around health issues.
- Vet the health education materials you use to ensure they do not reproduce stereotypes or assumptions about gender, class, race, disability, age or sexuality.
- Engage in action research in which researchers and the researched are partners.
- Develop a support network with like-minded health workers, where perspectives can be shared and issues discussed.
- Be honest to yourself and others about the limitations of your work role.

RESEARCH EXAMPLE 7.1
The Environmentally 'Woke' Nurse

There is a long history of nurses campaigning or advocating on behalf of a cause, and going beyond routine practice to embrace activism regarding women's suffrage, Black people's rights and women's right to birth control. As Fowler (2017, p. 4) writes, 'Nursing's social ethics has driven nursing's concerns for addressing structural injustices affecting…all socially marginalized, vulnerable, voiceless, stigmatized persons or groups'. In a study with nurse participants in the USA and the UK (Terry and Bowman, 2020) many nurses expressed concerns about environmental health issues in their practice and community. Although the International Council of Nurses issued a position statement in 2018 that it 'Strongly believes that nurses have a shared responsibility to sustain and protect the natural environment from depletion, pollution, degradation and destruction' (ICN, 2018, p. 3), many of the nurses experienced their activism as an additional emotional burden.

CONCLUSION

Politics, or the process and study of the distribution of power in society, underpins all human activities, including health promotion. The political scene is in a state of constant flux, with the 21st century witnessing neoliberalist ideology and globalization. These processes and values are embedded in the context in which health promoters practice. An understanding of, and engagement with, politics in its widest sense is necessary in order to practice reflectively and in accordance with one's personal values and beliefs.

There is often resistance to the idea that health promotion is a political activity. Accepting the premise that politics is involved in health promotion may be seen as muddying the waters, for it transforms a situation of relative certainty to one of uncertainty. It is no longer sufficient to rely on professional training to ensure effective health promotion. A whole range of different considerations needs to be taken into account, some of which threaten and call into question the whole notion of professional expertise.

However uncomfortable the process may be, an awareness of the political nature of health promotion is vital to its effectiveness (O'Neill, 1989). Accepting the status quo is not an apolitical position but a deeply political one. What exists is not inevitable, but is the result of complex forces and historical processes. Things might be otherwise. Health promotion is centrally concerned with a vision of better health for all. This vision may be informed by scientific knowledge and technical know-how, but its overall shape is determined by personal values and beliefs. Part of the task of health promoters is to uncover and hold up to scrutiny their values and beliefs. It is hoped that this chapter and Chapter 6 will help health promoters in this task.

REFLECTIONS ON PRACTICE

- To what extent do you regard your health promotion practice as a political activity?
- How have your political values and beliefs informed your practice?

SUMMARY

This chapter has examined the political implications of health promotion structures, organization, methods and content. The central proposition is that health promotion is a political activity, and to deny this lessens one's understanding and the possibility of effective action. This chapter has demonstrated that mainstream health promotion activity is predicated on certain political values. The late 20th and 21st centuries have witnessed a shift in the political values underpinning health promotion practice in England and many other countries, triggered by the growth of neoliberalist ideologies and the process of globalization. A non-interventionist role focused on individual advice and information giving sits alongside a commitment to tackle the social origins of health and illness.

The role of the practitioner is still crucial, although it could be argued that the practitioner's function needs to expand to include client advocacy and empowerment, with more emphasis on national and international networking and collaborative working across sectors and professions. Whether this shift in practice can occur, given increasing demands on healthcare services, is problematic. Some practitioners may feel that the broad political framework is now more supportive of health promotion. However, the task of practising in accordance with one's political beliefs remains a challenge.

FURTHER READING AND RESOURCES

Bambra, C., Smith, K., Kennedy, L., 2021. Politics. In: Naidoo, J., Wills, J. (eds.), Health Studies, fourth edn. Springer, Singapore.
Chapter 9 provides a clear overview of politics as a discipline, and applies its methodology and concepts to health issues.
Baggott, R., 2010. Public Health Policy and Politics, second edn. Wiley Blackwell, Oxford.
This book explores the UK political environment and addresses health promotion and public health issues.

FEEDBACK TO LEARNING ACTIVITIES

7.1. Aristotle thought that justice was giving each person their due or what they deserved. The purpose of the flute is to be played, and played well. Therefore, according to Aristotle, B should have the flute. However, other views produce different answers. If people's well-being is the priority, C should have the flute. If material ownership of goods is the priority (as in a capitalist state), then A should have the flute.

7.2. Free trade or trade liberalization may result in lower standards on food safety. Trade policy also affects the food chain, and may result in increased imports and a reduction in locally sourced food. This would impact on the environment as well as on the quality of food. Critics of free trade argue that it would increase corporate power and reduce the ability of governments to promote health through the regulation of markets or environmental protection.

7.3. Health is inextricably bound up with politics. For example, access to health services depends on political decisions such as funding and access criteria. In 1948 the National Health Service (NHS) was created in post-war England, the first national healthcare system available on the basis of need rather than wealth or fees. A Labour government was in power at this time. This political decision had the effect of freeing healthcare from politics, although socio-economic health inequalities persist in the UK. In contrast, in many other countries access to healthcare services varies according to wealth. In some countries, such as South Africa, the level of healthcare is largely dependent on ethnic status. People may want to take politics out of health because they want health services provided on the basis of need.

7.4. The political philosophies with which each statement most closely aligns are as follows:
- Most social democrats support a system of welfare.
- Conservatives believe in reducing taxation.
- The New Left has tried to encourage communitarianism.
- Neoliberalism, in its support for the free market, regards inequality as inevitable.
- Neoliberals and conservatives wish to roll back the state, partly to reduce dependency.
- A principle of socialism is that essential services, for example, railways and electricity, should be run by the state.
- Liberals, in particular, support ideas of localism.
- Equal opportunity is a key principle of liberalism.
- Conservatives are concerned that high levels of immigration threaten a country's stability, and want to support a nation-state.
- Conservatives believe that everyone has a chance to succeed.

You can identify your political compass and where you stand at www.politicalcompass.org/test.

7.5. Healthy choices, such as organic fruit and vegetables and daily physical activity, tend to be expensive and time-consuming. It can be argued that not everyone is able to make these choices. It may be a practitioner's role to advocate healthy choices, but unless your clients can afford these, this may be unethical. It might be more productive to find out what your clients believe to be healthy choices, and then discuss with them whether these are indeed healthy choices and, if so, how they may be put into practice.

7.6. It may be argued that individually negotiated methods are most used and valued by the relatively privileged, healthy and articulate sections of society. Those with the greatest need are least likely to be able to access this kind of health promotion intervention. The focus on the individual maintains the free-market consumerist ethos criticized in this chapter.

7.7. These initiatives reflect different views about the factors that contribute to sexual ill health or teenage pregnancy, and whether these relate to the individual or the social context in which young people live. They also reflect views about the extent to which individuals are responsible for their own health. Initiatives that rely on the individual or an accredited professional to achieve their goal (e.g., 4) or the provision of information to enable individual choice (e.g., 3) reflect conservative political values. Initiatives that rely on an enabling environment to achieve their goal (e.g., 5 to 8) are more in tune with left-wing political values. Initiatives that seek to empower people (e.g., 1 and 2) are more consonant with liberal political values.

7.8. The health promotion achievements of the 21st century include many that are legislative actions:
- the ban on smoking in public places (2007)
- the soft drinks industry levy on drinks with over 8g of sugar (2018)
- a minimum price for alcohol in Scotland (2018)
- the human papillomavirus (HPV) vaccine for girls (2008)
- the congestion charge (2003) and ultra-low emission zone (2019) in London
- decriminalization of abortion in Northern Ireland (2019)
- traffic light labelling on pre-packaged food (2013)
- ban on advertising of high fat, sugar and salt foods during television programmes aimed at children (2007).

7.9. These suggestions for radical health promotion practice are now 30 years old. But they reflect the core principles of health promotion: to strive for social justice, to work in partnership and to engage in co-production with patients, clients or the community. Depending on your role, you may be able to incorporate all or some of the suggestions for radical health promotion practice. Some of the suggestions (e.g., developing an equal relationship with clients) refer to everyday practice, whereas others (e.g., engage in action research) refer to activities over and above everyday practice. To ensure good practice, health promotion practitioners need to be aware that it is a political activity and that they work in a macro-political context.

REFERENCES

Abbasi, K., 2020. COVID-19: 'politicisation', 'corruption' and 'suppression of science'. Br. Med. J. 371, 24.

Adams, L., Slavin, H., 1985. Checklist for personal action. Rad. Health Promot. 2, 47.

Bambra, C., Fox, D., Scott Samuel, A., 2005. Towards a new politics of health. Health Promot. Int. 20 (2), 1–7. Available at: http://heapro.oxfordjournals.org/content/20/2/187.full.pdf+html.

Bambra, C., Scott-Samuel, A., 2005. The Twin Giants: Addressing Patriarchy and Capitalism. Politics of Health Group, UK. Available at: http://www.pohg.org.uk/.

Bambra, C., Smith, K., Kennedy, L., 2021. Politics. In: Naidoo, J., Wills, J. (eds.), Health Studies, fourth edn. Springer, Singapore.

Coveney, J., 1998. The government and ethics of health promotion: the importance of Foucault. Health Educ. Res. 13 (3), 459–468.

Department of Health, 1992. The Health of the Nation. HMSO (His/Her Majesty's Stationery Office), London.

Department of Health, 2003. Tackling Health Inequalities: A Programme for Action. Stationery Office (formerly HMSO), London.

Fowler, M., 2017. 'Unladylike commotion': early feminism and nursing's role in gender/trans dialogue. Nurs. Inq. 24, e12179.

Haines, A., Alleyne, G., Kickbusch, I., Dora, C., 2012. From the Earth summit to Rio+ 20: integration of health and sustainable development. Lancet. 379(9832), 2189–2197.

Heywood, A., 2015. Key Concepts in Politics, fourth edn Palgrave, Hampshire.

International Council of Nurses, 2018. Nurses, climate change and health. Available at https://www.icn.ch/sites/default/files/inline-files/ICN%20PS%20Nurses%252c%20climate%20change%20and%20health%20FINAL%20.pdf.

Jones, R., 2019. Climate change and indigenous health promotion. Global Health Promot. 26 (Supp. 3), 73–81.

Labonte, R., Schrecker, T., 2007. Globalization and social determinants of health: introduction and methodological background (Part 1 of 3). Global. Health 3, 5.

Marmot, M., 2010. Fair Society, Healthy Lives. Institute of Health Equity, London. Available at: http://www.instituteofhealthequity.org/resources-reports/fair-society-healthy-lives-the-marmot-review/fair-society-healthy-lives-full-report-pdf.pdf.

Marx, K., 1875. Critique of Gotha. International Publishers, New York, NY.

O'Neill, M., 1989. The political dimension of health promotion work. In: Martin, C.J., McQueen, D.V. (eds.), Readings for a New Public Health. Edinburgh University Press, Edinburgh, pp. 222–234.

Parkhurst, J., 2017. The Politics of Evidence: From Evidence Based Policy to the Good Governance of Evidence. Routledge, Oxon. Available at: https://eprints.lse.ac.uk/68604/1/Parkhurst_The%20Politics%20of%20Evidence.pdf.

Patrick, R., Capetola, T., Townsend, M., Nuttman, S., 2012. Health promotion and climate change: exploring the core competencies required for action. Health Promot. Int. 27, 475–485.

Raphael, D., 2008. Grasping at straws: a recent history of health promotion in Canada. Crit. Public Health 18 (4), 483–495.

Rootman, I., Pederson, A., Frohlich, K., Dupere, S., 2017. Health Promotion in Canada, fourth edn. Canadian Scholars, Toronto.

Scott-Samuel, A., Springett, J., 2007. Hegemony or health promotion: prospects for reviving England's lost discipline. J. R. Soc. Health 127, 210–213.

Smith, J., Crawford, G., Signal, L., 2016. The case of national health promotion policy in Australia: where to now? Health Promot. J. Australia 27, 61–65.

Swinburn, B.A., Kraak, V.I., Allender, S., Atkins, V.J., Baker, P.I., et al., 2019. The global syndemic of obesity, undernutrition, and climate change: The Lancet Commission report. The Lancet 393, 791–846.

Terry, L., Bowman, K., 2020. Outrage and the emotional labour associated with environmental activism among nurses. J. Adv. Nurs. 76, 867–877.

United Nations, Universal Declaration of Human Rights, 1948. United Nations Department of Public Information, Geneva. Available at: https://www.un.org/en/about-us/universal-declaration-of-human-rights.

Wilkinson, R.G., Pickett, K., 2009. The Spirit Level: Why More Equal Societies Almost Always Do Better. Penguin, London.

World Health Organization, 1978. Declaration of Alma-Ata, International Conference on Primary Health Care, Alma-Ata. World Health Organization, Geneva. Available at: https://www.who.int/publications/almaata_declaration_en.pdf.

Strategies and Methods

The Ottawa Charter for Health Promotion (World Health Organization, 1986) remains one of the most influential policy documents in the history of health promotion. It established the fundamental guiding principles and values of health promotion and described five key action areas:
1. Building healthy public policy.
2. Creating supportive environments.
3. Strengthening communities.
4. Developing personal skills.
5. Reorienting health services.

Each of these areas is the focus of a chapter in Part II. Together, these five areas encompass the goals of health promotion: to go 'upstream' and have an impact on the socio-economic and environmental determinants of health; to focus on population health; to emphasize prevention rather than treatment; and to build capacity in communities and individuals. But while social and physical determinants of health were highlighted in the Ottawa Charter, little attention was given to global, environmental and economic issues. This reflects the reality of the 1980s, when such issues were not on the agenda (Hills and McQueen, 2007). However, many of these issues can be addressed using the strategies outlined in the Ottawa Charter.

Improving the health of the population depends on many factors. Among the most important are:
- tackling socio-economic inequalities in health
- making health everybody's business
- making the healthy choice the easy choice.

These principles, and the values they encompass, underpin the Ottawa Charter's strategies. Tackling socio-economic inequalities in health promotes equity and moves upstream, away from a focus on blaming individuals to tackling the policies that shape environments.

The Ottawa Charter called for support for personal and social development through providing information, educating about health and enhancing life skills. This focus enables health promotion to increase the options available to people to exercise more control over their own health and their environments, and to make choices conducive to health. Individual skills therefore include not just knowledge about health issues, but also practical life skills such as negotiation, setting realistic and achievable targets, and building self-esteem, all of which have an impact on the ability to make lasting behavioural changes.

Because the Ottawa Charter emphasized a positive approach to health, disease prevention and health protection were not included as strategies. However, the COVID-19 pandemic has shown how important these elements are in the role of many health promoters who have been responsible for communicating about public health, identifying those at risk, and rolling out a vaccination programme.

Communication about health messages and one-to-one education play a central role in health promotion. The ways in which media are used to support campaigns or to lobby for policy change are the subject of Chapter 13.

Community development is a fundamental health promotion strategy cited in the Ottawa Charter. Community development draws on existing human and material resources in the community (assets) to enhance self-help and social support, and to develop flexible systems for strengthening public participation in, and direction of, health matters. Strengthening communities is a key strategy in moving upstream and provides a route to tackle the social determinants of health through, for example, improving access to education, employment and housing. The theoretical and policy base for community action has been the subject of recent research into community capacity building and concepts such as social capital and civic engagement.

Building health promoting public policy and ensuring health features in all policies is an increasingly important strategy for health promotion, and one that is currently being used in relation to an expanding number of issues, for example, tobacco control, active travel systems and food labelling. Health promoting public policy combines diverse but complementary approaches including legislation, fiscal measures, taxation and organizational change. It requires government intervention, practitioners' advocacy, and coordinated action by different sectors. Globalization presents new challenges for international action.

Reorienting the health services, from treatment towards prevention, is the subject of Chapter 9. In some respects, this strategy has proved most taxing and resistant to change. Demand always exceeds supply for health services, so trying to shift services away from immediate treatment to long-term prevention is extremely difficult. Treatment is high profile, media friendly and politically popular. Prevention is low profile, and its long timescale for effects to become evident makes it less prominent.

Creating supportive environments is the subject of Part III, where different environments are discussed in separate chapters.

The Ottawa Charter stated that all of the actions discussed in this chapter would be required to promote health. The skills of enablement, mediation and advocacy are central. Increasingly, health promotion activities combine a mix of strategies and multiple (national, regional, community) levels of action.

REFERENCES

Hills, M., McQueen, D.V., 2007. At issue: two decades of the Ottawa Charter. Promot. Educ. 14 (Suppl. 2), 5.

World Health Organization, 1986. Ottawa Charter for Health Promotion. Geneva. Available at: http://www.who.int/healthpromotion/conferences/previous/ottawa/en/.

8

Preventing Disease and Health Protection

LEARNING OUTCOMES

By the end of this chapter you will be able to:
- understand why health protection can be part of the health promotion role
- understand the principles of population-based programmes in the prevention and control of communicable diseases
- discuss the challenges associated with vaccination and screening programmes.

KEY CONCEPTS AND DEFINITIONS

Emerging infectious diseases (EIDs) Infectious diseases that are newly recognized in a population, for example, COVID-19 or which have existed but are rapidly increasing in incidence or geographic range. Many EIDs may be transmitted from animals to humans.

Health protection Activities designed to protect individuals, groups and populations from infectious disease incidents and outbreaks and non-infectious environmental hazards such as chemicals and radiation.

Immunization The process by which an individual is protected against a disease through vaccination.

Infection control The prevention of the spread of infections in healthcare settings or communities through contact, droplets or airborne transmission. It includes hand hygiene, the use of personal protective equipment, respiratory hygiene (controlling coughing and sneezing) and safety and sterilizing instruments and their safe disposal.

Primary prevention Primary prevention aims to prevent disease or injury before it occurs. This is done by preventing exposure to hazards that cause disease.

Screening Tests to check for the early identification of disease and health conditions before there are any signs or symptoms, enabling early and easier treatment.

IMPORTANCE OF THE TOPIC

Health promotion and disease prevention are separate concepts, as outlined by Nutbeam (1998, p. 115):

Disease prevention is essentially an activity in the medical field dealing with individuals or particularly defined groups at risk. It aims to conserve health. It does not represent a positive vision of health that moves ahead, but is concerned with maintaining the status quo. Health promotion on the other hand, starts out with the whole population in the context of their everyday lives, not selected individuals or groups. Its goal is to enhance health.

The key distinction is that health promotion includes positive definitions of health extending beyond the absence of disease, whereas disease prevention aims to avoid or eliminate diseases. Disease prevention cannot be achieved without health promotion, whether in the communication and promotion of screening or vaccination or because it aims to strengthen community action, which has proved to be crucial in dealing with outbreaks and pandemics.

During the Ebola crisis in 2015, Kickbusch and Reddy (2016, p. 76) argued that addressing a global pandemic threat (that actually emerged 5 years later with COVID-19) demands:

understanding socio-cultural values, prioritizing social relations, empowering citizens at the local level to deal with the threat, and respecting citizen ingenuity to deal with the unexpected. In particular, we highlighted the need for trusted relationships between the many actors and especially the trust in authorities and the state.

Descriptions of the global burden of disease include infectious diseases, non-communicable diseases (NCDs) and injuries. NCDs – which include cancer, diabetes, chronic obstructive pulmonary disease, cardiovascular disease and mental health conditions – were, until the COVID-19 pandemic, the leading cause of death worldwide. Infectious diseases remain, however, an important global problem in public health, causing over 13 million deaths each year and the pandemic accounted for a further 2,791,055 deaths by April 2021 (Table 8.1).

Changes in society, technology and the microorganisms themselves are contributing to the emergence of new diseases, the re-emergence of diseases that were previously controlled and the development of antimicrobial resistance (Fig. 8.1).

Until 2020 about 40% of mortality in developing countries was due to infectious, parasitic or respiratory disease, compared to 8% in developed countries. The year 2020, however, saw the start of the global COVID-19 pandemic and the introduction of measures to prevent citizens and health workers from getting infected – hand washing, wearing face masks and protective gloves and 'social distancing' (which should really be termed 'spatial distancing'). Other secondary prevention measures aimed to arrest the progress of coronavirus disease (COVID-19) through screening or 'test and trace' to identify people with COVID-19 and their contacts, and a vaccination programme started at the end of 2020.

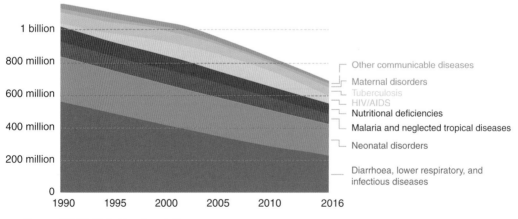

Disease burden from communicable, maternal, neonatal and nutritional diseases, World, from 1990 to 2016

Our world in data

Total disease burden from communicable, maternal, neonatal and nutritional diseases, measured in DALYs (Disability-Adjusted Lifer Years) per year. DALYs are used to measure total burden of disease – both from years of life lost and years lived with a disability. One DALY equals one lost year of healthy life.

Source: IHME, Global burden of disease

Fig. 8.1 The changing pattern of disease (Adapted from Global Burden of Disease Collaborative Network, 2018. Global Burden of Disease Study 2017 (GBD 2017) Results Tool. Institute for Health Metrics and Evaluation, Seattle, WA. Available at: http://ghdx.healthdata.org/gbd-results-tool.)

TABLE 8.1 The Global Burden of Infectious Diseases
2019
8.8 million have active tuberculosis
4 million die of respiratory disease
36 million have HIV with 5 million new infections recorded
350 million chronically infected with hepatitis B and 170 million with hepatitis C
350 million new cases of syphilis and gonorrhoea
875,000 children die from measles, 377,000 from tetanus and 295,000 from whooping cough
2.2 million die from diarrhoeal disease
300 million new cases of malaria
2020
1.78 million die from COVID-19

CHANGING PATTERN OF DISEASE

Communicable disease epidemics of diphtheria, typhus, cholera and tuberculosis were commonplace until the late 19th century, when the provision of clean water and safer disposal of sewage improved the sanitary conditions of town dwellers. The 20th century saw a further decline in mortality with the development of vaccination programmes and antibiotic therapies.

However, there has been considerable concern about communicable diseases in the past few decades due to:
- the emergence of previously unknown pathogens, for example, human immunodeficiency virus (HIV) and hepatitis C
- the re-emergence of diseases thought to have been eradicated, for example, tuberculosis
- the emergence of more virulent strains of known infections, for example, *Clostridium difficile*
- the increasing number of drug-resistant strains of bacteria, for example, methicillin-resistant *Staphylococcus aureus* (MRSA).

EIDs are either newly recognized diseases or diseases that are increasing in a specific place, or among a specific population. They can be transmitted in many ways, including by insects, water, animals or from person-to-person. Most emerging infections are zoonotic, meaning that they spread from animals to humans. Zoonotic diseases, such as COVID-19 or Ebola, pose significant threats due to their potential to become an epidemic, their high case fatality ratio and the absence of specific treatment and vaccines to control their spread.

The One Health concept encapsulates the idea that human and animal health are interdependent and bound to the health of the ecosystems in which they exist.

With increased global travel, population migration and the import and export of food products, it is easier for disease to travel, and 'developing' world viruses can be found in the 'developed' world. For example, in 1999 West Nile Virus was identified for the first time in New York, although it had previously only been found in Africa, Asia and Eastern Europe.

DISEASE PREVENTION

Public health focuses on the health of populations, and collective action is necessary in order to protect and improve the health and well-being of populations. This raises ethical issues, which are discussed in Chapter 6, about whether benefit for the greatest number outweighs individual concerns.

Protecting a population from infectious disease requires:
- prevention, for example, immunization and screening
- surveillance, for example, notification of cases or outbreaks, isolation/exclusion from workplaces, schools, etc.; and contact tracing
- regulation, for example, of water quality and the movement of people or animals
- public awareness.

A central question in disease prevention is whether to adopt:
- the population approach, in which the aim is to lower the average level of risk in the population, or
- the high-risk approach, in which people at particular risk are identified and offered advice and treatment.

Because most conditions follow a roughly normal distribution in the population as a whole, peaking in the middle years, most people with a risk factor or condition are to be found in the main body of the population. The prevention paradox (Rose, 2008) suggests that many people need to take protective action in order to prevent illness occurring in a few. There would be a greater improvement in population health if everyone reduced their risk, for example, lowering their cholesterol level, than if the few in the high-risk category reduced their cholesterol level to the mean. This supports the whole population approach rather than the targeted approach, which might initially appear to be the more logical choice.

In Chapter 1 we saw that there are many different meanings attached to the concept of health, but the notion that health is the 'absence of disease' is dominant. Different perceptions about the nature of health, and the factors contributing to it, underpin interpretations of health promotion. The shift from infectious and communicable diseases to chronic diseases in the 20th century highlighted the role of people's lifestyles in disease causation. Prevention therefore became much more important, often through targeting high-risk groups who have an increased likelihood of developing a specific disease.

Health promotion is often categorized as being concerned with primary, secondary or tertiary prevention, as shown in Fig. 8.2.

For those working in a clinical setting, primary or secondary prevention is the usual interpretation of health promotion, which often focuses on educating patients about the condition that triggered their contact with the health service.

INFECTION CONTROL

For those working in clinical settings, infection control is of central importance. For those in the community, understanding how infections are transmitted may also

be important as became apparent during the COVID-19 pandemic.

Infection occurs through a chain of links:

- *Infectious agent:* the pathogen is any microorganism (bacteria, virus, parasite) with the ability to cause disease.
- *Reservoir:* the site where infectious microorganisms reside and multiply, which includes people, food and equipment.
- *Site of exit:* route that provides a way for a microorganism to leave the reservoir, for example, when someone sneezes or coughs through the nose or mouth.
- *Method of transmission* by which the microorganism moves or is carried from one place to another. The principal routes of transmission are:
  - direct contact (human to human contact through, for example, touching, kissing and sexual intercourse; or from a pregnant woman to her foetus through the placenta)
  - via respiratory droplets when coughing, sneezing or talking
  - indirect contact (e.g., contact with contaminated surfaces touched by the infected person, or where droplets of bodily fluid have landed)

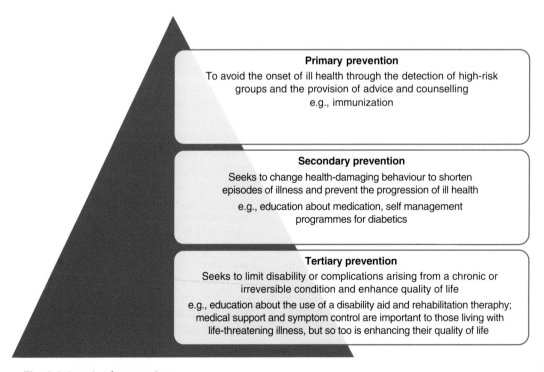

Fig. 8.2 Levels of prevention

CASE STUDY 8.1
Is COVID-19 Airborne?

In July 2020, 239 scientists signed an open letter appealing to the medical community and relevant national and international bodies to recognize the potential for airborne spread of COVID-19 (Morawska and Milton, 2020).

COVID-19 was identified as a respiratory virus. These can be transmitted in three main ways:

1. Through contact transmission where someone comes into direct contact with an infected person or touches a surface that has been contaminated.
2. Through droplet transmission of both large and small respiratory droplets that contain the virus, which would occur when near an infected person.
3. Through airborne transmission of smaller droplets and particles that are suspended in the air over longer distances and time than droplet transmission.

In the early stage of the COVID-19 pandemic an approach was adopted that combined reducing contact transmission through handwashing with reducing droplet transmission through social distancing, and airborne transmission through the wearing of a mask. The emphasis on the virus as potentially airborne is important as it begins to prioritize the importance of ventilation and new research into air conditioning and ventilation filtration systems.

- blood exposure
- consuming contaminated food/water
- parasite bites.

Understanding how a pathogen is transmitted is key to understanding how exposure can be reduced for individuals and populations. In the COVID-19 pandemic, the term 'super spreader' came to be used to describe those who may be asymptomatic but unwittingly transmit the virus.

Learning Activity 8.1 Reservoirs of Infection

What measures are taken to decrease contact with reservoirs of infection?

Fig. 8.3 is a visual produced by the microbiologist Siouxsie Wiles and the Spinoff company in New Zealand (https://thespinoff.co.nz/media/04-09-2020/the-great-toby-morris-siouxsie-wiles-covid-19-omnibus/) to illustrate the explanation of exponential spread, and

CASE STUDY 8.2
Quarantine as a Control Measure

Mary Mallon, in New York at the turn of the 20th century, was a super-spreader before the term existed, a disease carrier so notorious she acquired a celebrity nickname: Typhoid Mary. Mallon was a cook for affluent families. She showed no symptoms but was infected with typhoid and triggered multiple outbreaks. In 1907 a medical researcher identified her as the disease spreader, leading to Mallon being forcibly quarantined for the rest of her life on North Brother Island, a containment site on New York's East River. She died in 1938, aged 69, labelled in the press as 'the most dangerous woman in America'.

The practice of quarantine – the separation of those with a disease from those who are apparently healthy – has been around for a long time. The term comes from the Latin for 'forty' and refers to the 40 days that ships were required to lie at anchor before unloading in Venice.

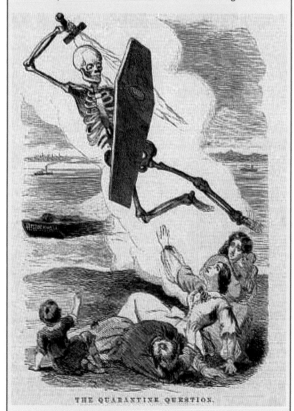

THE QUARANTINE QUESTION.

Appeared in *Harper's Weekly* in an 1858 issue as a Dr Anderson saying, 'While the Angel of Death rides on the fumes of the iron scow, and infected airs are wafted to our shores from the anchorage, we shall have no security against these annual visitations of pestilence'.

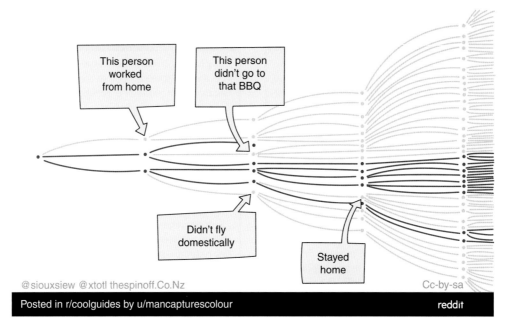

This person
worked
from home

This person
didn't go to
that BBQ

Didn't fly
domestically

Stayed
home

Fig. 8.3 The spread of infection (Adapted from Spinoff, 2021. The bumper Toby Morris and Siouxsie Wiles Covid-19 box set. Available at: https://thespinoff.co.nz/media/04-09-2020/the-great-toby-morris-siouxsie-wiles-covid-19-omnibus.)

how one small decision can make a big difference. This visual ended up being adopted by official communications channels in New Zealand, Argentina, Australia, Germany and Scotland.

- Site of entry through which the microorganism enters its new host and causes infection, for example, inhalation, ingestion, sexual contact, breaks in the skin, medical devices.
- Susceptible host. The infectious agent's ability to reproduce depends on the degree of the host's resistance.

Different individuals are not equally susceptible to infection, for a variety of reasons. Factors that increase the susceptibility of a host to the development of a communicable disease are called risk factors. Some risk factors may be individual, for example, having a pre-existing condition that results in low immunity to infectious agents. Analysis of why people from Black and Minority Ethnic groups are more likely to have severe COVID-19 infection has pointed to risk factors that are associated with greater exposure from employment, and less ability to isolate when infected (Public Health England, 2020).

Learning Activities 8.2 and 8.3 ask you to think about ways to encourage handwashing in practice.

 Learning Activity 8.2   Handwashing Campaign for Healthcare Staff
The Clean Your Hands campaign encouraged staff to wear badges inviting patients to ask them if they have washed their hands. What might be the advantages and disadvantages of this approach?

VACCINATIONS

Vaccinations fall into the category of primary prevention as they aim to prevent the onset of infectious disease that can have serious consequences. Vaccination programmes intend to give lasting active immunity against infection and in the UK there are comprehensive vaccination programmes for:

- diphtheria, tetanus, pertussis, polio, Hib (DTap/IPV/Hib), given at 2, 3 and 4 months
- measles, mumps, rubella (MMR) given at 12–15 months

Learning Activity 8.3 Handwashing Campaign for Public

Handwashing is taken as an everyday activity (where facilities are available) but the COVID-19 pandemic highlighted the importance of it being carried out carefully. Look at the example of a communication on how to wash your hands from the National Autism Association in USA. Do you think it is clear? Do you think it is accurate? What are the essential aspects of washing hands carefully?

 Wash hands

1		Turn on the warm water
2		Wet your hands
3		Turn off the water
4		Get soap
5		Wash and scrub for 20 seconds
6		Turn on the warm water and rinse off the soap
7		Dry your hands with a paper towel
8		Turn off the water with the paper towel
9		Throw the paper towel in the trash

RESEARCH EXAMPLE 8.1
Evidence on Handwashing

Evidence shows that handwashing practice in hospitals is sometimes poor. A study of 71 healthcare professionals (Jenner et al., 2006) found a discrepancy between self-reported and observed behaviour – many healthcare staff do not wash their hands as often as they think they do, and do not use appropriate products. Compliance is greatest where there is obvious contamination by blood or faeces. A systematic review (Erasmus et al., 2010) found compliance was lower in intensive care units (30%–40%) than in other settings (50%–60%); lower among physicians (32%) than among nurses (48%); and lower before (21%) rather than after (47%) patient contact. The widespread introduction in 2005 of alcohol hand rubs sought to address the barriers of time and environment, where a sink may not be nearby.

A systematic review of interventions to improve hand hygiene (Gould et al., 2017) identified the following strategies: increasing the availability of alcohol-based hand rubs, different types of education for staff, reminders (written and verbal), different types of performance feedback, administrative support and staff involvement. Studies that have examined the reasons for non-compliance have tended to focus on levels of knowledge about guidelines and awareness of the risks of contamination (Huis et al., 2012). Being observed has also been found to be strongly predictive of handwashing intent. An early study in the USA suggested that minimizing perceived 'deterrents' – especially detrimental effects on skin – would be more likely to increase compliance than emphasizing the importance of handwashing (Larson and Killien, 1982).

In rural communities where sanitation is a high priority there may be different motives for handwashing. The SuperAmma-project in India (Biran et al., 2014) identified that key drivers of handwashing with soap among rural mothers were likely to be:

- disgust of contaminated hands
- affiliation (the desire to adhere to local norms of behaviour)
- nurture, where mothers care about instilling good manners in their children.

- seasonal influenza recommended for at-risk groups and those aged over 65 years
- pneumoccocal infection recommended for at-risk groups and those aged over 65 years.

These vaccination programmes have significantly reduced mortality and morbidity rates, as shown in Table 8.2.

An immunization programme may be:
- selective: protecting those at highest risk, for example, Bacille Calmette-Guérin (BCG) for infants in high-risk areas for tuberculosis
- universal: eradicating, eliminating or containing disease, for example, mass infant immunization for childhood diseases or vaccination against COVID-19.

TABLE 8.2	Vaccination Successes	
Pre-Vaccine Cases per Year	Vaccine (Year)	Post-Vaccine Cases per Year (2019)
50,804	Diphtheria (1942)	10
92,407	Pertussis (1957)	3681
460,407	Measles (1960)	810
862	Hib (1992)	741
883	MenC (1999)	525

TABLE 8.3	The Challenges of Vaccination Uptake
Convenience	• Availability of vaccines • Health personnel to deliver services • Access, e.g., timing of appointments
Complacency	• Communication about risk and likelihood of getting disease • Perceived severity of the disease
Confidence	• Side-effects • (Rapid) development and safety • Constituents • Suitability, e.g., allergies, pregnancy • Efficacy

Herd immunity, the term given to the resistance to infection of groups of people, is dependent upon the percentage of the population that have been vaccinated. Herd immunity does not necessarily require 100% of the population to be vaccinated, because immune people will shield susceptible people from exposure to infected people. In order to obtain herd immunity for measles the percentage of the population that require vaccination is 90%.

Despite vaccines being available in many countries, they are not always accepted, as shown in Table 8.3. This may, at the simplest level, be due simply to inconvenience and difficulties accessing the place or time of the vaccination. Vaccine resistance may also be due to individual or community views about the disease being vaccinated against and its severity, and the perceived risk of becoming infected. As was the case with the COVID-19 vaccine, there may also be scepticism about the vaccine itself.

Vaccine hesitancy is not new and may be fuelled by any or all of these factors but needs to be distinguished from those who object to vaccination – now known as anti-vaxxers – as shown in Fig. 8.4. In the context of the 2009 H1N1 vaccine an analysis of those not accepting the vaccine found that 67% were 'disengaged sceptics', 19% were 'informed but unconvinced' and 14% were 'open to persuasion' (Ramanadhan et al., 2015), suggesting the need to use segmentation techniques and tailor engagement and communication. Online social media activity in 2020 led to an estimated 31 million people following anti-vaxx groups on Facebook. Media and social media are widely associated with low vaccine uptake. Learning Activity 8.4 asks you to consider and discuss how best to frame and tailor communications to encourage vaccine uptake. You may wish to read the

Vaccine hesitancy is not new

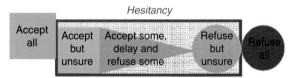

- **A delay in acceptance** or **refusal of vaccines,** despite availability of vaccination services
- **Complex and context** specific, varying across time, place and vaccine

Fig. 8.4 Vaccine hesitancy (From Report of the Sage Working Group on Vaccine Hesitancy. Available at: https://www.who.int/immunization/sage/meetings/2014/october/1_Report_WORKING_GROUP_vaccine_hesitancy_final.pdf.)

evidence in Research Example 8.2 about public perceptions in 2020 of COVID-19 and vaccines.

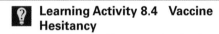

Learning Activity 8.4   Vaccine Hesitancy

How would you address vaccine hesitancy in your communications?

The role of the media and social media in influencing attitudes towards vaccination is discussed in the following research study (Research Example 8.3) in relation to measles.

Learning Activity 8.5 asks you to consider and discuss if the encouragement of vaccine uptake could be better be undertaken in communities.

RESEARCH EXAMPLE 8.2
Public Perceptions of COVID-19 Conspiracies and Vaccination

A study of 4860 adults in the UK between 21 November and 22 December 2020 conducted by Kings College London and the University of Bristol (https://www.kcl.ac.uk/policy-institute/assets/coronavirus-conspiracies-and-views-of-vaccination.pdf) found:

- 27% of the public believe 'the real truth about coronavirus is being kept from the public', which rises to 64% among people who say they're unlikely to, or definitely won't, get vaccinated against the virus.
- 21% believe 'an impartial, independent investigation of coronavirus would show once and for all that we've been lied to on a massive scale' – compared with 51% of the vaccine-hesitant who say the same.
- 20% believe that 'the authorities want us to think that coronavirus is much more dangerous than it really is'.
- 27% of ethnic minorities say they suspect that 'reporters, scientists, and government officials are involved in a conspiracy to cover up important information about coronavirus' – almost twice as high as the 14% of people from White ethnic groups who say the same.
- People from Black, Asian and minority ethnic (BAME) groups (25%) are also twice as likely as White people (13%) to state that 'the only reason a coronavirus vaccine is being developed is to make money for pharmaceutical companies'.
- 41% of White people say potential concerns about how quickly a vaccine was developed would be likely to persuade them not to take it, compared with 58% of people from other ethnic groups.
- 41% of people from BAME groups say concerns about not wanting to overload their immune system would probably convince them not to get vaccinated – almost twice as high as the 22% of White people who feel the same.

Learning Activity 8.5   Increasing the Uptake of Flu Immunization

How would you organize an effective local influenza immunization programme to ensure high uptake in all relevant groups?

SCREENING

Screening has been defined as 'a public health service in which members of a defined population, who do not

RESEARCH EXAMPLE 8.3
Media Publicity and Vaccine Uptake

In November 2013 an outbreak of 700 cases of measles was reported in Wales, when 45% of children in the Swansea area had not been vaccinated. A detailed analysis of media coverage of the measles, mumps and rubella (MMR) vaccine following Dr Wakefield's invalid claims of the link between MMR and autism showed a clear link with the drop in vaccination (Boyce, 2007).

The South Wales Evening Post (SWEP) was one newspaper that started an 'MMR Parents' fight for facts' campaign. During the period July to September 1997 the paper published five headline articles, three opinions and at least 18 other articles on the MMR vaccine. Subsequently at least six further front page main headlines, six opinions and 22 other articles have been published. A detailed local analysis (Mason and Donnelly, 2000) demonstrates that while a drop in the uptake of the MMR vaccine occurred in the whole of Wales, there was a statistically significant greater decline within the distribution area of the SWEP.

The study by Walsh et al. (2015, p. 559) concludes:

The proliferation of information on the internet means that communities are increasingly exposed to bad science and interest-driven scare stories. To counteract this, public health communication strategies need to be more sophisticated and monitoring trends in parental attitudes to immunization should be considered an important component of public health surveillance.

---

necessarily perceive they are at risk of, or are already affected by a disease or its complications, are asked a question or offered a test, to identify those individuals who are more likely to be helped than harmed by further tests or treatment to reduce the risk of a disease or its complications' (www.screening.nhs.uk).

Screening is used to select people at higher risk of developing a disease and offer an appropriate intervention.

- Primary prevention: preventing development of disease, for example, screening for high cholesterol levels.
- Secondary prevention: preventing serious outcomes of existing disease, for example, breast cancer screening.

It is also used for other purposes:

- selection of people for a particular job, for example, health checks for army recruits;

- containment of infection, for example, screening new staff for tuberculosis, or food handlers for Salmonella, or screening school staff for COVID-19.

Population screening programmes should contribute to the reduction of disease and disability by identifying those at an early stage of disease progression, when treatment is beneficial. Understandably many people will only seek medical advice with the onset of signs and symptoms. Screening aims to identify those individuals who have developed disease pathology before the onset of obvious symptoms.

For screening to be effective in containing a condition or disease there are certain criteria that need to be fulfilled (Wilson and Jungner, 1968):

- the disease should have a long pre-clinical phase, so a screening test will not miss its signs
- earlier treatment of the condition or disease should improve outcomes
- the test should be sensitive, i.e., it should detect all those with the condition or disease
- the test should be specific, i.e., it should detect *only* those with the condition or disease
- it should be cost-effective, i.e., the number of tests performed should yield a number of positive cases, making it an economically sound intervention.

There are various approaches to population screening:

Selective Screening

Screening is restricted to groups identified by behaviour or risk, for example, hepatitis C screening of intravenous drug users (IVDU). The aim of selective screening is to identify a specific disease or predisposing condition in those with a known risk factor.

Mass Screening

Everyone is invited, regardless of their risk level, to attend for testing in a systematic programme which covers the whole population over a defined period of time, for example, breast screening. The aim is to test large numbers of people for a condition regardless of their individual risk factors.

Anonymous Screening

Screening is carried out in order to establish the prevalence of a disease or condition in a given population. For example, the Unlinked Anonymous Monitoring Survey of people who inject drugs (PWID) aims to measure the distribution of unrecognized (undiagnosed) infection and associated risk factors for HIV, hepatitis B and hepatitis C.

Routine Screening

Routine screening is carried out pre- and postnatally and throughout childhood. For example, prenatal screening can be used to assess risk and to inform decisions regarding the continuation of the pregnancy and to help prepare psychologically for any physical or mental limitations that the infant may have.

Genetic Testing

Screening is carried out to identify individuals at risk of an inheritable condition. Genetic screening is not population-based but is carried out among some groups, for example, Ashkenazi Jews, among whom 1 in 25 carry Tay-Sachs – a genetic disease that leads to progressive neurodegeneration.

A screening test does not reduce the risk of, or prevent, ill health. Screening tests identify signs of potential problems and flag up individuals who have an increased risk of having or developing a health-related problem. Not all screening tests are diagnostic, for example, a nuchal translucency scan, taken between 11 and 13 weeks of pregnancy, measures the risk that the baby has Down's syndrome. The diagnostic test used to confirm the presence of Down's syndrome is chorionic villus sampling.

Any screening test intended to screen a population needs to be evaluated for its efficacy as part of a screening programme. To appraise the viability, effectiveness and appropriateness of a screening programme, the test and the screening programme need to be scrutinized. Learning Activity 8.6 asks you to consider and discuss why screening is not appropriate for certain conditions.

Learning Activity 8.6   Applying Screening Criteria

If you were to apply Wilson and Junger's classic criteria as described above, would you recommend a national screening programme for:
- asthma
- depression?

Despite rigorous criteria, screening is not foolproof or an unambiguously good thing (Table 8.4). False positive results can give rise to unnecessary and painful investigations such as biopsies, increase needless anxiety and deter future programme participation. False

TABLE 8.4   Benefits and Disadvantages of Screening

Benefits	Disadvantages
Improved prognosis for some individuals with identified conditions	Over-treatment of some insignificant or minor abnormalities
Less radical treatment	Expensive
Reassurance for those with negative results	False reassurance for those with false negative results
	Unnecessary anxiety for those with false positive results

negative results give false reassurance of being disease free, and if symptoms do develop, may deter individuals from seeking medical advice.

Population screening programmes require a high level of participation for three reasons:

1. To reduce levels of morbidity and mortality.
2. To ensure adequate evaluation.
3. To be cost-effective.

There are groups of people who are less likely to participate in population screening programmes, for example, those not registered with a GP, those from a lower socio-economic group, those who are deaf and those with learning disabilities. It is also significant that individuals from the highest risk groups have the highest non-participation rates. Public Health England (https://www.gov.uk/government/publications/breast-screening-programme-supporting-women-with-learning-disabilities/supporting-women-with-learning-disabilities-to-access-breast-screening#:~:text=Evidence%20has%20shown%20that%20breast,being%20able%20to%20access%20screening) has recognized that women with learning disabilities may find it difficult to access breast screening tests due to a number of factors including:

- practical barriers, including mobility issues, difficulty using appointment systems and a lack of accessible information and resources
- lack of knowledge among professionals of the needs of people with learning difficulties
- lack of family members or carers to support attendance at screening services
- communication barriers between women and health professionals, which could be reduced by pre-screening visits

- a negative attitude towards health promotion and screening, or a lack of knowledge, among people with learning disabilities
- difficulties around consent for people with learning disabilities
- lack of awareness among screening staff about easy to read information.

Measures to increase the uptake of screening in the population include:

- Personalized letter of invitation to the person due to be screened stating why, where and when plus a brief but understandable description of the process.
- Ensuring that screening takes place in accessible venues and at various times.
- Advertising the health gains from the screening procedure, and where and when screening takes place, using a wide range of methods to share information.
- Monitoring screening uptake by sex, ethnicity and socio-economic group to identify if the screening programme is differentially accessed by different population groups.

SURVEILLANCE

The UK Health Security Agency, formed in April 2021, as part of the Department of Health and Social Care (DHSC) is responsible for the surveillance of infectious diseases and emergency responses and preparedness. Surveillance is a key activity for an effective infection control and disease prevention programme. As we saw in Chapter 3 there are many sources of information, for example,

- primary care reports on asthma consultations
- blood lead level measurement reports from pathology services
- disease registers (e.g., congenital anomaly registers, cancer registers, GP asthma registers)
- analyses of hospital episode statistics (e.g., acute asthma admissions)
- environmental tracking (e.g., radon measurements, air quality monitoring reports, measurements of lead levels in local water supplies).

Surveillance systems have been brought into sharp focus during the COVID-19 pandemic. A key aspect of controlling the pandemic is contact tracing so that a person testing positive for COVID-19 isolates themselves, as do their close contacts, thereby breaking the chain of transmission. Contact tracing requires adequate laboratory facilities and public trust in the process.

ANTIMICROBIAL RESISTANCE

Antibiotic resistance is a global health threat and recently there has been a rise in drug-resistant infections. Resistance arises when antimicrobial drugs, most commonly antibiotics but also antivirals, antifungals and medicines that are active against parasites (such as antimalarial drugs), fail to eliminate infections completely. This allows the spread of any microbes that have become resistant to the antimicrobial drug being used. This process is accelerating, encouraged by widespread use of antimicrobials, especially in animal production, and by treatment regimes that are not completed, and prescribing for inappropriate virus conditions. Responsible prescribing requires a major educational effort among healthcare practitioners, particularly GPs who are responsible for 70% of prescribed antibiotics, and also among the public, who often view antibiotics as a 'magic bullet'. The first part of the COVID-19 pandemic saw a dramatic drop in antibiotic prescribing as infections dropped due to better hand hygiene, reduced travel and social distancing.

■ CONCLUSION

A key part of public health is health protection, and for the health promoter, being able to communicate about risk at an individual and population level is an important part of their work. The Public Health Knowledge and Skills Framework used in the UK (https://assets. publishing.service.gov.uk/government/uploads/system/ uploads/attachment_data/file/584408/public_health_ skills_and_knowledge_framework.pdf) states that practitioners should be able to:

- assess and manage outbreaks, incidents and single cases of contamination and communicable disease;
- target and implement nationwide interventions designed to offset ill health, for example, screening and immunization programmes;
- plan for emergencies and develop local and national resilience to a range of potential threats.

REFLECTIONS ON PRACTICE

- Did you observe good hand hygiene in your practice area? Did you practice good hand hygiene?
- Would you expect to be prescribed antibiotics for a cough, a cold or an ear infection?
- How would you explain a screening test to a patient or member of the public?

■ SUMMARY

This chapter has discussed screening and vaccination as initiatives to protect the public's health. Many healthcare practitioners play a vital role in discussing risk with their patients and promoting the uptake of preventive measures such as vaccination. The importance of being up to date with policies and guidelines has been emphasized. The underpinning principle is that in order to protect the health of populations, individual choice may be eroded. This poses ethical dilemmas, as we saw in Chapter 6.

FURTHER READING AND RESOURCES

Ghebrehewet, S., Stewart, A.G., Baxter, D., Shears, P., Conrad, D., 2016. Health Protection Principles and Practice. Oxford University Press, Oxford.
 A practical guide covering communicable disease control, emergency preparedness, resilience, response and environmental public health. The book includes lots of practice examples and case studies.
Van den Broucke, S., 2020. Why health promotion matters to the COVID-19 pandemic, and vice versa? Health Promot. Int. 35 (2), 181–186.
The website of the UK Health Security Agency at https:// www.gov.uk/government/organisations/uk-health-security-agency.
Resources to support screening professionals at https://www. gov.uk/guidance/nhs-population-screening-education-and-training.
The e-learning for healthcare hub has various programmes including on vaccination at https://www.e-lfh.org.uk/.

FEEDBACK TO LEARNING ACTIVITIES

8.1. Measures that might be taken to decrease contact with reservoirs of infection include:
- Condom use to prevent transmission of HIV and other sexually transmitted infections (STIs).
- Use of insecticide-treated nets (ITNs) over the bed at night, insect repellants and wearing protective clothing to prevent diseases transmitted by insect vectors.
- Wearing surgical or very clean gloves and clean protective clothing while examining patients, particularly if they have wounds, or if the examination involves the genital area.
- Maintaining personal hygiene, like taking a daily bath and washing your hands frequently. Hand washing with soap and water is the simplest, and one of the most effective, ways to prevent transmission of many communicable diseases.

8.2. Involving patients in this aspect of their care is not without challenges. It may cause patients anxiety if they are left worrying that not to ask staff to wash their hands will result in their contracting an infection. Equally, some staff may find it difficult to accept being challenged by patients, which could have a negative effect on their relationships with them.

8.3. The WHO's nine-step procedure for proper handwashing is:
- Step 1: Wet your hands....
- Step 2: Apply soap to your hands....
- Step 3: Rub your palms together....
- Step 4: Rub your hands over each other....
- Step 5: Interlace your fingers....
- Step 6: Scrub your thumbs....
- Step 7: Rub fingertips against palms....
- Step 8: Rinse your hands.

These do not include how to dry hands or the importance of not touching a tap.

8.4. Addressing vaccine hesitancy may require presenting vaccinations as part of a package of health behaviours designed to promote health and well-being in adults and older adults, rather than being seen primarily as measures to prevent transmission of disease from specific pathogens that people may not identify as severe.

8.5. The steps to implement a local immunization campaign that would encourage high uptake include:
- Identify the different potential target groups (elderly, those with chronic health conditions, children [as 'super-spreaders'], pregnant women, certain occupations such as health/social care staff).
- Information/education targeted to specific groups to increase awareness (including media, printed materials, training of health/social care staff).
- Identify registers of individuals within the target group – primary care/population registers, disease registries, school roll, occupational records.
- Identify, setup and/or review appropriate systems for call/recall and uptake monitoring. Identify, set up and/or review appropriate and accessible routes for access to immunization services, including primary care, district nursing, midwifery, school/children's services, occupational services, etc.
- Engage immunization service providers through normal service planning and delivery mechanisms or set up a stakeholder group.
- Develop and implement an action plan with SMART objectives. Monitor and evaluate implementation of the plan.

8.6. Asthma would not be recommended for a national screening programme as there is not a phase in which early detection would lead to a better outcome with treatment. Additionally, once symptoms are apparent, asthma can be readily diagnosed on clinical examination and be adequately managed.

Depression would not be recommended as there is no validated test or assessment for depression at a population level and there is no reliable demarcation of depression from social and situational unhappiness. Current guidelines (NICE, 2009) do not recommend anti-depressants as the primary intervention for mild/moderate depression, which accounts for the majority of cases. Furthermore, it is likely that a national screening programme would not be socially acceptable.

REFERENCES

Biran, A., Schmidt, W.P., Varadharajan, S.K., Rajaraman, D., Kumar, R., et al., 2014. Effect of a behaviour-change intervention on handwashing with soap in India (SuperAmma): a cluster-randomised trial. Lancet Glob. Health 2 (3), e145–e154.

Boyce, T., 2007. Health, Risk and the News. Peter Lang, London.

Erasmus, V., Daha, T.J., Brug, H., Richardus, J.H., Behrendt, M.D., et al., 2010. Systematic review of studies on compliance with hand hygiene guidelines in hospital care. Infect. Control Hosp. Epidemiol. 31 (3), 283–294.

Gould, D.J., Moralejo, D., Drey, N., Chudleigh, J.H., Taljaard, M., 2017. Interventions to improve hand hygiene compliance in patient care. Cochrane Database Syst. Rev. 9, CD005186.

Huis, A., van Achterberg, T., de Bruin, M., Grol, R., Schoonhoven, L., et al., 2012. A systematic review of hand hygiene improvement strategies: a behavioural approach. Implement. Sci. 7, 92.

Jenner, E.A., Fletcher, B.C., Watson, P., Jones, F.A., Miller, L., et al., 2006. Discrepancy between self-reported and observed hand hygiene behaviour in healthcare professionals. J. Hosp. Infect. 63 (4), 418–422.

Kickbusch, I., Reddy, K.S., 2016. Community matters: why outbreak responses need to integrate health promotion? Glob. Health Promot. 23 (1), 75–78.

Larson, E., Killien, M., 1982. Factors influencing handwashing behavior of patient care personnel. Am. J. Infect. Control 10 (3), 93–99.

Mason, B.W., Donnelly, P.D., 2000. Impact of a local newspaper campaign on the uptake of the measles mumps and rubella vaccine. J. Epidemiol. Community Health 54 (6), 473–474.

Morawska, L., Milton, D.K., 2020. It is time to address airborne transmission of COVID-19. Clin. Infect. Dis. ciaa939.

Nutbeam, D., 1998. Health promotion glossary, Health Promotion International 13 (4), 349–364.

Public Health England, 2020. Disparities in the risk and outcomes of COVID-19. Available at: https://assets. publishing.service.gov.uk/government/uploads/system/ uploads/attachment_data/file/908434/Disparities_in_ the_risk_and_outcomes_of_COVID_August_2020_ update.pdf.

Ramanadhan, S., Galarce, E., Xuan, Z., Alexander-Molloy, J., Viswanath, K., 2015. Addressing the vaccine hesitancy continuum: an audience segmentation analysis of American adults who did not receive the 2009 H1N1 vaccine. Vaccines 3 (3), 556–578.

Rose, G., 2008. The Strategy of Preventive Medicine, second edn. Oxford University Press, Oxford.

Walsh, S., Thomas, D., Mason, B., Evans, M., 2015. The impact of the media on the decision of parents in South Wales to accept measles-mumps-rubella (MMR) immunization. Epidemiol. Infect. 143 (3), 550–560.

Wilson, J.M.G., Jungner, G., 1968. Principles and Practice of Screening for Disease. World Health Organization, Geneva. Available at: http://www.who.int/bulletin/ volumes/86/4/07-050112BP.pdf.

Reorienting Health Services

IMPORTANCE OF THE TOPIC

Many agencies, services and practitioners contribute to the promotion of health, and this chapter outlines the role of different stakeholders and occupational groups. A reorientation of health services towards prevention was one of the key action areas of the Ottawa Charter (World Health Organization, 1986), yet it has not been successfully implemented. Health promotion poses several ambitious challenges for the healthcare sector: to extend the core focus of health services from clinical outcomes to quality of life; and from patients and relatives to staff and the wider community; and to integrate prevention into care and cure practices. These goals can only be achieved through organizational and funding changes. This chapter discusses these challenges, and how practitioners' and agencies' contribution to health promotion can be mainstreamed and validated. The provision of healthcare and social care services differs widely from country to country, and this chapter focuses on the UK.

INTRODUCTION

Historically, the cure and treatment of illness has taken precedence over the prevention of ill health or the promotion of positive health. For most people, health services conjures up thinking about hospitals and family doctors, a focus on treatment, developments in surgery, new techniques and more effective medicines. There is widespread acceptance that prevention is better than cure, and is the only rational way forward for public health. A survey of National Health Service (NHS) decision makers by the Faculty of Public Health in 2019 found a majority agreed that the NHS should spend more of its current budget on prevention, but did not see prevention as part of their remit. The reluctance to invest in prevention is due in part to the fact that benefits accrue over time. With limited resources and pressure to demonstrate immediate results, the focus of health services thus becomes skewed towards care.

While the contribution of health services to longevity is obvious, as we saw in Chapter 2 many other factors have a profound impact on health. However, health services do make a unique and significant contribution towards population health. This chapter argues that health services, defined as 'all the activities whose primary purpose is to promote, restore, or maintain health' (World Health Organization, 2000), are critically important in progressing health and human development. Learning Activity 9.1 asks you to consider and discuss whether and how health services address the social determinants of health and what more they could do.

 Learning Activity 9.1   Health Systems and Equity

The WHO Commission on the Social Determinants of Health (2007, p. viii) considered the contribution of health systems to equity. Do you agree with the following statement? What evidence is there to support your view?

'[Health systems] fail to apply their expertise to address the social determinants of health; fail to contribute to social empowerment in the interests of health equity; institutionalize healthcare arrangements that create financial and geographic barriers to access for disadvantaged groups; alienate disadvantaged groups through culturally insensitive and sometimes antagonistic health worker and institutional practices; and impoverish the poor whilst allowing the rich to capture greater levels of public healthcare spending.'

Chapter 4 outlined the case made for health promotion by the Ottawa Charter of 1986, which stated that healthcare should encompass traditional education, disease prevention and rehabilitation services but also 'health enhancement by empowering patients, relatives and employees … enabling people to increase control over, and to improve, their health'. Not only would this involve 'the opening of channels between the health sector and broader social, political, economic and physical

environmental components', but it would also demand a 'change of attitude and organization of health services which refocuses on the total needs of the individual as a whole person'. Learning Activity 9.2 asks you to consider and discuss whether you agree that prevention is a neglected part of health services.

Learning Activity 9.2   Reorienting Health Services

Of the Ottawa Charter's key action areas, reorienting health services is the least successfully applied (Wise and Nutbeam, 2007). What might be the reasons for this?

There is some evidence of change in the NHS, and a recognition of the need to move the NHS away from being a sickness service and towards becoming an NHS. The focus has shifted from treatment for acute conditions to management of chronic conditions and the maintenance of optimum health. In recent years concepts such as 'self-management', 'collaborative' care, 'shared decision-making' and 'the expert patient' have become integrated into the management of chronic conditions such as diabetes. Case Study 9.1 outlines a recent policy document in England that makes a commitment to prevention and health promotion.

A major incentive for the reorientation of health services is economics. Increased longevity and expectations, coupled with the rising costs of health services, have led to a concern about the cost-effectiveness of services. There is growing economic evidence for shifting the focus from treatment to health promotion. A major UK review to examine healthcare funding needs (Wanless, 2002) concluded that the 'fully engaged scenario', in which people self-manage their health and the NHS embraces prevention, is the most cost-effective. However, this review found that in many countries less than 4% of the health budget is allocated to public and primary health.

The goals of reorienting health systems are:
- to achieve a better balance between prevention and treatment
- to focus on population health outcomes alongside the focus on individual health
- to achieve a better health status for the population as a whole
- to achieve more cost-effective services
- to integrate services and maximize the contribution of the entire workforce.

The NHS Long-Term Plan and Prevention

The NHS Long-Term Plan launched in 2019 (www. longtermplan.nhs.uk) makes a clear commitment to health promotion, supporting people to live longer and healthier lives, being able to make healthier lifestyle choices, and with early treatment of avoidable illnesses. The plan includes commitments on tackling smoking, obesity, alcohol, air pollution, antimicrobial resistance and health inequalities in order to:

- make sure that everyone who has to stay overnight in hospital is given help to stop smoking
- make sure that every pregnant woman is offered face-to-face support to stop smoking, which will benefit both her and her unborn child
- help people using outpatient services for conditions that are made worse by smoking (e.g., cancer) to quit smoking
- make sure that more people are able to access support to help control their diabetes
- support more people to attend weight management services, especially those who are obese and have another condition such as high blood pressure
- make sure that people admitted to hospital with alcohol-related problems can be cared for by specialist Alcohol Care Teams
- continue to use antibiotics sensibly so that they will still be available and effective for future generations
- provide digital tools, such as smartphone apps, to enable more people to access online NHS services and to support self-management of health conditions.

PROMOTING HEALTH IN AND THROUGH THE HEALTH SECTOR

In addition to its obvious role of providing healthcare services, the NHS plays a major role in promoting health.

- The NHS is a major employer, employing 1.3 million people in the UK (NHS Confederation at www.nhs-confed.org/resources/key-statistics-on-the-nhs).
- The NHS purchases a wide range of goods and has the potential to support local economies. The purchasing power of the NHS is estimated as £27 billion per year, spent on, among other things, food, furniture, medical supplies, cleaning and office equipment, road vehicles and building materials (Health Foundation, 2019, chap. 4, p. 24).

- The NHS is a major user of energy and producer of waste and carbon emissions. NHS emissions are equivalent to 4% of England's total carbon footprint. About 2.4 million tonnes of resources, excluding water and oxygen, are consumed in the NHS, with about 15% being discarded as waste and 1% remaining as stock. The annual carbon footprint of the NHS is 25 million tonnes of carbon dioxide equivalents in procurement, building, energy and travel (NHS England, 2020).
- The NHS is a direct provider of health promotion services.
- The NHS enables communication with large numbers of people, whether as patients, family members, carers, employees, policymakers, suppliers or health professionals. The NHS has contact with a million people every 24 hours (NHS England, 2019, p. 34).
- The NHS provides social cohesion and is a highly valued social institution, now called an 'anchor institution', as shown in Fig. 9.1.

The NHS is a social setting, like a school (see Part III). The NHS has its own organizational procedures, values and ethos and cultural norms. For the NHS to embrace the promotion of health (rather than the treatment of disease), as its goal requires a change in all these elements.

The health service is an important setting for health promotion because it offers a range of health professionals the opportunity to integrate health promotion into their practice, fulfilling the early promise of a comprehensive and health promoting health service.

There are several unique characteristics of the health service setting that make it ideal for promoting health. Use of health services is universal – everyone at some point in their lives comes into contact with health service providers. For many more vulnerable groups, such as people with long-standing limiting illness, contact is long term and frequent. In the UK 97% of the population are registered with a GP, and 70% consult their GP at least once a year. Health practitioners enjoy high levels of trust and credibility among the general population, and thus are able to affect people's knowledge, attitudes and beliefs. The NHS is the country's largest single employer, so workplace initiatives may affect a significant percentage of the UK workforce and their families. All these factors provide good reasons for prioritizing the health services as a setting for health promotion. Chapter 18 discusses the hospital as a health promoting setting.

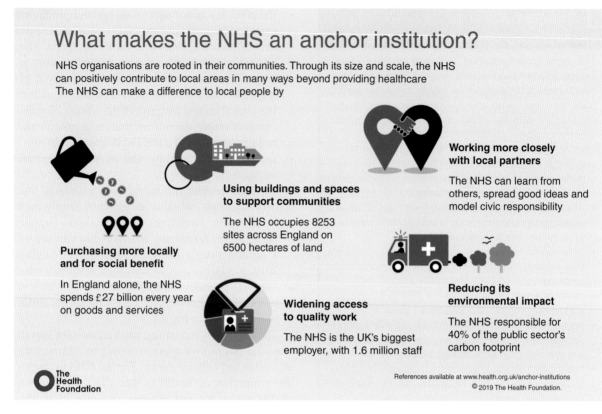

Fig. 9.1 The NHS as an anchor institution (Adapted from The Health Foundation, 2019. The NHS as an anchor institution. Available at: https://health.org.uk/news-and-comment/charts-and-infographics/the-nhs-as-an-anchor-institution.)

The Royal Society of Public Health developed impact pathways for healthcare professionals with high levels of contact with the public: allied health professionals (AHPs), nurses and midwives, pharmacists and dentists, and encourages healthcare professionals to record their everyday interactions, for example, around dementia (https://www.rsph.org.uk/static/uploaded/2c2132ff-cdac-4864-b1f1ebf3899fce43.pdf).

PRIMARY HEALTHCARE AND HEALTH PROMOTION

The 1978 Alma Ata Declaration (World Health Organization, 1978) defined primary care:

Primary health care seeks to extend the first level of the health system from sick care to the development of health. It seeks to protect and prevent the problems at an early stage. Primary health care services involve continuity of care, health promotion and education, integration of prevention with sick care, a concern for population as well as individual health, community involvement and the use of appropriate technology.

Primary care is often used interchangeably with primary medical care, as its focus is on clinical services provided predominantly by GPs, as well as by practice nurses, primary/community healthcare nurses, early childhood nurses and community pharmacists.

Primary healthcare (PHC) incorporates primary care, but has a broader focus. PHC is a comprehensive range of generalist services provided by multidisciplinary teams including GPs, nurses, AHPs and other health workers. PHC services operate at a community level. The Royal College of General Practitioners (www.rcgp.org.uk) identifies the functions of the PHC team as:

- diagnosis and management of acute and chronic conditions and treatment in emergencies, when necessary in the patient's home
- antenatal and postnatal care, and providing access to contraceptive advice and provision
- prevention of disease and disability
- follow-up and continuing care of chronic and recurring disease
- rehabilitation after illness
- care during terminal illness
- the coordination of services for those at risk, including children, those with mental illness, the bereaved, the elderly, those with a disability and those who care for them
- helping patients and their relatives to make appropriate use of other agencies for care and support, including hospital-based specialists.

Learning Activity 9.3 asks you to reflect on the role of primary care in the contribution of health services to health improvement.

> ### Learning Activity 9.3 Primary Care Provision
>
> There are 60,000 primary care physicians in France, about 1.7 per 1000 people, which is double the number in the UK. There are just over two primary care nurses, including health visitors, per doctor in France, which is about half the ratio of the UK.
>
> What effect might this have on the promotion of health in France and the UK?

The reorientation of health services towards prevention requires:

- A holistic understanding of health as well-being, rather than the absence of disease.
- Recognition that good health depends on multiple determinants – health services are important, but so too are housing, education, agriculture and other services.
- Health services reflect local needs and involve communities and individuals at all levels of service planning and provision.
- Services and technology are affordable, accessible and acceptable to communities.
- Health services strive to address inequity and prioritize services for the most needy.

Gaining control over health is the goal of health promotion. For individuals this will mean a partnership with healthcare professionals, with more person-centred care in which, as the NHS Long-Term Plan (NHS England, 2019, p. 24) states: 'what matters to someone is not the same as what's the matter with someone'. Much of the health promotion practised in PHC settings is carried out by nurses, and much of this is opportunistic which you are asked to consider in Learning Activity 9.4. For example, a client has a consultation or is referred to a member of the PHC team and is identified as 'at risk'. The practitioner takes the opportunity to offer advice, information or a further referral on a health-related issue – this process of Ask, Advise, Assist is known as 'making every contact count'. In some cases the practitioner may start a series of brief interventions using motivational interviewing to identify the client's readiness to change (see Chapter 10).

> ### Learning Activity 9.4 Opportunistic Health Promotion
>
> What are the advantages and disadvantages of opportunistic health promotion?

The emphasis of recent policy has been on developing more planned and proactive health promotion activities. The need for a risk assessment becomes a key skill enabling PHC practitioners to target health promotion. For example, only a minority of those at risk of a sexually transmitted infection (STI) attend genitourinary medicine clinics, whereas the great majority of adults will access primary care in any one year. This suggests that GPs are likely to encounter patients from across the risk spectrum for STIs, and should develop planned ways of raising the issue of sexual health risks with all patients. Case Study 9.2 describes an initiative in England in which people aged over 40 are invited through the health system to be 'checked' for health indicators such as blood pressure and be offered lifestyle advice.

The reorientation of health services requires systemic change. In England there is a move towards Integrated Care Systems (ICS) with the explicit aim of addressing locally identified needs and shifting the focus from treatment to prevention and early intervention, thus improving population health and well-being outcomes. ICS will try to join up the different hospital and community-based providers of physical and mental health and social care. ICS will be locally based, close to the places where people live and work, easy to access and free at the point of delivery

CASE STUDY 9.2
NHS Health Checks

Public health policy identifies a small number of health risk factors: poor diet, smoking, high blood pressure, obesity, physical inactivity, alcohol use and high levels of cholesterol. These are addressed through therapeutic, behavioural and structural interventions. Finding and managing those with high-risk factors is the first stage. The NHS Health Check is a population-wide approach which was introduced in 2009 and became part of the public health function of local authorities in 2014. The Health Check is a face-to-face risk assessment for cardiovascular disease, stroke and type 2 diabetes. The aim of the Health Check is to be an easily available means of screening to identify those at risk. Although it was anticipated that about 75% of eligible adults would take up this screening offer, in the 5-year cycle starting in 2013, only 45.6% of eligible adults across England have attended an NHS Health Check (Martin et al., 2018).

CASE STUDY 9.3
The Peckham Experiment

The Pioneer Health Centre was started in the 1930s by two doctors concerned about the health of poor people living in south London. The health centre tried to address health in a holistic way, and incorporated a fitness club, theatre, gym, swimming pool, billiards table, children's nursery, a cafeteria serving healthy, cheap food, a library and medical consulting rooms. One shilling (5 p) a week per family gave access to all of the centre's facilities. In 1938, 600 families belonged to the centre. The centre closed during the Second World War, reopening in 1946 when it added a nursery school, youth club, marriage advisory service, Citizens' Advice Bureau and child guidance. The centre closed in 1950 because it did not fit into the structure of the emerging NHS. The centre has been revived as Pulse Health and Leisure – a partnership between Southwark Council and Lambeth, Lewisham and Southwark health authorities, funded by £3.2 million of lottery money. Its aim is 'to provide a unique leisure, health and fitness resource that encourages local people to invest in their own health and well-being'. The new partnership thus places the responsibility for health squarely on the individual.

and able to provide prompt assessment, response, referral and continuity of care for people throughout all levels of the healthcare system. There is an increasing percentage of people, including frail older people, with chronic and complex health conditions that require care in the community. One benefit of an ICS is that more specialized hospital-based services are unnecessary. For example, proper management and monitoring of chronic conditions such as diabetes and asthma should help prevent the development of crises which require hospitalization.

Traditionally it would be the family doctor who would gain a detailed knowledge of patients over time and develop a personalized care pathway. This has become less possible as general practice consultations in the UK tend to be short (8 to 9 minutes) compared to other countries, populations are more transient, and a wide range of psychosocial problems are experienced by disadvantaged population groups. About 20% of GP visits are for social issues such as loneliness, leading many organizations to advocate social prescribing as an important way to expand the options for GPs and provide more individualized care (Husk et al., 2019). Like 'exercise on prescription' or 'exercise referral' social prescribing, the evidence for which is outlined in Research Example 9.1 provides GPs with a non-medical referral option linking individuals to community-based resources such as hobby groups, nature-based activities or volunteering in a planned and organized way through link workers.

RESEARCH EXAMPLE 9.1
The Effectiveness of Social Prescribing

In 2017 Bickerdike et al.'s systematic review suggested of the 15 extant studies 'Most were small scale and limited by poor design and reporting. All were rated as having a high risk of bias. Common design issues included a lack of comparative controls, short follow-up durations, a lack of standardised and validated measuring tools, missing data and a failure to consider potential confounding factors. Because most services are small and local there is often no budget for evaluation, but positive outcomes are reported'. Nevertheless, based on evidence from this review, the authors claim that the enthusiasm for social prescribing is unwarranted. Evidence that social prescribing may minimize the burden on GP services is also not borne out, with individuals' heightened awareness of their health needs leading to greater use of GP services (Loftus et al., 2017; Rempel et al., 2017). Woodall et al. (2018) also question the sustainability of third sector providers in delivering health and social care activities and the potential dangers in overburdening small-scale organizations through social prescribing.

Participation, collaboration, empowerment and equity are core health promotion principles, but incorporating them into health services is a challenge.

PARTICIPATION

It is now accepted that the public have the right to be consulted and to have a say in the policymaking process and in decisions about their own care and treatment. Patient and Public Involvement and Engagement (PPIE) is also a cardinal principle in the planning, designing, implementation and dissemination of research. Involvement, participation and engagement can range from being formal to informal, one-off events to ongoing contact and reactive to proactive. Any of the following activities undertaken to increase public participation and involvement could be said to be public health interventions.

- Supporting patient participation groups in general practice and including lay people's views in community health profiles.
- Seeking feedback from the community on service provision, and using this to change practice.
- Supporting self-help groups in the community.
- Working with community groups on health issues.

EQUITY

As we saw in Chapter 2, there is a strong argument for advocating greater social and economic equity as a means of promoting health. Equity refers to both material resources and power (the ability to achieve desired goals). Equity, or being fair and just, is not the same as equality, which is the state of being equal. While equality may be impossible to achieve, equity, or providing equal services for people with equal needs and working to reduce known inequalities in health, is a realistic goal. Learning Activity 9.5 asks you to reflect on your own practice and what you can do to promote equity.

 Learning Activity 9.5   Promoting Equity

What can you do in your health promotion role to promote equity?

COLLABORATION

Partnership working or collaboration is based on the understanding that individual and community well-being is determined by social, environmental and economic systems as much as by healthcare provision. It follows that the promotion and maintenance of health does not belong to one professional group or sector. Partnership working has been a central feature of health promotion and a cornerstone in the development of healthy public policy. There is a long history of partnership working to deliver health improvements in England, for example, through local strategic partnerships and community budgets and more recently through ICS.

Some of the challenges associated with partnership working across organizational boundaries arise from differences in priorities, organizational ethos, funding arrangements, competition for contracts and geographical boundaries. Enabling factors include committed individuals, joint funding and pooling of resources, shared education and training opportunities and existing projects which span different agencies.

NHS Health Scotland has developed a framework to support the development of a health promoting service, as shown in Fig. 9.2. The roots of the tree show the necessity of understanding the underlying conditions that determine health and ill health:

- biological inheritance
- physical environment
- cultural, social, political and economic circumstances.

This understanding of who is affected, and when and where, enables possible interventions to be identified. The trunk of the tree illustrates the importance of organizational commitment to improving health. The branches describe key areas for health promotion activity and those aspects of the setting that contribute to health, for example, organizational policy and public involvement.

The England Public Health Outcomes framework sets out objectives in four domains, with over 75 indicators for measuring progress (https://fingertips.phe.org.uk/profile/public-health-outcomes-framework). There are 14 indicators in relation to smoking that include:

- smokers who have successfully quit for 4 weeks
- smoking prevalence at age 15
- smokers setting a quit date
- smoking prevalence in adults employed in routine and manual occupations
- smoking prevalence in adults with serious mental illness.

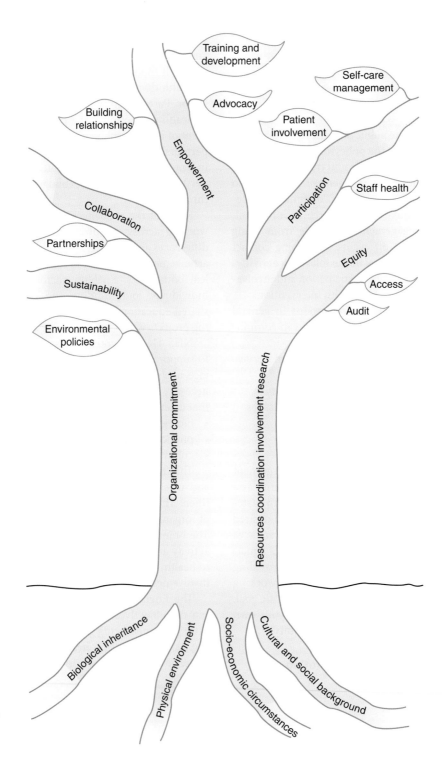

Fig. 9.2 The tree of health promotion

WHO PROMOTES HEALTH?

This section discusses the organizational system that seeks to promote health. Learning Activity 9.6 asks you to identify those organizations and roles.

> ### Learning Activity 9.6   Who Promotes Health?
> Health is a state of complete physical, social and mental well-being, not merely the absence of disease or infirmity (World Health Organization, 1946). Using this well-known definition of health, make a list of who is involved in promoting and protecting the nation's health.

Fig. 9.3 illustrates the sectors and range of agencies that can be involved in promoting health. These span international and global interests and national, regional and local levels. Many of these agencies would not regard health as their core business, but their activities can make a significant contribution to the promotion of good health in society. Reorienting the work of such agencies and organizations would mean making explicit their health goals and impact.

Numerous international organizations, such as the World Health Organization, have health promotion as a core function. Other organizations, such as the World Trade Organization, which is responsible for free trade and investment agreements between nations, can have an impact on resource consumption, environmental stress and wage rates, and thereby on the efforts of countries to reduce inequities. The World Bank provides financial assistance to low-income countries and is a major funder of health projects, including mass-immunization campaigns and anti-malaria projects. Case Study 9.4 highlights how many issues such as wars brought about by nation states and organizations impact on population health.

National

A range of government agencies have a remit for aspects of health, for example, Food Standards Agency – regulation of food labelling, food safety:

- National Institute for Health and Care Excellence – gathering of evidence on effective interventions
- UK Health Security Agency – management of health threats, including infectious disease; radiation, chemical and environmental hazards; and emergency response.

> ### CASE STUDY 9.4
> **War and Public Health**
>
> Increasing global interdependence has meant that wars are more likely to affect countries geographically far removed from the conflict, through economic repercussions, emigration patterns and even direct forms of action such as terrorism. Almost all wars since the Second World War have been fought in developing countries, which has allowed the West to consider war as an exceptional event rather than a mainstream concern for public health. This is despite the fact that in 1990 war was the 16th largest cause of the total global burden of disease (Murray and Lopez, 1997). In 2017 it was estimated that almost 30 million civilian deaths were indirectly attributable to global armed conflict between 1990 and 2017, two-thirds of which were due to communicable, maternal, neonatal and nutritional diseases (Jawad et al., 2020). Armed conflict has been highlighted by the United Nations as a major barrier to the implementation and attainment of the Sustainable Development Goals. Beyond the direct and immediate casualties, armed conflict can produce enduring political instability and the destruction of health systems and key infrastructures. This in turn can contribute to a toxification of the environment that can have an adverse impact on clean water and food supplies, further elevating the risk of communicable disease. Wars have also had a dramatic impact on the spending of low-income countries, which buy approximately 85% of world arms and weaponry. Many of these countries spend more on arms and weapons than on education or health (Levy and Sidel, 2002). The five major developed powers (China, France, Russia, the USA and the UK) produce 90% of the world's arms, and the arms trade plays a role in the perpetuation of conflict (Bunton and Wills, 2005).

In England the lead agency for health promotion is now the Office for Health Improvement and Disparities (OHID) which sits in the Department of Health and Social Care. Health Scotland, the NHS Public Health Agency for Northern Ireland and Public Health Wales take on this role in the other UK countries. In other countries there are national centres which may coordinate research and knowledge, contribute to policy advocacy and provide a voice for public health and health promotion practitioners, for example, the Public Health Agency for Canada.

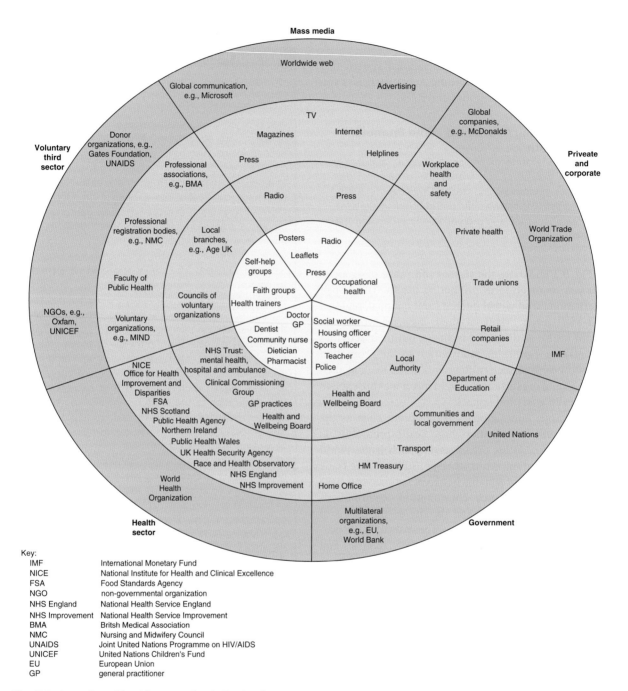

Mass media

Worldwide web

Global communication,
e.g., Microsoft

Advertising

Voluntary
third
sector

Donor
organizations, e.g.,
Gates Foundation,
UNAIDS

TV

Internet

Global
companies,
e.g., McDonalds

Priveate
and
corporate

Magazines

Helplines

Professional
associations,
e.g., BMA

Press

Workplace
health
and
safety

Radio

Press

Professional
registration bodies,
e.g., NMC

Local
branches,
e.g., Age UK

Posters

Radio

Private health

World Trade
Organization

Leaflets

Self-help
groups

Press

Faculty of
Public Health

Faith groups

Occupational
health

Trade unions

Councils of
voluntary
organizations

Health trainers

NGOs, e.g.,
Oxfam,
UNICEF

Voluntary
organizations,
e.g., MIND

Dentist

Doctor
GP

Social worker

Community nurse

Housing officer

Retail
companies

Sports officer

IMF

NHS Trust:
mental health,
hospital and ambulance

Dietician

Teacher

Pharmacist

Police

Local
Authority

NICE
Office for Health
Improvement and
Disparities
FSA
NHS Scotland
Public Health Agency
Northern Ireland
Public Health Wales
UK Health Security Agency
Race and Health Observatory
NHS England
NHS Improvement

Clinical Commissioning
Group

GP practices

Health and
Wellbeing Board

Department of
Education

Health and
Wellbeing Board

Communities and
local government

United Nations

Transport

HM Treasury

Home Office

World
Health
Organization

Multilateral
organizations,
e.g., EU,
World Bank

Health
sector

Government

Key:
IMF   International Monetary Fund
NICE   National Institute for Health and Clinical Excellence
FSA   Food Standards Agency
NGO   non-governmental organization
NHS England   National Health Service England
NHS Improvement National Health Service Improvement
BMA   British Medical Association
NMC   Nursing and Midwifery Council
UNAIDS   Joint United Nations Programme on HIV/AIDS
UNICEF   United Nations Children's Fund
EU   European Union
GP   general practitioner

Fig. 9.3 Agencies of health promotion in England

Local

The NHS is locally organized within a centralized policy framework. Currently the NHS in England comprises 209 clinical commissioning groups which commission community-based and hospital services from 251 provider organizations of acute trusts, mental health trusts, community providers and ambulance trusts and 8000 GP practices.

Key areas that impact on health, such as housing, transport and sport and leisure, are all local government responsibilities. Prior to the 1970s public health was located in local government, but was transferred to the NHS in 1974. The public health function reverted back to local government in 2013. Local government is now responsible for improving the health of the local population and for public health services, including sexual health services and drug and alcohol services. Health and well-being boards are local authority committees that link health and care systems with the aim of reducing inequalities and improving health. In 2015 local government took responsibility for 0 to 5-year-olds, and school nursing and health-visiting services became public health responsibilities.

PUBLIC HEALTH AND HEALTH PROMOTION WORKFORCE

Public health services require a balance between health promotion, preventive care and illness treatment. This is best achieved through the use of teams drawn from a variety of disciplines, including not only medical and nursing health professionals but also community workers, public health information workers and educators.

The Report of the Chief Medical Officer's Project to Strengthen the Public Health Function (Department of Health, 2001) provided a framework for assessing the contribution of the broader public health workforce to the public health function. The document referred to three main categories of employees.

1. Wider contributors
2. Practitioners
3. Specialists

Reorienting the workforce means identifying health promotion opportunities that arise within one's work and encouraging a way of working which is empowering and enables people to take control over their health issues. Fig. 9.4 illustrates the range of professionals associated with public health and health promotion as mapped by the Centre for Workforce Intelligence in 2014.

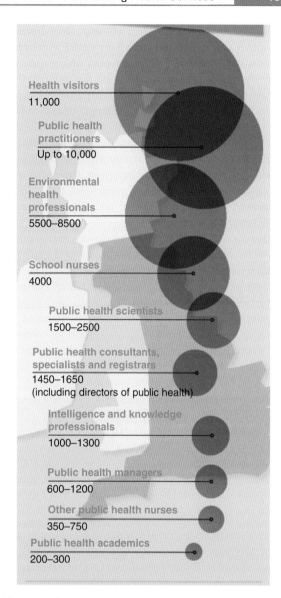

Health visitors
11,000

Public health practitioners
Up to 10,000

Environmental health professionals
5500–8500

School nurses
4000

Public health scientists
1500–2500

Public health consultants, specialists and registrars
1450–1650
(including directors of public health)

Intelligence and knowledge professionals
1000–1300

Public health managers
600–1200

Other public health nurses
350–750

Public health academics
200–300

Fig. 9.4 Core public health roles (From Centre for Workforce Intelligence, 2014. Mapping the core public health workforce. London. Available at: https://assets. publishing.service.gov.uk/government/uploads/system/ uploads/attachment_data/file/507518/CfWI_Mapping_ the_core_public_health_workforce.pdf.)

Wider Contributors

Wider contributors are professionals who, through their work, have an impact on public health but may not recognize this, for example, teachers and social services employees. Wider contributors are important because they can reach people who are not in contact with health services and refer them on to sources of advice and support. To maximize their contribution the public health aspects of their work need to be recognized and foregrounded. Teachers provide an example of this failure to recognize the importance of public health and health promotion: although schools are seen as key settings for health promotion in many countries, with national standards and key roles to strengthen the social and emotional well-being of both pupils and staff, health promotion is not part of initial teacher education in many countries (Chapter 14).

There is also a huge informal workforce that contributes to health, and Case Study 9.5 describes the roles of health trainers and health champions. Voluntary groups and non-governmental organizations act as service providers, self-help groups, pressure groups and sources of education and information. They are involved in planning and consultation exercises, such as community plans. Voluntary organizations are important in providing specialized information, and being close

to communities and isolated and vulnerable groups. Voluntary groups can reflect people's experiences of a service and give an indication of other needs, acting as a catalyst for change. The precarious funding of many voluntary organizations means they have to expend a great deal of time and effort securing grants and funding, which can make long-term planning difficult and lead to low morale.

Practitioners

The term 'public health practitioner' is used to describe about 10,000 members of the core public health workforce employed in various areas of public health including health improvement, health protection and health and social care quality. They may work in the public, private and voluntary and community sectors. Although they work in different areas of public health, all public health practitioners contribute to public health outcomes and the improvement of health and well-being.

Changing contracts and more specific definitions of roles and competencies mean that job remits in primary and social care are in a state of constant flux. Any account of working practice is in danger of being both context-specific and out-of-date in the near future. Increasingly roles are becoming generic, such as those within 'the children's workforce' where the skills, competencies and knowledge required are similar regardless of professional background or role, and apply to a very wide range of workers including personal advisers, health visitors, midwives, youth workers, family workers, substance misuse workers, nursery nurses, educational welfare officers, community children's nurses, school nurses and support staff such as learning mentors working in schools. An example of a generic and extended community role for health is described in Case Study 9.6.

A brief description of some other key roles follows. It illustrates the importance of health promotion in many job remits, but also the challenges faced and why, for many individual practitioners, health promotion often slips to the bottom of a busy workload.

SPECIALIST COMMUNITY PUBLIC HEALTH NURSES

Health promotion is a priority in the role of specialist community public health nurses such as health visitors and school nurses:

CASE STUDY 9.5
Health Trainers and Health Champions

Health trainers, also called health ambassadors, were introduced as a new kind of workforce in the document Choosing Health (Department of Health, 2004). Their role is to support people to make healthier choices and change their health-related behaviours. Health trainers are drawn from local communities, so they understand the health concerns and experiences of those they support, and have a stake in improving health in the areas where they live. Health trainers may be paid workers or volunteers.

Health champions are people who, with training and support, voluntarily use their ability to relate to people and their own life experience to transform health and well-being in their communities. Health champions share their learning with patients, resulting in better self-management of health, increased engagement and less reliance on services. The Altogether Better project (www.altogetherbetter.org.uk/health-champions) claims they 'transfer knowledge into the system and increase the intelligence held by services of community issues and assets, identifying opportunities for redesign that services are receptive to because they know and trust our Champions'.

CASE STUDY 9.6
A Community Well-Being Officer

This case study comes from examples of the work of public health practitioners on the NHS Careers website (https://www.healthcareers.nhs.uk/explore-roles/public-health/roles-public-health/public-health-practitioner):

I am based in a GP practice and work with colleagues and other community agencies to support the health and well-being of patients and the local population. The practice has an action plan, informed by the local joint strategic needs assessment (JSNA) and in turn this helps to guide the priorities for my role.

I help people to find their way through 'the system' and reach the services they need to make improvements to their own personal situation; this may relate to poor health or social problems such as debt or isolation.

Many of my clients face challenges that go hand in hand with living in deprivation, such as poor health and well-being levels, debt, poor housing or relationship problems. I work with individuals to design holistic interventions that help them to develop the skills and knowledge to improve their own well-being, and

to become resilient in the face of difficulties. If I don't have the skills or knowledge to personally deal with an issue, or there is a specialist agency that could better help, then I will refer clients on to other services. If necessary, I can continue to support them whilst they build up their confidence levels and achieve their goals.

In addition to one-to-one work my role also involves delivery or design of various training courses. For example, we offer a long-term health conditions programme for people with on-going health issues who may also have problems associated with their social health such as debt or isolation. There is often an overlap between health and social issues and we try to address this in the courses we offer.

As a CWO we support individuals to build up their confidence to a point where they want to become a volunteer or a well-being champion. This involves us working together to develop a personal development plan (PDP) where individuals can pass on the message of well-being to others in the wider community.

Specialist community public health nursing aims to reduce health inequalities by working with individuals, families, and communities promoting health, preventing ill health and in the protection of health. The emphasis is on partnership working that cuts across disciplinary, professional and organizational boundaries that impact on organized social and political policy to influence the determinants of health and promote the health of whole populations (www.nmc-uk.org).

Increasingly, community nurses are expected to use a population focus, adopting community development methods (see Chapter 11), identifying local needs and supporting community and voluntary groups. Health visitors, family nurses and school nurses are now part of the public health workforce and work closely with other community nurses, GPs and social workers. However, health promotion may not always be coordinated or prioritized because health and social care workers tend to concentrate on their own caseload.

Community nurses visit people in their own homes and are able to build a strong relationship with their clients over a period of time. This enables community nurses to carry out one-to-one education, counselling and opportunistic health education. District nurses, for example, visit people with chronic sickness or disability in their homes. Much of their work is with older people (one in four people over 75 are on a district nurse caseload), and they carry out opportunistic health education as well as liaising between people living in the community and other relevant health and welfare workers. The individualized basis of patient care offers opportunities for health promotion, but is also a constraint, limiting time and separating district nursing from a population perspective. Learning Activity 9.7 asks you to identify the health promotion role of a district nurse. Reflecting on this aspect of a role or job is helpful to identify the types of activities that may be undertaken, the approach and priority given to prevention and promotion of health and well-being and therefore, what should be included in the education and training for this role.

Learning Activity 9.7   Professional Roles

What is the health promotion role of a district nurse?

MENTAL HEALTH NURSES

Promoting mental health requires a collaborative approach from a diverse and wide-ranging group of stakeholders. Mental health promotion is often associated with the health and social care services involved in delivering care and treatment to people experiencing mental ill health. While treating mental illness is an important component, mental health promotion is concerned with the mental health and well-being of the whole population throughout their life course. Mental health promotion is delivered in a variety of settings including schools, the workplace, care homes, prisons and the community at large.

SCHOOL NURSES

School nurses are part of the community nursing service and their role varies enormously. Originally the role of the school nurse was to focus on the detection and treatment of poor hygiene, infestations and malnutrition, but it has since evolved to become routine health surveillance and screening. In common with health-visiting, the current role for school nurses is to move away from routine surveillance towards identifying needs and targeting support, for example, support for children with chronic diseases or the provision of education and counselling on specialized topics such as sexual health. School nurses may also implement the national Child Measurement Programme on obesity. Some areas adopt a life-course approach, with the school nurse acting as a navigator for children throughout their school journey. The school is recognized as a setting for health promotion and school nurses are a school-based service. Yet there are challenges and barriers facing school nurses who wish to extend their role, particularly within schools, where they may not feel part of the organization.

MIDWIVES

Hospital midwives are involved in antenatal education and the delivery of babies. Community midwives visit all new mothers in their area and provide support and education as well as monitoring the health of mothers and babies.

A review of public health interventions by midwives (McNeil et al., 2012) identified several effective actions which are already recommended as routine practice, for example, education about folic acid supplementation and pelvic floor muscle training to prevent or reduce the risk of urinary incontinence. However, guidelines have not been routinely applied. Other effective interventions were identified which could easily be implemented by a midwife and could potentially impact on public health, such as education programmes for parents of pre-term infants and implementation of specific strategies to reduce caesarean section rates. Case Study 9.7 is similar to the previous one but this time asks you to consider the health promotion role of a midwife.

 CASE STUDY 9.7
The Midwife's Role in Health Promotion

A Royal College of Midwives (RCM, 2017, p. 25) report on the public health role of midwives describes the scope of involvement in these examples:

In my current role I am involved in public health in the areas of smoking cessation & carbon monoxide exposure for pregnancy women & babies, healthy diet & avoidance of obesity, food hygiene & the avoidance of food poisoning, avoidance of alcohol in pregnancy, the health benefits of breastfeeding for both mother & baby & the signs & symptoms of Group A strep infection in pregnancy & the puerperium leading to sepsis. Contraceptive choices to enable healthy family spacing, prevention of SIDS & the promotion of pelvic floor exercises postnatally are also within my role.

The public health role that midwives undertake tends to depend on the health complexities of their clientele and thus is a dynamic concept and truly hard to define completely. I suppose if you consider the health issues that are relevant to all childbearing women in the first instance such as: promoting breast feeding, advising on cervical cytology/breast screening, diet and exercise to reduce obesity and diabetes and perinatal mental health to then move onto more specific issues pertinent to the individual woman. These may include smoking, alcohol and substance misuse, homelessness, physical and mental abuse, including forced marriages etc.

I have experienced promoting health issues in all aspects of my training – mental health, screening, vaccines, breastfeeding, smoking and alcohol, diet (we try and discuss throughout but it's often missed).

GENERAL PRACTITIONERS

General practice has traditionally been a private and personal consultation between doctor and patient. Health promotion consisted of opportunistic advice or information, often limited by time or a concern not to be 'intrusive'. The contracting of GP services provides additional payments to GPs to carry out preventive work such as immunizations, health checks to identify risk and giving advice. Opportunities for planned interventions have increased, and there are numerous examples of exercise referral schemes and lifestyle management programmes.

PRACTICE NURSES

Practice nurses are directly employed by GPs. Practice nursing is a relatively new profession, although there are now over 25,000 practice nurses in the UK. Their health promotion role has been largely confined to immunization, taking bloods, cytology, lifestyle and travel health advice and health checks, but increasingly they are staffing minor-illness centres.

DENTISTS AND DENTAL THERAPISTS

There is an increasing emphasis on prevention in dentistry, particularly with children. Dentists receive a capitation fee per child, and so have an interest in keeping that child's teeth healthy. Many practices employ a hygienist or dental therapist who gives advice on dental health. They may advise on smoking cessation, healthy diet and alcohol intake. Health authorities also have a community dental service which may offer dental health promotion to schools and residential homes.

EYE HEALTHCARE PROFESSIONALS

These include ophthalmologists, optometrists and opticians. Nearly a hundred people start to lose their sight every day and at least 50% of this is preventable if detected and treated in time (Access Economics, 2009). Smoking, obesity and diabetes are all risk factors for eye problems.

Although there is a recognition of the importance of health promotion in the role of eye healthcare professionals (Rowe and Henshall, 2005), a systematic review found no studies of eye healthcare professionals and health promotion (Needle et al., 2011). Although it is recommended that all eye care professionals advise patients to quit smoking, a survey of optometrists in 2013 in the UK found that only one in three regularly assessed patients' smoking status and advised on smoking cessation (Lawrenson and Evans, 2013).

There are a number of barriers to eye healthcare professionals taking a more active health promotion role. There may be a lack of knowledge of lifestyle health promotion and a lack of the broader skill of engaging in healthy conversations. Time is also a barrier as an eye healthcare professional may only have 10 minutes of contact time with a patient. A further barrier is that health promotion advice is not part of opticians' NHS contract.

PHARMACISTS

The potential of community pharmacies to promote health has been recognized in a national strategy (Department of Health, 2008). Pharmacy staff advise the public on the safe use of medicines, minor ailments and healthy lifestyles. They may also provide specific public health interventions as part of a broader NHS service, for example, weight-loss clinics, specialist smoking cessation advice or drug misuse services (see Chapter 18). To maximize their potential, all pharmacies should have areas set aside where members of the public can have a private consultation with the pharmacist.

ENVIRONMENTAL HEALTH WORKERS

The role of environmental health is particularly wide-ranging, encompassing statutory powers relating to food hygiene and pollution (of noise and air), specialist work on safety in the workplace and places of entertainment and work on sustainability and recycling. Because environmental health officers have wide-ranging statutory powers, their work in health promotion is mainly giving advice on legislation and enabling people to conform to regulations. Their work may thus involve offering training courses or one-to-one advice.

ALLIED HEALTH PROFESSIONALS

Many other professions allied to medicine, such as speech and language therapists, chiropodists, physiotherapists, radiographers and dietitians (known as

AHPs), have a part to play in health promotion, especially patient education.

Many health professionals have been encouraged to work flexibly and extend their roles to include promoting health and well-being, educating patients and viewing every patient contact as an opportunity for health promotion. Health promotion is a routine component of AHP practice, but is not necessarily thought through or well delivered. The evidence points to a variation between professions, with physiotherapists and dietitians engaging in more highly developed health promotion practice (https://www.rsph.org.uk/static/uploaded/58510d9a-c653-4e7a-a90133fc4c7b192e.pdf).

CARE WORKERS

Population projections indicate a rapid ageing of the population. People aged 85 and over will comprise 3.8% of the UK population by 2031, and the majority of these will need residential care. Care workers have a key health promotion role to improve fitness and nutrition and thereby minimize illness and dependence. Care workers also have a role in positive mental health promotion and empowering older people to have a degree of control over their lives. Preventing ill health in the frail aged is important, for example, the prevention of falls and pressure sores. Residential care workers liaise with GPs, social workers, physiotherapists, chiropodists and catering staff.

SPECIALISTS

Specialist advisers in public health are usually public health consultants and specialists working at a strategic or senior-management level. They play a role in developing public health programmes and often have specific scientific expertise and accreditation. In many countries they are physicians. Multiprofessional health workers first appeared in Finland, Ireland, the USA and the UK. Alongside specialists in public health are public health practitioners, who work in a variety of settings and have varying remits, from health improvement to health protection and health intelligence. These practitioners are mainly employed in public health departments, which are now part of local government, and are usually accountable to the Director of Public Health (DPH). Public health departments vary widely in size,

from a handful to 50 staff. They have the lead role in initiating, coordinating and supporting health education and health promotion activity (termed health improvement – see Chapter 4) within their areas. Activities include:

- assessing local health needs
- contributing to the operational and strategic plans of the local authority
- reviewing service agreements to ensure that they seek to promote health
- coordinating the plans and services of different agencies.

Provider activities include:

- managing health promotion programmes on specific issues such as HIV/AIDS, smoking cessation or coronary heart disease
- providing advice and consultancy to the public and policymakers
- providing training, support and advice to all health promoters and agencies that provide health promotion.

■ CONCLUSION

Reorienting health services is a challenging task, and to date little progress has been made. There are many reasons for the intransigence of the health services to change. Both primary and acute care are social systems with their own structures and cultures which determine the ways in which they tackle health and ill health. Partnerships tend to be client rather than population focused, and though primary care is based in communities, there may be little engagement with communities. Health services are driven by a medical model of health rather than a social model, and evaluation is still often measured in terms of reduced morbidity and mortality rather than in terms of health-gain processes and outcomes. The priority is treatment, which means that often patient compliance is valued above patient autonomy and participation. Although progress has been made in prioritizing health promotion, it is still 'bolted on' to core tasks instead of being integral to everyone's work and service delivery. Key health promotion activities, such as addressing health inequalities, are replaced by the need to respond to client demands, which may paradoxically have the effect of reinforcing inequalities by providing more services for more educated and articulate patients. Perhaps the biggest barrier is the growing burden of non-communicable diseases, which leads to health promotion focusing on lifestyle changes.

A policy paper from the UK government in spring 2021 (https://www.gov.uk/government/publications/transforming-the-public-health-system/transforming-the-public-health-system-reforming-the-public-health-system-for-the-challenges-of-our-times) proposed a new Office for Health Promotion (later renamed as OHID) led by the Chief Medical Officer:

> *The Office for Health Promotion will be a dynamic, multi-disciplinary unit that will oversee policy development, expert advice and implementation on prevention of ill-health. It will house a range of skillsets and expertise, spanning functions such as policy making and delivery, data and actuarial science. This office will lead a new age of health promotion. It will set direction on prevention and will work to support and drive prevention across national government, local government, the NHS and the wider health system*

Chapter 18 discusses what is meant by a health promoting health service and draws attention to some of the challenges highlighted here in enabling patients to engage with the design, implementation and evaluation of health information and services. Reorienting health services and promoting health mean addressing the diverse needs of populations and the ways in which their health is shaped by social determinants.

On the plus side, there is a large pool of potential health promoters, including many practitioners in primary, secondary and tertiary care services. The effective delivery of health promotion would, in the long run, ease the workload of most practitioners, as well as enabling people to enjoy better health and increased longevity. Health promotion underpins many of the activities already being undertaken by practitioners, for example, collaboration and partnership working. The economic argument for reorienting health services is robust, and provides a compelling case for action. Combining all these positive factors is a long-term and daunting task, but many small steps have already been taken. The challenge is to keep the reorienting health services agenda in the foreground and to identify ongoing strategies to progress this goal. This chapter draws from examples from the UK but the challenges of reorient health services to prevention are echoed across the world.

REFLECTIONS ON PRACTICE

Think of a health promotion intervention you have made concerning the health of a service user.
- Reflect on the reasons for your action.
- Could you have done something different?
- Would other health promoters have done the same as you?
- If you adopted a public health approach to your work what, if any, aspects of this intervention would change? How could you:
- increase participation?
- promote equity?
- increase collaboration and partnership working?
- What can be done to reorient the healthcare sector to take greater responsibility for health promotion? What in your work experience are the prospects and problems of collaboration with others to promote health?
- How can public health and health promotion professionals engage with the wider workforce to build their capacity and promote health?

SUMMARY

This chapter has discussed the potential of the healthcare sector to promote health, and the challenges posed by the medical paradigm. It has outlined the contribution of different agencies and practitioners to health promotion.

FURTHER READING AND RESOURCES

DHSC (Department of Health and Social Care), 2018. Prevention is better than cure. Available at: https://assets.publishing.service.gov.uk/government/uploads/system/uploads/attachment_data/file/753688/Prevention_is_better_than_cure_5-11.pdf.

Masters, R., Anwar, E., Collins, B., Cookson, R., Capewell, S., 2017. Return on investment of public health interventions: a systematic review. J. Commun. Health 71, 827–834.

Scriven, A. (ed.), 2005. Health Promoting Practice: The Contribution of Nurses and Allied Health Professionals. Palgrave Macmillan, Basingstoke.
Discussion of how different roles conceptualize health promotion, and examples of practice.

The King's Fund is a source of commentary about the health services. It has made a short animated film about the current structure of the NHS. www.kingsfund.org.uk/projects/nhs-65/alternative-guide-new-nhs-england.

The UK's Faculty of Public Health describes the public health function. www.fph.org.uk/what_is_public_health.

FEEDBACK TO LEARNING ACTIVITIES

9.1. Health systems can help to level the health gradient, but they can also inadvertently contribute to inequality. Access to, and utilization of, services should not depend on socio-economic status, yet people in equal need do not receive equal treatment. Those on higher incomes are more likely to receive specialist, preventative and dental services. The EU Survey on Income and Living Conditions found that financial factors are the most important reason why people miss out on healthcare when they need it (www.cso.ie/en/media/csoie/releasespublications/documents/silc/2012/silc_2012.Pdf). There are geographic barriers for older people and those with limited ability. Limited health literacy can also be a barrier.

9.2. Resistance to reorienting health services is primarily due to the organizational tradition and culture, particularly within the state-funded NHS, of providing treatment and care. This acute-care paradigm means that all too frequently health practitioners view their role as patching people up and sending them home. Prevention is seen as 'helping people to get better by doing what is good for them', with patient compliance an important objective. Patients who do not follow advice may be seen as demanding and, in some cases, may be refused treatment if they do not follow recommended behaviour change. In countries funded by social contributions, practitioners who are paid a fee for service have little incentive for prevention or activities such as managing chronic disease or health education, which are time-consuming and bring no financial reward.

9.3. The NHS provides excellent access and opportunities for health promotion. Every day over 835,000 people visit a GP; 50,000 visit accident and emergency; 49,000 have an outpatient consultation; 94,000 are admitted to hospital as emergencies; and 36,000 people are in hospital for planned treatment (HSCIS, 2013). In terms of credibility and competence, the 2013 Care Quality Commission satisfaction survey found that 64.2% of people definitely had confidence and trust in the last GP they had seen (www.england.nhs.uk/statistics/statistical-work-areas/gp-patient-survey/). In many countries, such as France, there has been a move away from PHC in favour of a centralized hospital system. Community care is delivered by medical practitioners with much less involvement in providing a broad PHC with health promotion at its core.

9.4. You may have included some of the following disadvantages of opportunistic health promotion.
- Opportunistic health promotion relies on the decisions of individual practitioners. This leads to patchy and uneven implementation, on a basis of chance rather than proven need.
- Health promotion remains a marginalized luxury, to be tacked on to the end of a consultation if there is time. Lack of time is an important factor limiting the amount of health promotion undertaken by both GPs and nurses.
- Doubts as to the ethics of opportunistic health promotion have been expressed, for example, raising the subject of smoking with patients consulting for unrelated problems. You may have included some of the following advantages of opportunistic health promotion.
- Immediate relevance of information.
- Highly motivated patients.
- The ability to adapt and modify the input to suit individual needs.

9.5. Most practitioners see the promotion of equity as a political task beyond their role or competence. However, even small steps contribute to greater equity. For example, ensuring that clients know their benefit entitlement and claim it, helping clients to fill out the necessary forms and supporting the case for a welfare benefits advisory service to receive health authority funding are all aspects of working to improve material circumstances and to promote equity. Identifying inequities in local services, such as people not registered with general practices, and supporting such groups to gain access to services, is also working for equity. Targeting areas of deprivation for more intensive interventions is another example which is frequently found.

9.6. Identifying who promotes health depends on how it is defined. If you adopt a fairly narrow medical model of health, you may have included a range of health professionals such as GPs and health visitors. If, however, your definition is wider and health is seen as socially and economically determined, then a much wider range of partners (e.g., local authorities, businesses) can be seen to promote health.

9.7. The roles of the district nurse include the following.
Building community intelligence:
- sharing information about older patients and their needs
- broad public health approach to health needs assessment, for example, transport to shops, street safety
- access to private accounts of health.

User participation strategies:
- access to the most vulnerable and least heard
- access to a large population, of both well and ill people.

Working in partnership with individual patients:
- the expert patient and the contribution of district nurses to patients managing their own conditions and educating others.

REFERENCES

Access Economics, 2009. Future sight loss UK (1): The economic impact of partial sight and blindness in the UK adult population. Available at: https://www.rnib.org.uk/sites/default/files/FSUK_Report.pdf.

Bickerdike, L., Booth, A., Wilson, P.M., Farley, K., Wright, K., 2017. Social prescribing: less rhetoric and more reality; a systematic review of the evidence. BMJ Open 7, e013384.

Bunton, R., Wills, J., 2005. War and public health. Crit. Public Health 15, 79–81.

Department of Health, 2001. The Report of the Chief Medical Officer's Project to Strengthen the Public Health Function. Department of Health, London. Available at. http://webarchive.nationalarchives.gov.uk/+/www.dh.gov.uk/en/Publicationsandstatistics/Publications/PublicationsPolicyAndGuidance/DH_4062358.

Department of Health, 2004. Choosing Health. Available at: https://webarchive.nationalarchives.gov.uk/+/http://www.dh.gov.uk/en/Publicationsandstatistics/Publications/PublicationsPolicyAndGuidance/DH_4094550.

Department of Health, 2008. Pharmacy in England: Building on Strengths – Delivering the Future Cm 7341. TSO (The Stationery Office), London. Available at. www.gov.uk/government/uploads/system/uploads/attachment_data/file/228858/7341.pdf.

Health Foundation, 2019. Building healthier communities: the role of the NHS as an anchor institution. Available at: https://www.health.org.uk/publications/reports/building-healthier-communities-role-of-nhs-as-anchor-institution.

HSCIS (Health and Social Care Information Centre), 2013. Monthly Hospital Episode Statistics for Admitted Patient Care, Outpatients and Accident and Emergency Data, April 2012–March 2013. Information Centre, London.

Jawad, M., Hone, T., Vamos, E.P., Roderick, P., Sullivan R., et al., 2020. Estimating indirect mortality impacts of armed conflict in civilian populations: panel regression analyses of 193 countries, 1990–2017. BMC Med. 18, 266.

Husk, K., Elston, J., Gradinger, F., Callaghan, L., Asthana, S., 2019. Social prescribing: where is the evidence? Br. J. Gen. Pract. 69 (678), 6–7.

Lawrenson, J.G., Evans, J.R., 2013. Advice about diet and smoking for people with or at risk of age-related macular degeneration: a cross-sectional survey of eye care professionals in the UK. BMC Public Health1 3, 564.

Levy, S.B., Sidel, W., 2002. The health and social consequences of diversion of economic resources to war and preparation for war. In: Taipale, I. (ed.), War or Health? A Reader. Zed Books, London.

Loftus, A., McCauley, F., McCarron, M., 2017. Impact of social prescribing on general practice workload and polypharmacy. Public Health148, 96–101.

Martin, A., Saunders, C.L., Harte, E., Griffin, S.J., MacLure, C., et al., 2018. Delivery and impact of the NHS Health Check in the first 8 years: a systematic review. Br. J. Gen. Pract. 68 (672), e449–e459.

McNeil, J., Lyn, F., Alderdyce, F., 2012. Public health interventions in midwifery: a systematic review of systematic reviews. BMC Public Health 12, 955. Available at. http://www.biomedcentral.com/1471-2458/12/955.

Murray, C.J., Lopez, A.D., 1997. Mortality by cause for eight regions of the world: Global Burden of Disease study. Lancet 349, 1269–1276.

NHS England, 2019. The NHS Long Term Plan. Available at: https://www.longtermplan.nhs.uk/wp-content/uploads/2019/08/nhs-long-term-plan-version-1.2.pdf.

NHS England, 2020. Delivering a 'Net Zero' National Health Service. Available at: https://www.england.nhs.uk/greenernhs/wp-content/uploads/sites/51/2020/10/delivering-a-net-zero-national-health-service.pdf.

Needle, J., Petchey, R., Benson, J., Scriven, A., Lawrenson, J., et al., 2011. The Allied Health Professions and Health Promotion: A Systematic Literature Review and Narrative Synthesis. Final report NIHR Service Delivery and Organisation programme.

Rempel, E.S., Wilson, E.N., Durrant, H., Barnett, J., 2017. Preparing the prescription: a review of the aim and measurement of social referral programmes. BMJ Open7 10, e017734.

RCM, 2017. Stepping Up to Public Health: A New Maternity Model for Women and Families, Midwives and Maternity Support Workers. Royal College of Midwives, London.

Rowe, F., Henshall, V., 2005. Orthoptists and their Scope in Health Promotion. In: Scriven, A. (ed.), Health Promoting Practice: The Contribution of Nurses and Allied Health Professionals. Palgrave Macmillan, Basingstoke, pp. 270–282.

Wanless, D., 2002. Securing Our Future Health. Taking a Long Term View. HM Treasury, London. Available at. http://webarchive.nationalarchives.gov.uk/+/http:/www.hm-treasury.gov.uk/consult_wanless_final.htm.

WHO Commission on the Social Determinants of Health, 2007. Challenging Inequity Through Health Systems. Final report, Knowledge Network on Health Systems. Available at: https://www.who.int/social_determinants/resources/csdh_media/hskn_final_2007_en.pdf.

Wise, M., Nutbeam, D., 2007. Enabling health systems transformation: what progress has been made to re-orienting health services? Promot. Educ. 14 Suppl. 2, 23–28.

Woodall, J., Trigwell, J., Bunyan, A.M., Raine, G., Eaton, V., et al., 2018. Understanding the effectiveness and mechanisms of a social prescribing service: a mixed method analysis. BMC Health Serv. Res. 18, 604. Available at: https://doi.org/10.1186/s12913-018-3437-7.

World Health Organization, 1946. Constitution. WHO, Geneva. Available at: http://www.who.int/governance/eb/who_constitution_en.pdf.

World Health Organization, 1978. Declaration of Alma Ata. International Conference on Primary Health Care, Alma Ata, 6–12 September. World Health Organization, Geneva. Available at: http://www.who.int/publications/almaata_declaration_en.pdf.

World Health Organization, 1986. Ottawa Charter for Health Promotion. Journal of Health Promotion 1, 1–4. Available at: http://www.who.int/healthpromotion/conferences/previous/ottawa/en/.

World Health Organization, 2000. World Health Report: Health Systems; Improving Performance. Available at: https://www.who.int/whr/2000/en/whr00_en.pdf.

10

Developing Personal Skills

LEARNING OUTCOMES

By the end of this chapter you will be able to:
- discuss the relative roles of knowledge, attitudes and skills in health behaviours and behaviour change
- describe the key theoretical frameworks that underpin a psychological approach to promoting health
- describe the role of regulation, information and incentives in changing health behaviours.

KEY CONCEPTS AND DEFINITIONS

Attitudes How a person feels about something, including affective and cognitive components.

Behaviour change Actions to change health-related behaviour, for example, smoking. Action may be at the individual, household, community or population level.

Brief intervention A short, time-limited intervention to raise awareness of a lifestyle issue and assess a person's willingness to address it.

Empowerment A process through which people gain greater control over their lives and health.

Health psychology A discipline that seeks to understand the psychological and behavioural processes in health, illness and healthcare.

Locus of control A person's belief in the control they have over their life.

Motivational interviewing A counselling technique used to assess motivation to change.

Self-efficacy A person's belief in their ability to succeed.

Social norms The behaviours and beliefs appropriate for a social group.

IMPORTANCE OF THE TOPIC

Health behaviours are any behaviours that are related to the health status of the individual. These can be behaviours that have a negative impact on health, such as smoking, eating foods high in fat, sugar or salt, drinking large amounts of alcohol, having a sedentary lifestyle and having unsafe sex. Health behaviours may have a positive effect, for example, tooth brushing, wearing seat belts, seeking health information, having regular check-ups, taking medication, sleeping an adequate number of hours per night, having a healthy diet and being physically active.

Certain health behaviours and unhealthy lifestyles are regarded as risk factors for many modern diseases,

so a main focus of health promotion has been on modifying behaviours known to have a negative impact on health. In previous chapters we have argued that such an approach is unlikely to be effective unless it acknowledges how people's behaviour may be a response to, and maintained by, the environment in which they live. However, many health promoters see their role as helping people to live their lives to their best potential, which may involve some changes in their health behaviour.

This chapter is concerned with those aspects of health behaviour that people can control. Understanding why people behave in certain ways, and how they can be helped to maintain chosen behaviours, is central to self-empowerment. This chapter explores the usefulness of health psychology, which offers several theoretical models that identify the determinants of behaviour change. These can contribute to an understanding of how people make decisions about their health, and can be a useful tool in planning health promotion interventions. The influence of specific factors, such as individual self-esteem or people's perceptions of control over their lives, needs to be taken into account by the health promoter in order to offer practical support and positive experiences in making choices.

Empowerment is a much used term in health promotion. It is a complex concept that encompasses various levels of working for change:

- individual empowerment, working with people to develop confidence and control
- community empowerment (see Chapter 11), working to create healthy and independent communities
- organizational empowerment (see Part III), working to create supportive environments.

Enabling people to change is often assumed by health promoters to mean health education about health behaviours or factors that the health promoter regards as important to change, for example, smoking or unhealthy diets, with behaviour change as the goal. Client-centred health promotion, by contrast, focuses on promoting and maintaining a person's independence in decision-making. Such an approach acknowledges that people can take some control over their lives through gaining knowledge, skills and confidence. It is also important for people to identify structural barriers and facilitators to their health. This kind of empowering education was described by Paolo Freire in his approach to radical adult literacy pedagogy (see Chapter 11). Frequently, however, developing personal skills is equated with helping people to change, drawing on psychological theories of behaviour change, motivation and self-efficacy. Increasingly, techniques such as motivational interviewing (MI), which draw upon such theories, are used.

Several theories have attempted to explain the influence of different variables on an individual's health-related behaviour:

- the health belief model (Becker, 1974)
- the theory of reasoned action (Ajzen and Fishbein, 1980)
- the stages of change model (Prochaska and DiClemente, 1984).

This chapter explores the application of these models of behaviour change to health, and considers how an understanding of cognition and decision-making can be incorporated into empowerment and education strategies.

DEFINITIONS

According to health psychology theories of behaviour change, people's behaviour is partly determined by their attitude towards that behaviour: an individual's attitude to a specific action and the intention to adopt it, motivation which comes from a person's values, attitudes and drives or instincts and social norms.

Beliefs

A belief is based on the information a person has about an object or action. For example, a person may believe or attribute their overweight to their genetic inheritance and believe that this is not controllable. If this person is encouraged to believe that their diet may contribute to their overweight, then they may change aspects of their behaviour. So information can influence attitudes and beliefs, which will in turn influence behaviour. This simple model is referred to as the knowledge–attitudes–behaviour model. However, behaviour change is never quite as simple as that. Information alone is neither necessary nor sufficient for behaviour change. The health risks of smoking are well known, yet nearly 30% of the UK population continue to smoke.

Values

Values, acquired through socialization, are emotionally charged beliefs which are important to someone. A person's values influence a whole range of feelings about family, friendships, career and society. For example, values relating to sex and gender give rise to attitudes towards motherhood, employment of women, body image, breastfeeding and sexuality.

Attitudes

Attitudes are more specific than values, and describe relatively stable feelings towards particular issues. There is no clear association between people's attitudes and their behaviour. Changing attitudes may stimulate a change in behaviour, and behaviour change may influence attitudes. For example, many people continue to smoke despite society's negative attitude to smoking, while ex-smokers often hold the most vehement anti-smoking views.

People's attitudes are made up of two components:
1. Cognitive – knowledge and information.
2. Affective – feelings and emotions and evaluation of what is important.

Although resistant to change, attitudes can be changed by providing more or different information, or by increasing a person's skills. For example, providing information about different types of physical activity and their effects on the body might influence a person's attitude towards the benefits of exercise. Attitudes might also be influenced by improved performance, which motivates the person and encourages them to think of exercise as enjoyable.

Festinger (1957) used the term cognitive dissonance to describe a person's mental state when new information is given which is counter to that already held. This prompts the person to either reject the new information (as unreliable or inappropriate) or adopt attitudes and behaviour which comply with it.

Many of the learning activities in this chapter ask you to reflect on your own health behaviours and those of individuals with whom you have worked and what contributes to behaviour change. Learning Activity 10.1 focuses on the role of information-giving in health promotion.

Learning Activity 10.1   Health Risks and Behaviour
How do people respond to information about the risks to their health from particular behaviours?

Drives

The term 'drive' is used in the health action model (Green et al., 2019) to describe strong motivating factors such as hunger, thirst, sex and pain. It is also used to describe motivations which can become drives, such as addiction. Addiction is the result of frequently repeated acts which become a habit, and is based on a psychological fear of withdrawal. Social learning theory (Bandura, 1977) uses the term instinct to describe behaviours which are not learned but are present at birth. Instincts can override attitudes and beliefs. Hunger, for example, can easily override a person's favourable attitude and intention to diet.

Understanding the impact of people's beliefs regarding their behaviour is key to addressing behavioural issues. Using smoking as an example:

- If you regard smoking as an addiction (50% of smokers have a cigarette within 30 minutes of waking), then the aim is to help the individual gain control.
- If you regard smoking as a learned behaviour which smokers associate with specific actions and rewards (social belonging, confidence, less stress), then the aim is to restructure thinking and activities to avoid potentially stressful situations, or to develop alternative means of dealing with stress, for example, relaxation.
- If you regard smoking as having a social meaning (e.g., young women seeing smoking as providing status), then the aim is to clarify and challenge such associations, and develop alternative means of achieving the social goal.

Motivation

The term 'motivation' refers to our reasons for action and to our enthusiasm for doing it (how much do you want to do it?). The strength of the motivation is sometimes referred to as our intention. Different factors influence motivation including conscious and subconscious processes, internal and external drivers, different beliefs about the consequences of their current behaviour, the expected outcomes of the new behaviour and perceptions of social norms including others attitudes and behavioural approval.

Learning Activity 10.2 focuses on the skills that individuals may need in order to change behaviours.

Learning Activity 10.2   Skills and Behaviour Change
What personal skills are needed to take greater control over one's health? Consider this in relation to a change of behaviour you have made.

Practitioners need to understand what contributes to people's decision-making about health and what makes some people more amenable to change than others. The following social cognition models highlight these factors as important.
- People's views about the cause and prevention of ill health.
- The extent to which people feel they can control their life and make changes.
- Whether people believe change is necessary.
- Whether people perceive change to be beneficial in the long term, outweighing any difficulties and problems which may be involved.

Learning Activity 10.1 asked you to consider the role of information-giving in health promotion. Learning Activity 10.3 follows up on this, asking you to explain why individuals may not necessarily act on their knowledge about unhealthy behaviours they engage in.

Learning Activity 10.3   The Gap Between Knowledge and Behaviour

How do you explain consistent findings in many studies that show a gap between knowledge and behaviour change? For example, there is a high awareness of the impact of transport on climate change, yet only a small minority act on this knowledge by, for example, giving up their cars.

The following theoretical models try to unpack the relative importance of different factors involved in decision-making, recognizing that what people say is not necessarily what they will do, and that numerous antecedent and situational variables impact on decision-making.

THE HEALTH BELIEF MODEL

The health belief model is probably the best-known theoretical model highlighting the function of beliefs in decision-making (Fig. 10.1). This model, originally proposed by Rosenstock (1966) and modified by Becker (1974), has been used to predict protective health behaviour, such as screening or vaccination uptake and compliance with medical advice.

The model suggests that whether or not people change their behaviour is influenced by an evaluation of the change's feasibility and its benefits weighed against its costs. In other words, people considering changing their behaviour engage in a cost–benefit or utility analysis. This may include their beliefs concerning the likelihood of the illness or injury happening to them (their susceptibility), the severity of the illness or injury and the efficacy of the action or how likely it is to protect the person from illness or injury.

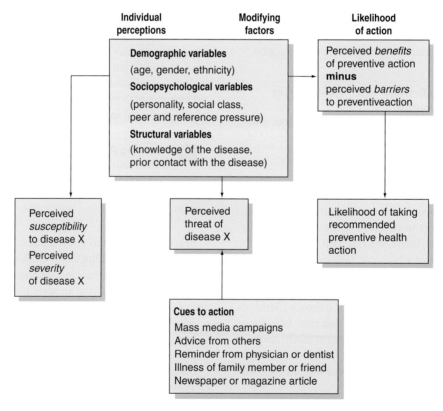

Fig. 10.1 The health belief model (From Becker, M.H. (ed.), 1974. The Health Belief Model and Personal Health Behaviour. Slack, Thorofare, New Jersey.)

For a behaviour change to take place, individuals must:

- have an incentive to change
- feel threatened by their current behaviour
- feel a change would be beneficial in some way and have few adverse consequences
- feel competent to carry out the change.

 Learning Activity 10.4   Applying the Health Belief Model to Vaccination Intentions

Consider the following situation, and then try to apply the health belief model to see if you can predict how the woman might respond.

A mother of three children under five receives a card from her GP informing her that her oldest child should receive a pre-school booster against diphtheria, tetanus, whooping cough and polio. The woman works full time at a local factory as an hourly paid packer. Her mother cares for the children while she is at work, but has no transport.

Most learning theories are based on the premise that people's behaviour is guided by consequences. If these are deemed to be positive, the person is more likely to engage in that behaviour. These explanations, which see behaviour as a simple response to positive or negative rewards, do not account for the persistence of health behaviours which have negative consequences, such as smoking or drinking and driving. However, it is frequently the case that short-term gratification is a greater incentive than the possibility of long-term harm.

Becker (1974) suggests that individuals are influenced by how vulnerable they perceive themselves to be to an illness, injury or danger (their susceptibility) and how serious they consider the illness, injury or danger to be (severity). People's perception and assessment of risk are central to the application of this model. Most people make a rough assessment about whether they are at risk, influenced by four factors:

1. Personal experience.
2. Ability to control the situation.
3. A feeling that the illness or danger is rare.
4. Any outcomes are in the distant future.

Where a situation is not familiar people tend to have an unrealistic optimism that 'it won't happen to me' (Weinstein, 1984).

 Learning Activity 10.5   Applying Behavioural Insights to Safer Driving

There are over 250,000 traffic accidents each year with 30,000 casualties, of which 3400 are fatalities. Excess speed is a contributory factor in a significant number of road accidents. There are over 2 million recorded speeding offences each year. The current response to speeding is:

- traffic calming
- police enforcement
- media campaigns, for example, 'speed kills'.

How might an understanding of social cognitions help to target a strategy for safer driving?

Since beliefs may be affected by experience, direct contact with those who have a condition can powerfully affect attitudes, exposing stereotypes and prejudice. For example, contact with a person who is human immunodeficiency virus (HIV) positive, or who is living with acquired immunodeficiency syndrome (AIDS), can change beliefs about the fatality of the disease, and about who is affected and how. Those who work with young people find perceptions of risk are very different among this age group. For adolescents, risk taking is an important task marking their development and separation from their family. It is hard for young people to appreciate the long-term effects of, for example, smoking when being 25 can seem distant and old.

Many health education campaigns have attempted to motivate people to change their behaviour through fear or guilt. Drink-drive campaigns at Christmas show the devastating effects on families of road accident fatalities and smoking-prevention posters urge parents not to 'teach your children how to smoke'. Increasingly, hard-hitting campaigns are used to raise awareness of the consequences of binge drinking, smoking and drug use. Whether such campaigns do succeed in shocking people into changing their behaviour is the subject of ongoing debate (see, e.g., Hill et al., 1998). Although fear can encourage a negative attitude and even an intention to change, such feelings tend to disappear over time and when faced with a real decision-making situation. Being very frightened can also lead to denial and avoidance of the message. Protection motivation theory (Rogers, 1975) suggests that fear only works if the threat is perceived as serious and likely to occur if the person does not follow the recommended advice.

The health belief model suggests that people need a cue to change a behaviour or make a health-related decision. The issue needs to become salient or relevant.

The cue could be noticing a change in one's internal state or appearance. For example, a pregnant woman stops smoking when she feels the baby move. The trigger can be external, such as altered circumstances resulting from a change in job or income, or the death or illness of someone close. The trigger might be a comment from a 'significant other', or reading a newspaper article. Healthcare workers can be significant others, for example, GPs have expertise, are trustworthy and have authority, leading patients to want to comply with their advice. The effects of persuasive communications on attitudes are discussed more fully in Chapter 13.

❓ Learning Activity 10.6 Applying the Health Belief Model to Sexual Health Behaviour

According to surveys in several countries including Scotland (Sigma Research, 2014 – http://gaymen-survey.sphsu.mrc.ac.uk/home.html) and China (Wu et al., 2014), about 50% of sexually active gay men had unprotected anal sex in the previous year and most men were unaware of their own HIV status.

- Consider how the health belief model could be used to explain this health behaviour.
- What reasons could you offer for individuals not carrying out their intentions to act in ways that are perceived as beneficial?

The health belief model has been widely criticized. Some of these criticisms relate to its lack of weighting for different factors – all cues to preventive action, for example, are seen as equally salient. It may appear that complex behaviours and actions are informed and chosen via analysis of independent conceptual components.

However, behaviour appears to be more nuanced, with many different interwoven arguments and scripts. The health belief model may not be very helpful in predicting behaviour or identifying those elements that are important in influencing people to change, but it does highlight the range and complexity of factors involved.

THEORY OF REASONED ACTION AND THEORY OF PLANNED BEHAVIOUR

According to the theory of reasoned action (Ajzen and Fishbein, 1980), behaviour depends on two variables:

1. Attitudes – beliefs about the consequences of the behaviour, and an appraisal of the positive and negative aspects of making a change.
2. Subjective norms – what 'significant others' do and expect, and the degree to which the person wants to conform and be like others.

These two influences combine to form an intention.

Ajzen and Fishbein (1980) acknowledge that people do not necessarily behave in a way that is consistent with their intentions. The ability to predict behaviour is influenced by the stability of a person's belief. Stability is determined by many factors: the strength of belief, how long it has been held, whether the belief is reinforced by other groups to which the individual belongs, whether it is related to, and integrated with, other attitudes and beliefs held by the individual, and how clear or structured the belief is. The theory of reasoned action differs from the health belief model in that it places importance on social norms as a major influence on behaviour.

Fig. 10.2 shows the significance of social norms in the theory of reasoned action. Social pressure may be

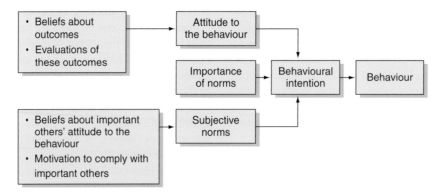

Fig. 10.2 The theory of reasoned action (From Ajzen, I., Fishbein, M., 1980. Understanding Attitudes and Predicting Social Behaviour. Prentice Hall, Englewood Cliffs.)

exerted through societal norms (such as those relating to weight and body image), community norms, peer groups and the beliefs of 'significant others' (such as parents or partners).

The motivation to comply with perceived social pressure from 'significant others' could cause individuals to behave in a way that they believe these other people or groups would think is right. The influence of peer-group pressure (even if it is not overt pressure) can be very powerful if an individual values, or is seeking, membership of, a group. Young people are susceptible to social pressures which are exacerbated by internet websites such as Facebook, which exposes them to marketing and advertising that may encourage the early adoption of a teen lifestyle.

SOCIAL LEARNING AND MODELLING

All behaviour is learned through the three key mechanisms of modelling (watching others), reinforcement (any reward) and association (linkage with internal factors such as mood, or external environmental factors). Positive and negative health behaviours can be acquired from watching those around us.

The role of modelling has been particularly important in health promotion. Concern has been expressed that there is indirect modelling of behaviour depicted in the media (Rutger et al., 2009). Direct modelling is sometimes assumed to be less influential, but people who have status and credibility, such as musicians and sports people, have been used as role models to present health promotion messages. Learning Activity 10.7 asks you to reflect on whether health promotion practitioners may themselves be exemplars and whether taking care of their own health should be a professional duty.

> **Learning Activity 10.7   Health Promoters as Role Models**
> - Should health promoters 'practise what they preach'?
> - Think of some examples where practitioners' behaviour may be at odds with the health improvement they wish to promote. How do you think this impacts (if at all) on their health promotion activities?

Some health promotion programmes use the influence of peer groups to promote positive health.

The rationale is that peers may have more credibility, are able to communicate in appropriate ways and are models to follow, although there may be doubts about the skills and information that peer educators possess (Wilton et al., 1995; Harden et al., 1999).

The previous learning activities in this chapter have considered aspects of behaviour change. Research Example 10.1 shows how behavioural science and insights can explain public behaviours in relation to recycling and waste management.

A behaviour is always more likely to recur if it is reinforced or rewarded in some way, for example, through the form of stickers that save money. Positive reinforcement is more effective than criticism, which often just lowers people's self-esteem or mood rather than enabling changes in their behaviour. The following example (Research Example 10.2) focuses on how reinforcement of unhealthy or risky behaviours can take place online among youth.

> ### RESEARCH EXAMPLE 10.1
> **Applying Behavioural Insights in Recycling**
>
> There are three barriers to recycling:
> 1. Structural/environmental, for example, limited space for storage.
> 2. Informational, for example, lack of knowledge about what can be recycled.
> 3. Motivational, for example, not believing recycling to have a positive impact.
>
> A systematic review (Varotto and Spagnolli, 2017) identified information, feedback, incentives, commitment, behaviour modelling and environmental alterations as psychological strategies to encourage greater recycling. In addition to making recycling easier by having more kerbside collections, or conversely by limiting household waste capacity, addressing social norms was found to be successful. Social norms are the beliefs that people hold about health behaviours, how they are practised and how common they are in society or among family and friends. What is important is the individual's beliefs about what other people do, not people's actual behaviour. Currently, positive recycling norms are often 'invisible' to the public as recycling is a mainly private activity, which takes place within the household. Sticking 'gold stars' on bins has been trialled as a way of indicating a good recycling household and a means of generating social pressure to follow suit. Stigmatizing poor recycling behaviour by, for example, appealing to community responsibility has also been suggested.

RESEARCH EXAMPLE 10.2
Non-suicidal Self-Injury

Non-suicidal self-injury (NSSI), or self-harm, is an increasingly prevalent health behaviour among adolescents. Considerable research has been conducted to understand potential risk factors that may motivate or reinforce adolescents' engagement in NSSI. This research refers to 'peer contagion' effects related to a variety of other health-risk behaviours. Given the salience of peer relationships in adolescence, peer influence may be implicated in the emergence and maintenance of NSSI. Discussions of NSSI, its methods and associated feelings are popular on the internet, and serve as an information source. Social learning theory predicts that individuals may conform to behaviours that they believe will earn them high status among their peers. NSSI is seen as a means of emotional regulation and, if associated with high-status peers, may be adopted by others seeking advancement among their peers (Heilbron and Prinstein, 2008).

RESEARCH EXAMPLE 10.3
Drug Use and Young People

A review of research studies (Frisher et al., 2007) found that the key predictors of drug use are not psychological factors but parental discipline and family cohesion. Male gender and older age are associated with higher levels of drug use. Pupils' school behaviour (e.g., truancy, poor attendance) is linked to drug use. What is clear from the many studies included in the review is the diversity of factors influencing drug use, reflecting the complexity of the social environment and situational determinants. There appears to be little consensus on the value of drug education.

Group techniques, such as those used by Alcoholics Anonymous, appear to have some success in getting clients to identify with the group through personal testimony and a public commitment, which encourages group members to support each other.

Bandura's (1977) social learning theory suggests that the health choices people make are related to:
- expected outcomes (whether an action will lead to a particular outcome)
- self-efficacy (whether people believe they can change).

Perceptions of self-efficacy are based on people's assessment of themselves – whether they have the knowledge and skills to make changes in their behaviour, and whether external factors such as time and money will allow such changes. Learning Activity 10.8 asks you to reflect on how self-efficacy can be developed.

 Learning Activity 10.8   Self-Efficacy

How might observing others' behaviour influence our own behaviour? To what extent does believing we can do something enable us to do it?

Self-efficacy is determined by:
- previous experiences of success and failure (e.g., having lost weight before)
- relevant vicarious experiences (e.g., seeing someone else lose weight)
- verbal/social persuasion (e.g., being told you can do it)
- emotional arousal (e.g., being scared of the consequences of not losing weight).

Personal judgement of worth, expressed in the attitudes people hold towards themselves, also contributes to one's self-efficacy, for example, we refer to high or low self-esteem, or feeling more or less worthwhile and valued. Self-concept refers to the beliefs people have about themselves, their abilities and attributes. Self-concept includes individuals' ideas about their appearance, intelligence and physical skills. Self-concept is built and modified through our perceptions of how other people behave towards us, how we are accepted and affirmed, or rejected and criticized. Ideally self-concept is built upon a network of social support.

The development of self-concept and self-esteem has been central to work in health education and promotion. It is assumed that people with high self-esteem will feel confident about themselves and have social and life skills which will enhance their feelings of personal efficacy. Many health education programmes, particularly those targeted at young people, have been based on the premise that there is a relationship between low self-esteem and harmful health behaviours. Research Example 10.3 discusses the evidence from reviews of the contributory factors to drug use among youth.

As shown in the research studies of drug use among young people, personal or 'micro' factors are played out in many situations involving choices, and real-life decision-making is often not a rational process. A study of HIV-positive people (Ridge et al., 2007) found that

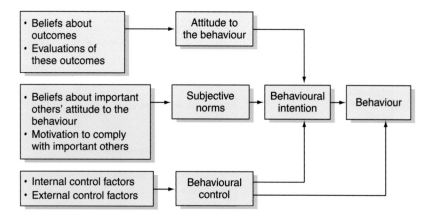

Fig. 10.3 The theory of planned behaviour (From Ajzen, I., 1991. The theory of planned behaviour. Organisational Behaviour and Human Decision Processes 50, 179–211.)

although there may be an intention to use a condom, 'irrational feelings' such as intimacy, trust and desire could all influence perceptions of risk and resulting sex behaviour.

Ajzen (1991) further developed the theory of reasoned action, and recast it as the theory of planned behaviour (Fig. 10.3).

The theory of planned behaviour incorporated another variable – that people's behaviour is a consequence of their perceived control. People differ in the extent to which they think they can make changes in their lives. Social learning theory suggests that the ways in which people explain what happens to them are a product of their childhood experiences. Those who are rewarded for their successes, and punished consistently and fairly, will come to believe that they are in control of their lives. Those who have inconsistent rewards, or punishments irrespective of their behaviour, are more likely to see events as resulting from chance, and perceive their own role to be irrelevant (Rotter, 1954).

Control in the context of health can be understood in terms of:
- internal locus of control (the extent to which individuals believe that they are responsible for their own health)
- external locus of control (the extent to which people believe that their actions are influenced by powerful others, chance, fate or luck).

Research has focused on categorizing attitudes to health by using a locus of control measure such as a multiple-choice inventory. It has been assumed that those who have a strong internal locus of control will see themselves as better able to cope and more able to act decisively and appropriately, and will undertake preventive health actions or change to more healthy behaviours. To date, only a weak relationship between feelings of control and specific behaviours has been found. However, associations have been found between smoking cessation and weight loss, and the propensity to use preventive medical services (Wallston et al., 1978). A lifestyle survey of 9000 adults found that 'unhealthy' behaviours are more likely to be associated with an internal locus of control (Blaxter, 1990). At the same time, those who recorded positive or responsible attitudes to health were also more likely to have a high internal locus of control. This confirms the argument made earlier in this chapter that specific behaviour cannot necessarily be predicted from attitudes.

People who register as 'externals' on the multidimensional health locus of control scale are those with lower levels of education and of lower socio-economic class – in other words, people who have reasons to believe that they do not have much control over their lives or health status.

Fig. 10.4 is a diagrammatic representation of some of the influences on a person's decision to take up an exercise programme. It shows how confidence to participate in physical activity can be built through positive attributions such as fitness, weight loss and successful physical performance. Social support networks are also crucial in maintaining commitment.

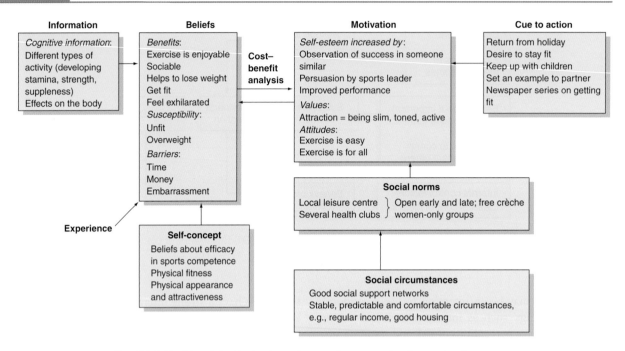

Fig. 10.4 Health-related behaviour change: the example of exercise in women

THE STAGES OF CHANGE MODEL

So far in this chapter we have discussed the factors influencing the decisions people make in relation to their health.

Prochaska and DiClemente's (1984, 1986; Prochaska et al., 1992) transtheoretical model is important in describing the process of change. The model derived from their work on encouraging change in people with addictive behaviours, although it can be applied to most people who go through stages when trying to change or acquire behaviours.

Learning Activity 10.9 asks you to reflect on your own life and a time when you have made a health behaviour change and whether this has been maintained.

❓ Learning Activity 10.9   Making a Change

Many people have had the experience of knowing what they ought to do and not doing it. Most people have tried and failed at some point in their lives to change their health behaviour, for example, give up smoking or lose weight. Identify one of your experiences of failing to make a change. What factors contributed to your failure to change?

Now think about a change you have managed to make. Why do you think you were able to stick to this decision?

Fig. 10.5 illustrates this process and identifies the following stages.

Pre-contemplation

Those in the pre-contemplation stage have not considered changing their lifestyle or become aware of any potential risks in their health behaviour. When they become aware of a problem, they may progress to the next stage. A readiness to change is a key first step in behaviour change.

Contemplation

Although individuals are aware of the benefits of change, they are not yet ready to instigate change, and may be seeking information or help to make that decision. This stage may last a short while or several years. Some people never progress beyond this stage.

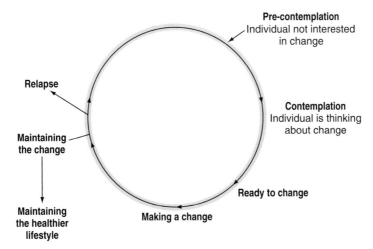

Fig. 10.5 The stages of change model (Adapted from Prochaska, J.O., DiClemente, C., 1984. The Transtheoretical Approach: Crossing Traditional Foundations of Change. Don Jones/Irwin, Harnewood, IL.)

Preparing to Change

When the perceived benefits seem to outweigh the costs, and when the change seems possible as well as worthwhile, the individual may be ready to change, perhaps seeking some extra support.

Making the Change

The early days of change require positive decisions by the individual to do things differently. A clear goal, a realistic plan, identified support and rewards are features of this stage.

Maintenance

The new behaviour is sustained and the person adopts a healthier lifestyle. Some people find maintaining the new behaviour is difficult, and they may revert or relapse back to previous stages.

Change is not a smooth process. While few people progress through each stage in an orderly way, if they make a change they will have gone through each stage. This insight has proved helpful for many healthcare workers, who find it reassuring that a relapse on the part of a client is not a failure. Individuals can go backwards and forwards through a series of cycles of change – like a revolving door. Thus, a smoker may stop smoking many times before finally giving up completely. Temporary smoking cessation shows the client that change is possible, and can contribute to permanent cessation. While

individuals may not have an awareness of contemplating, actioning and maintaining change, their intention will be based on deciding that it is in their best interests to change. The key to successful interventions is thus for a client to be motivated. Health promoters must bear in mind that their clients may not share their perceptions about the worthiness of a particular behaviour.

The Com-B model (Michie et al., 2011) as shown in Fig. 10.7 later in this chapter is a simple model to facilitate the understanding of behaviour which identifies the following:

- Capability: the psychological or physical ability to enact the behaviour. Capability can be encouraged by education or modelling.
- Motivation: the reflective or automatic mechanisms that activate or inhibit the behaviour. Motivation can be encouraged by incentives, persuasion and training.
- Opportunity: the physical and social environment that enables the behaviour. Opportunity can be provided by fiscal measures, regulations or service provision.

Helping People to Change

As we have seen in this chapter, health promoters may use a range of methods to support individuals to change:

- information-giving
- education
- counselling.

The aim of all these methods is to discuss:

- any concerns people may have about their health
- what needs they have, for information or for support
- what other influences there may be on their health, which may be barriers to change
- what changes they wish to make.

If people feel more in control of their lives, they are more likely to feel enabled to make health choices and empowered to take part in decision-making regarding their health. Poor information-giving is a common source of patient dissatisfaction. A health promoter has to be able to give information in a manner that is relevant, acceptable, understandable, coherent, contemporaneous and evidence-based. Written information may be used to reinforce verbal information, and should be understandable, accurate, acceptable, visually appealing, clear and precise.

MI, originally developed for use with addictive behaviours, is a specific technique with a non-directive counselling style. It starts with an exploration of the client's readiness to change (in keeping with the transtheoretical model of change) and how important change or the behaviour is to the person (Miller and Rollnick, 2002). Central to this technique is the view that motivation is enhanced if the person articulates for themselves the costs and benefits of change. The person's confidence that change can happen is bolstered by support, discussion of barriers and negotiated action plans.

The health promoter uses open questions and interventions borrowed from counselling techniques to encourage the person to develop their motivation to change, often in brief interventions of 5 to 10 minutes. Table 10.1 illustrates some of the core techniques that should be adopted.

MI follows a series of stages.

- Establishing rapport

  The health promoter uses questions to encourage patients to examine their knowledge about their health behaviour and the extent to which they want to change. There may be a discrepancy between what is happening at present and what the person wishes for the future, which can emphasize the importance of a change.

- Exploring ambivalence

  MI focuses on the notion of cognitive dissonance and the discomfort people feel when there is a mismatch between how they see themselves and how they are behaving, for example, you see yourself as

TABLE 10.1 Using Client-Directed Counselling Techniques

Do	Don't
• Summarize your understanding of the client's thoughts and feelings	• Interrupt or finish sentences
• Look and sound interested	• Advise or tell the client what to do
• Keep eye contact and use positive body language	• Disagree or contradict (raise alternatives)
• See things from the client's point of view	• Project your own beliefs or feelings onto the client
• Ask open questions to get more information	• Assume your experiences are the same as the client's
• Be curious rather than intrusive	• Constantly repeat the same paraphrases, e.g., 'it sounds like' or 'you feel like'
• Give the client time to think as well as talk	• Pretend you understand if you don't – ask for more explanation
• Respond to what the client is saying rather than trying to lead the conversation	

Based on Michie, S., Rumsey, N., Fussell, A., Hardeman, W., Johnston, M., et al. 2008. Improving Health: Changing Behaviour; NHS Health Trainer Handbook. British Psychological Society. Available at: https://webarchive.nationalarchives.gov.uk/ukgwa/20130123194224/ http://www.dh.gov.uk/en/Publicationsandstatistics/Publications/PublicationsPolicyAndGuidance/DH_085779.

an active and available grandparent, but are too obese to play with your grandchildren on the floor. Instead of reassurance, MI tries to expose the dissonance so that an individual may change what they do in order to be more closely aligned with their beliefs and behaviours. This is achieved by asking people to describe the costs and benefits of their behaviour and then feeding these back to them so that they can see the gap between one set of beliefs about themselves and what they are actually doing. There is a common and natural experience of feeling torn between wanting and not wanting to do something, for example, the desire to give up smoking and the desire not to put on weight. Resolving ambivalence can be a key to change. Attempts to force a person in a particular direction through direct persuasion, or by making them frightened of the consequences, can lead to a paradoxical response and even strengthen the

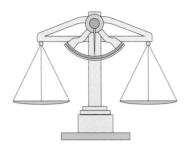

	Advantages	Disadvantages
Changing my behaviour	Might lose weight Feel healthier Save a bit of money	Friends might think I'm boring Might get bored
Not changing my behaviour	Feel relaxed Something to do Be with my friends Sleep well	Put on weight Feel paranoid sometimes Argue with friends and family Smoker's cough

Fig. 10.6 Exploring ambivalence about cannabis use

problematic behaviour. One way of helping a person to become clearer about their intentions is to use a decision–balance matrix in which the person works out the costs and benefits of changing or not changing their behaviour for themselves. Fig. 10.6 illustrates this in relation to cannabis use.

- Assessing the patient's readiness to change
  This assessment is based on the cost–benefit analysis and how important a change is to the person, and their confidence in being able to make the change, for example, do the advantages outweigh the disadvantages? A scaling question might be used: 'On a scale of one to ten how able do you feel to make a change?' Sometimes the person may be willing but not feel able to make a change.
- Developing an action plan
  Even when the person accepts the importance of a change and has the confidence to make the change, it may not be top of their priorities: 'I want to make the change, and will do so, but not now'. Having low readiness can be viewed as the person needing information about what the next step is towards change. MI is about negotiation and working with people to devise a health action plan if they are ready for change.
- Setting goals
  MI is about goal setting, which should be realistic, specific and measurable and not too ambitious or unrealistic in its outcomes. For example, a person's aim may

be to drink sensibly; their objectives may be that they reduce the number of times a week that they consume alcohol and the amount of alcohol they drink.

Such client-centred approaches arguably require specific characteristics, which Carl Rogers (1951) called core qualities, on the part of the health promoter. These core qualities help clients to have a therapeutic relationship with the health promoter, and include the following:

- Unconditional positive regard – acceptance of people irrespective of their condition, age, gender, culture, ethnicity, socio-economic background, expressed thoughts, behaviours or beliefs. The person should not be judged by any set of rules or standards. Health promoters must set aside their own values and beliefs, biases and prejudices in order to help their patients. This acceptance should not be confused with liking or approval.
- Genuineness or congruence – being oneself or being true and sincere, being non-defensive and free in behaviour and being real. The health promoters would therefore use their own language and own behaviour and be genuine.
- Empathy – being able to appreciate meanings and understand the world as seen through the eyes of the patient or client.

Thus the focus of the intervention is to take on board the person's 'frame of reference', endeavour to understand them and their circumstances and enable and encourage the patients to take responsibility for their own health decisions and actions. Self-empowerment approaches have at their core the principle of participation. These techniques allow people to examine their own values and beliefs, explore the factors that affect the choices they make and develop the skills to act upon their intentions. Rogers (1951) argues that if all this is in place behaviour change is more likely to happen.

Case Study 10.1 describes an initiative that has been adopted in the UK that mirrors some of the principles and techniques of MI and counselling. It is termed 'Making Every Contact Count (MECC)'.

Helping people to change may also mean designing interventions. The Com B model described above points to the importance of understanding behaviours as comprising capabilities (skills and knowledge), opportunities (social or environmental factors that are external to an individual and allow change to occur) and motivation which is guided by reflective or emotional processes. The COM-B Model forms the hub of the Behaviour Change Wheel (BCW) framework and nine types of intervention

surround this hub (Fig. 10.7). This illustrates a range of possible interventions: training, education, modelling, environmental restructuring, enablement, persuasion, coercion, incentivism and restrictions. To determine which intervention may be appropriate the model suggests the following criteria:

- Affordability: Can it be delivered within an acceptable budget?
- Practicability: Can it be delivered as designed and to scale?
- Effectiveness/cost: How well does it work and is it worth the cost?
- Acceptability: Is it appropriate to relevant stakeholders (policy makers, practitioners, the public) and does it engage potential users?
- Side-effects/safety: Does it have unwanted side-effects or unintended consequences?
- Equity: Will it reduce or increase disparities in health/well-being/standard of living?

THE PREREQUISITES OF CHANGE

All the models of behaviour change discussed in this chapter suggest that people are involved in a rational assessment of information when they make a decision. However, people are not usually so consciously rational, as a study of the health beliefs of working-class mothers in south Wales illustrates:

> In the subjects we studied there was little evidence of a rational approach to the personal decision-making process, i.e. a weighing up of the advantages and disadvantages of a particular change followed by a decision to act. Instead any change was a consequence not just of thought but also a mix of emotion, habit, impulse, social influences and bolshie lack of forethought, which is so typically human.
> **Pill and Stott (1990)**

Pill and Stott's (1990) study of self-initiated change shows the importance of key life events and the minor part played by health concerns. For example, women who gave up smoking did so to save money, and those who took up exercise did so to join in with their children. The importance of considering the social context and everyday life is made clear by this study, which showed that eventually most women reverted to their original behaviours because of the influence of partners

CASE STUDY 10.1
Making Every Contact Count

MECC is an English national initiative originally developed in 2009 by National Health Service (NHS) Yorkshire and Humber to radically extend the delivery of public health advice to the public. MECC works by training non-specialist staff from a wide range of service organizations in the basic skills of health promotion and prevention, thus creating an 'extended sales force for healthier living' (Ion, 2011). For example, in Wigana 'Making Health Everyone's Business' workstream has been embedded within key organizations, including Bridgewater community healthcare, children's centre and nursery provision, Greater Manchester Fire and Rescue, Greater Manchester Police, Wigan Council's Adult Social Care, Economic Regeneration and Environmental Services departments and a range of voluntary sector partners.

A range of training materials is available for those wishing to develop skills to practice MECC. They enable participants to:
- recognize opportunities to deliver key messages about adopting a healthy lifestyle and overcome any personal barriers to MECC
- confidently provide appropriate lifestyle advice
- understand the relevance of MECC to their role
- understand where to find additional information.

From www.makingeverycontactcount.com (accessed 20.08.21).

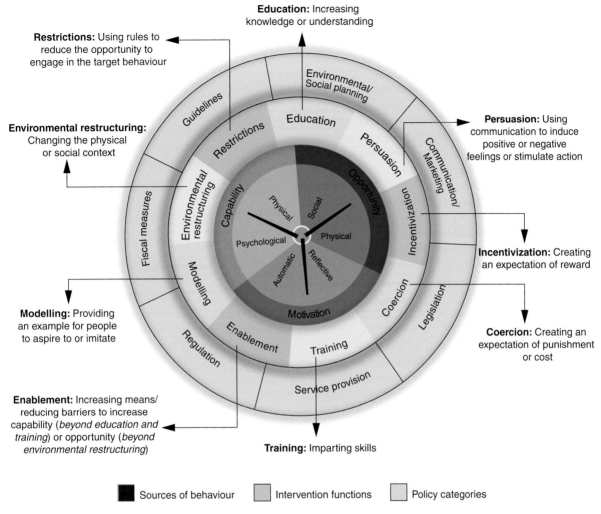

Fig. 10.7 The behaviour change wheel and intervention development (With permission from Michie, S., Van Stralen, M., West, R., 2011. The behaviour change wheel: a new method for characterizing and designing behaviour change interventions. Implementation Science 6, 42.)

or children, or because it was too difficult to juggle personal and family priorities.

The evidence from people who have changed their health behaviour suggests that there are certain minimum conditions required for change to take place.

- The change must be self-initiated
  Some people react adversely or wish to contain any attempt to look at their 'unhealthy behaviour'. To some people their behaviour may not seem unhealthy at all, but may constitute a clear source of well-being, its benefits far outweighing its risks. There is a clear

message here for those health promoters who work with individual clients and are sometimes accused of 'telling people what to do': people will only change if they want to.

- The behaviour must become salient
  Most health-related behaviours, including smoking, alcohol use, eating and exercise (or lack of it), are habitual, and built into the flow of everyday life such that the individual does not give them much thought. For a change to occur, that behaviour or habit must be called into question by some other activity or

event. For example, a smoker going to live with a non-smoker triggers a reappraisal of their smoking behaviour; or the death of a relative from breast cancer may prompt a woman to go for breast cancer screening.

- The new behaviour must become part of everyday life
  The habitual behaviour needs to become difficult to maintain while the new behaviour needs to become part of everyday life. For example, one reason why people on diets often resume their previous eating pattern is because they are constantly made aware of the diet and so it is never allowed to become a habit. Similarly, exercise is often not maintained because it requires effort; hence the advice to reluctant 'couch potatoes' to build physical activity into their daily life by walking to work or running up stairs rather than going out to exercise at a pool or gym.
- The behaviour is not part of the individual's coping strategies
  People have various sources of comfort and solace, and will resist changing these behaviours. Sometimes clients can be enabled to identify alternative coping strategies. For example, a person who eats chocolate when depressed may be encouraged to become physiologically aroused by taking up jogging.
- The individual's life should not be problematic or uncertain
  There is a limit to a person's capacity to adapt and change. For example, those living on low incomes will be stretched by coping with poverty and its uncertainties. Having to make changes in their health behaviour may be too much to expect for people whose lives are already problematic.
- Social support is available
  The presence and interest of other people provides reinforcement and keeps the behaviour salient. Changing one's behaviour can be stressful, and individuals need support. The influence of peer-group pressure and support is not given sufficient weight in psychological theories of change.

Learning Activity 10.10 returns you to reflecting about a behaviour change that you have made.

Think about an attempt you have made to enhance your health, for example, giving up smoking or losing weight.
- Were you successful in the change?
- What influenced you to make the change?
- Can you identify any specific triggers that prompted you to make the change?
- How do your family and friends regard the behaviour?
- What were the costs and benefits of making the change?

Look at the list of minimum conditions above. Do any of these factors help to explain your success or failure in making the health-related behaviour change?

CONCLUSION

What is clear from this outline of psychological theories of behaviour change is that none of them provides a full explanation. However, the variables identified by these models do appear in people's accounts of their health behaviour:

- perceptions of risk and vulnerability
- perceptions of the severity of the disease
- perceived effectiveness of the behaviour in contributing to better health
- perception of one's ability to make a change
- perception of how 'significant others' evaluate the behaviour.

While these models may not help to predict who will adopt preventive or protective health practices, they can help to plan education programmes by clarifying which factors influence decisions.

The client-centred approaches described reflect a shift away from traditional didactic and persuasive methods. Their aim is to enable clients to have the understanding and skills to translate intention into practice. Those most likely to benefit, however, are people with good education and literacy, social support and personal and economic resources. For this reason, such approaches must be accompanied by broader programmes that make the healthier choice the easier choice, and which will reach out to more disadvantaged people.

REFLECTIONS ON PRACTICE

- Do these theories help you to understand the reasons why people may or may not change their health behaviour?
- Think about a time when you encouraged a client to change their health behaviour. What aspect of their behaviour – capability, opportunity or motivation – did you think was most important to change?
- Think of a time in your life when you had a habit (e.g., diet, smoking, exercise) and then realized that this habit had changed. Identify what triggered this change in your behaviour and reflect upon what factors helped you make and sustain this change.

▌ SUMMARY

This chapter has reviewed the role of psychosocial factors in health behaviour and discussed three theoretical models. These models have been used to explain and predict health-related decisions, such as screening or compliance with medical advice. All the models identify some common variables which influence the likelihood of people adopting 'healthy' behaviours: beliefs about the efficacy of the new behaviour; motivation and whether they value their health enough to change; and normative pressures and the influence of significant people. The limitations of the role of social psychology in health promotion are outlined, but it is concluded that an understanding of those factors influencing individual behaviour can help in planning appropriate health promotion interventions.

FURTHER READING AND RESOURCES

Dixon, A., 2008. Motivation and Confidence: What Does It Take to Change Behaviour?. Kings Fund, London, Available at: https://www.kingsfund.org.uk/sites/default/files/field/field_document/motivation-confidence-health-behavious-kicking-bad-habits-supporting-papers-anna-dixon.pdf.
A useful guideto the theory and practice of behaviour change and the role of motivation and confidence. Others in the series explores the evidence for financial incentives (https://www.kingsfund.org.uk/sites/default/files/field/field_document/paying-the-patient-kicking-bad-habits-supporting-paper-karen-jochelson.pdf) and using information (https://www.kingsfund.org.uk/sites/default/files/field/field_document/information-promote-healthy-behaviours-kicking-bad-habits-supporting-paper-ruth-robertson.pdf).
Mason, P., 2018. Health Behaviour Change: A Guide for Practitioners, third edn. Elsevier, London.
Auseful guide for practitioners using brief interventions with clients. The book describes techniques and includes case study material.
Nice, 2006. Behaviour Change: The Principles of Effective Interventions PH6. Available at: www.nice.org.uk/guidance/ph6.
Nice, 2014. Behaviour Change: Individual Approaches. NICE, London, Available at: www.nice.org.uk/guidance/ph49.
Current guidance on behaviour change approaches and evidence on what works.
Ogden, J., 2019. Health Psychology: A Textbook, sixth edn. Open University, Buckingham.
An accessible textbook on psychological theory which integrates case studies and examples of research studies.

◄ FEEDBACK TO LEARNING ACTIVITIES

10.1. Some people may become concerned and make changes when presented with information about health risks. Others may make some change, such as switching to a lower-risk substitute (e.g., low-fat spread). Others may deny their risk, perhaps by underestimating the frequency or amount of their current potentially health-damaging behaviour.

10.2. Practitioners often prioritize knowledge and information as necessary to take control over one's health. Also relevant is self-confidence and a belief that change is possible, as well as a willingness and motivation to make a change.

10.3. Such findings illustrate the fact that knowledge of health benefits is only loosely associated with behaviour change. Equally, self-reported motivation is often unrelated to propensity to change. Although opportunities to change are greatest in most affluent areas, little action is taken. Understanding that wider cultural frameworks, such as pleasure, comfort and convenience, underpin decision-making is essential to motivating individuals and groups to make changes.

10.4. If we use the health belief model for predicting health behaviour, we would see the mother as a rational problem-solver who would be aware of not only the causes of childhood diseases but also the risks of contracting them (the child's susceptibility and the severity of diseases). We would assume that the mother would have been made aware of the efficacy of the vaccine and its role in increasing the child's protection following their routine vaccination as a baby. She would also be aware of any possible side-effects or contraindications. If the mother has had this child or other children immunized against other diseases, with no adverse effects, then she is more likely to view this vaccination favourably and have confidence in its effectiveness. In using this model as a predictor of behaviour, we need to take into account the perceived barriers and costs to taking this action. The mother would need to ask her own mother to take the child to the doctor. The child's grandmother may be unwilling or unable to take three children on public transport; or the mother would have to take the children and take time off work with consequent loss of earnings.

10.5. Although responses to road traffic accidents and speeding tend to focus on the adaptation of the environment or enforcement through speed cameras, driver-offender training is becoming more common (Wood et al., 2012). In relation to changing people's attitudes, you may have considered people's beliefs about:
- the consequences of accidents
- likelihood of being stopped by police
- likelihood of putting people at risk
- social disapproval
- perceived control over driving.

10.6. Factors associated with HIV-positive men having unprotected sex were:
- being in a serodiscordant (only one partner HIV-positive) or unknown-status relationship
- having 30 or more sexual partners
- having a high self-rating for attractiveness
- drug or alcohol use.

10.7. Being a role model usually refers to an individual who engages in positive health behaviours, for example, someone who is a healthy weight and a non-smoker. It is often assumed that nurses can be more effective in encouraging behaviour change among their patients if they themselves embody the desired behaviours. A counter-argument suggests that an idealized role model may be off-putting for patients.

There is a growing expectation that nurses should be role models for healthy behaviours, the rationale being that there is a relationship between nurses' personal health and the adoption of healthier behaviours by patients. This may be due to patients being motivated by, and modelling, the visible healthy lifestyle of the nurse, or that nurses are more willing to promote their patients' health by offering health promotion advice and referring the patient to support services. A systematic review (Kelly et al., 2017) found that the proposed causal relationship between nurses' health behaviours and patients' adoption of public health messages is not borne out by the research evidence.

10.8. Observing others who are similar to ourselves doing something can be encouraging. For example, if a friend quits smoking, this may well encourage you to quit. One's own experience of success with previous attempts to change behaviour can also build self-belief and self-efficacy.

10.9. There are many reasons why people are unable to change a health-related behaviour, for example:
- lack of motivation
- lack of support
- a social environment that encourages the unhealthy behaviour
- lack of time or other resources
- psychological inability to enact a change.

Overcoming any of these barriers can trigger a behaviour change.

10.10. Reflection on whether all the minimum conditions for behaviour change were met, and the relative weighting of each of the conditions, will help clarify the importance of these factors for you. It might be helpful to do this exercise with a friend or colleague and then compare notes, especially regarding the relative importance of different factors and triggers for behaviour change.

REFERENCES

Bandura, A., 1977. Social Learning Theory. Prentice Hall, Englewood Cliffs, NJ.

Blaxter, M., 1990. Health and Lifestyles. Tavistock/Routledge, London.

Festinger, L., 1957. A Theory of Cognitive Dissonance. University Press, Stanford.

Frisher, M., Crome, I., Macleod, J., Bloor, R., Hickman, M., 2007. Predictive Factors for Illicit Drug Use Among Young People: A Literature Review. Home Office, London. Available at: dera.ioe.ac.uk/6903/1/rdsolr0507.pdf.

Green, J., Tones, K., Cross, R., Woodall, J., 2019. Health Promotion. Planning and Strategies, fourth edn. Sage, London.

Harden, A., Weston, R., Oakley, A., 1999. A review of the appropriateness of peer delivered health promotion interventions for young people EPPI Centre Social Science Research Unit, Institute of Education. University of London, London. Available at: https://eppi.ioe.ac.uk/cms/LinkClick.aspx?fileticket=bCmFZQRwu-o%3D&tabid=255&mid=1071.

Heilbron, N., Prinstein, M.J., 2008. Peer influence and adolescent nonsuicidal self-injury: a theoretical review of mechanisms and moderators. Appl. Prev. Psychol. 12, 169–177. Available at: http://mitch.web.unc.edu/files/2013/10/Heilbron-Prinstein-2008-APP.pdf.

Hill, D., Chapman, S., Donavan, R., 1998. The return of scare tactics. Tob. Control 7, 5–8. Available at: http://m.tobaccocontrol.bmj.com/content/7/1/5.full.pdf.

Ion, V., 2011. Making every contact count: a simple but effective idea. Perspect. Public Health 131 (2), 69–70.

Kelly, M., Wills, J., Sykes, S., 2017. Do nurses' personal health behaviours impact on their health promotion practice? A systematic review. Int. J. Nurs. Stud. 76, 62–77.

Michie, S., Van Stralen, M., West, R., 2011. The behaviour change wheel: a new method for characterizing and designing behaviour change interventions. Implement. Sci. 6, 42. Available at: www.implementationscience.com/content/pdf/1748-5908-6-42.pdf.

Miller, W., Rollnick, S., 2002. Motivational Interviewing: Preparing People to Change, second edn. Guildford Press, London.

Pill, R.M., Stott, N.C.H., 1990. Making Changes: A Study of Working Class Mothers and the Changes Made in Their Health Related Behaviour over Five Years. University of Wales College of Medicine, Cardiff.

Prochaska, J.O., DiClemente, C.C., 1986. Towards a comprehensive model of change. In: Miller, W.R., Heather, N. (eds.), Treating Addictive Behaviours: Processes of Change. Plenum, New York.

Prochaska, J.O., DiClemente, C., Norcross, J.C., 1992. In search of how people change. Am. Psychol. 47, 1102–1114.

Ridge, D., Ziebland, S., Anderson, J., Williams, I., Elford, J., 2007. Positive prevention: contemporary issues facing HIV positive people negotiating sex in the UK. Soc. Sci. Med. 65, 755–770.

Rogers, C., 1951. Client Centred Therapy. Houghton Mifflin, Boston.

Rogers, R.W., 1975. A protection motivation theory of fear appeals and attitude change. J. Psychol. 91, 93–114.

Rosenstock, I., 1966. Why people use health services. Millbank Mem. Fund Quart. 44, 94–121.

Rotter, J.B., 1954. Social Learning and Clinical Psychology. Prentice Hall, Englewood Cliffs.

Rutger, C.M.E., Hermans, E.R., van Baaren, R.B., Hollenstein, T., Sander, M.B., 2009. Alcohol portrayal on television affects actual drinking behaviour. Alcohol and Alcoholism 44 (3), 244–249.

Varotto, A., Spagnolli, A., 2017. Psychological strategies to promote household recycling. A systematic review with meta-analysis of validated field interventions. J. Environ. Psychol. 51, 168–188.

Wallston, K.A., Wallston, B.S., DeVellis, R.F., 1978. Locus of control and health: a review of the literature. Health Educ. Monogr. 6, 107–117.

Weinstein, N., 1984. Why it won't happen to me; perceptions of risk factors and susceptibility. Health Psychol. 3, 431–457.

Wilton, T., Keeble, S., Doyal, L., Walsh, A., 1995. The Effectiveness of Peer Education in Health Promotion: Theory and Practice. HEA, London.

Wood, S., Bellis, M., Watkins, S., 2012. Road traffic accidents: a review of evidence for prevention. Available at: http://www.cph.org.uk/wp-content/uploads/2012/08/road-traffic-accidents-a-review-of-evidence-for-prevention.pdf.

Wu, J., Hu, Y., Jia, Y., Su, Y., Cui, H., et al., 2014. Prevalence of unprotected anal intercourse among men who have sex with men in China: an updated meta-analysis. PLoS One 9 (5), e98366.

11

Strengthening Community Action

LEARNING OUTCOMES

By the end of this chapter you will be able to:
- define community/communities
- understand theories of empowerment and social action
- understand the processes involved in a community development approach
- discuss the challenges presented by a community development approach.

KEY CONCEPTS AND DEFINITIONS

Community The identification and sense of belonging attached to a group of people who may be defined by geography, culture, faith or interests.

Community action Involves campaigns and activities taken collectively by people who identify themselves as a community, in terms of geography or shared interests.

Community development A process whereby members of a community get together to address common problems and take collective action. Community development often leads to community well-being (material and social).

Community mobilization A process which helps communities to identify their own needs and respond to, and address, these needs.

Empowerment Individual or community action to gain control over life choices and the determinants of health.

Social capital The networks and relationships of people who have something in common (typically living in the same area, working for the same employer or sharing the same interests and beliefs).

IMPORTANCE OF THE TOPIC

We have seen in previous chapters how there are many different ways of working for health. Strengthening community action is one of the key action areas identified in the Ottawa Charter (World Health Organization, 1986). Community development has been seen as the central defining strategy for health promotion, which aims to empower people so that they gain control over the factors influencing their health (Green and Raeburn, 1990).

There has been an increased focus on working with communities in recent years, for different reasons. In the last couple of decades, the policy focus has been on devolved services and seeing individuals as consumers, expected to participate in deciding the nature of governmental services. The community is where needs are both defined and met. There is a recognition that some groups, such as migrants or older people, may be marginalized, harder to reach and excluded from mainstream services. Laverack and Mohammadi (2011) argue that strengthening community action is a key area for health promotion, and that particular attention should be given to engaging with socially marginalized and excluded minorities.

The first learning activity (Learning Activity 11.1) in this chapter begins the process of defining community by asking you to think about communities to which you belong.

> **Learning Activity 11.1   Belonging to a Community**
> - Which communities do you belong to?
> - Are these the same communities as those to which your parents belonged?
> - What are the key characteristics of the communities you belong to?

DEFINING COMMUNITY

The concept of community is frequently used in discussions about health and healthcare. The community is usually seen as a desirable context, for example, care in the community, community policing and community education are all seen as preferable to alternative (non-community) services. In contrast to services provided by the state or bureaucratic organizations, those provided by and in the community are often seen as more appropriate and sensitive. However, there is no consensus about the definition of community. There are many different ways of defining a community, with the most commonly cited factors being geography, culture and social stratification. These factors are seen as being linked to the subjective feeling of belonging or identity which underpins the concept of 'community'. Other characteristics of communities are social networks and communal resources such as people's skills or knowledge.

Geography

A community may be defined on a geographical or neighbourhood basis (see Chapter 17). A well-known example is the East End of London, but this use of community is not restricted to working-class or urban areas. It is this notion of community which gives rise to 'patch'-based work, where people such as social workers, police officers or health visitors are assigned a geographically bounded area. The assumption is that people living in the same area have the same concerns. This in turn rests on the assumption that the physical environment is a key factor influencing health and social identity.

Culture

Community may be defined in cultural terms, as in 'the Chinese community' or 'the Jewish community'. The underlying assumption is that common cultural traditions transcend geographical or class barriers and unite otherwise scattered and disparate groups of people.

There is an expectation that members of a cultural community will assist each other and share resources. The most commonly cited elements of a common cultural heritage are ethnic origin, language, religion and customs.

Social Stratification

A community may be based on common interests, which are usually the product of social stratification, for example, 'a working-class community' and 'the gay community'. This definition implies that members of a community share networks of support, knowledge and resources, which may transcend other boundaries, even national ones.

Most definitions of community tend to suggest that it is a homogenous entity. However, any geographical community will include people whose primary identity is based on different factors, for example, class, race, gender or sexual orientation. People who feel united by a shared interest, for example, pensioners or the unemployed, will also be members of other communities, geographical and otherwise. People may belong to several different communities, some of which may have more salience for the individual than others. People may find their allegiance to different communities shifting at different points in their life span. More recently, people may feel that they belong to virtual communities – online groups with common interests. Research Example 11.1 discusses a measure of community – the Sense of Community Index – and identifies the characteristics which it seeks to measure.

The meaning and significance of community varies across different communities. Definitions of community are important, because they influence how practitioners understand community dynamics and the challenges that may arise when working with communities. Practitioners feel more comfortable working with some communities than with others.

WHY WORK WITH COMMUNITIES?

Community action – the active involvement of people in formal or informal activities to bring about planned changes or improvements in community life, services and/or resources – has long been a central tenet of health promotion. Communities, whether geographically based or based on a common identity or affinity, have a vital contribution to make to health and well-being.

RESEARCH EXAMPLE 11.1
Sense of Community Index

A strong sense of community is seen as desirable because it fosters socially supportive behaviour which helps members deal with external challenges and threats, as evidenced during the COVID-19 pandemic. The UK government recognizes the importance of social relationships which support people and facilitate individual and collective access to resources and measures social bridges, social bonds and social links in its indicators of integration framework (https://assets.publishing.service.gov.uk/government/uploads/system/uploads/attachment_data/file/835573/home-office-indicators-of-integration-framework-2019-horr109.pdf). Relationships characterized by trust and reciprocity generate 'social capital' and enable people to use and exchange resources (Putnam, 2000). However, relationships may also flag up inequalities due to differences in access to power and/or resources and entrench social divisions.

The Sense of Community Index (SCI) is a measure used to gauge people's feelings of community based on membership, influence, the meeting of needs and shared emotional connection. The SCI is derived from McMillan and Chavis' (1986) theory that a feeling of community provides emotional safety and a sense of belonging for members. McMillan and Chavis (1986) argue that communities are cohesive and exert a degree of influence or conformity over members and that members must perceive belonging to the community to be rewarding. The more that people interact, the more likely they are to form close relationships and develop even stronger bonds. The SCI measures feelings such as: 'I want the same things as others in this group' and 'I get a lot out of being in this group'.

South (2015) identifies several reasons for working with communities:

- Participatory approaches directly address the marginalization and powerlessness caused by entrenched health inequalities.
- The assets within communities, such as skills and knowledge, social networks, local groups and community organizations, are building blocks for good health.
- Social connectedness and engagement with community life are not only good for mental health but also offer protection in times of adversity.
- The National Health Service (NHS), local government and their partners can create safe and supportive places, fostering the resilience of local communities.

APPROACHES TO STRENGTHENING COMMUNITY ACTION

There are different ways of working with communities. Many practitioners are community based, for example, they work in the community, organizing projects to meet people's health needs or doing outreach work, for example, extending professional services such as screening into the community to improve accessibility. These practitioners may have the term community in their title, for example, specialist community health nurses or community police officers. The shift to primary healthcare from the late 1970s in post-colonial and socialist countries such as China and Uganda saw the creation of community health workers (CHWs) to provide local basic services as an alternative to high-cost urban health systems and as a route to community transformation. These CHWs are similar to health trainers in England or doulas who may support women in childbirth:

> Community health workers should be members of the communities where they work, should be selected by the communities, should be answerable to the communities for their activities, should be supported by the health system but not necessarily a part of its organization, and have shorter training than professional workers.
> https://www.who.int/hrh/documents/community_health_workers.pdf.

There are numerous issues that arise from the deployment of CHWs (Lehman and Sanders, 2007):

- Who volunteers to be a CHW and does the selection process reinforce inequalities in the community?
- What knowledge, skills and characteristics are required for a CHW? What training do they receive?
- Should a CHW be paid? If they are paid, does this distance them from their local communities?
- What are the boundaries for their work – for example, do they have the expertise to give clinical advice?
- To whom is a CHW accountable? If they are part of government health services, they may struggle to achieve status and recognition, but if they are embedded in their local community, they may come into conflict with government services.

Table 11.1 illustrates some of the differences between community-based work carried out by a practitioner

TABLE 11.1 Characteristics of Community-Based Versus Community Development Models

Community Based	Community Development
• Problem, targets and action defined by sponsoring body	• Problem, targets and action defined by community
• Community seen as medium, venue or setting for intervention	• Community itself the target of intervention in respect to capacity building and empowerment
• Notion of 'community' relatively unproblematic	• Community recognized as complex, changing, subject to power imbalances and conflict
• Target is largely individuals within either a geographic area or a specific subgroup in a geographic area defined by sponsoring body	• Target may be community structures or services and policies that impact on the health of the community
• Activities largely health-oriented	• Activities may be broad-based, targeting wider factors which impact on health, but have indirect health outcomes (e.g., empowerment, social capital)

After Labonte, R., 1998. A Community Development Approach to Health Promotion: A Background Paper on Practice Tensions, Strategic Models and Accountability Requirements for Health Authority Work in the Broad Determinants of Health. Prepared for Health Education Board of Scotland, Research Unit on Health and Behaviour Change. University of Edinburgh.

who is place-based, and community development work in which a practitioner seeks to build capacity and self-sufficiency within communities.

South (2015) refers to a 'family of community-centred approaches':

1. *Patient/consumer involvement in development*. This involves engagement with community members in service development, including consultation or collaboration with the community about the intervention design or local plans (see Chapter 19).
2. *Peer- or lay-delivered interventions*. This involves engagement with communities or their representatives to deliver interventions. In this model, the credibility, expertise or empathy of the community member enables the intervention, for example, health trainer

RESEARCH EXAMPLE 11.2

Community Engagement Approaches and Evidence of Outcomes

A systematic review of community engagement approaches (O'Mara-Eves et al., 2013) found that these interventions are effective in improving health behaviours, health consequences, participants' self-efficacy and perceived social support for disadvantaged groups. There also appear to be gains to human and social capital, and there is evidence of benefits for those engaged in community activities, including skills acquisition and future employment. The review did not find one approach to be more effective than another, although it did suggest that peer- or lay-delivered interventions had greater effectiveness than interventions taking an empowerment approach or those involving community members in the intervention's design. The review concluded by suggesting that community engagement in public health is more likely to require a 'fit-for-purpose' rather than a 'one-size-fits-all' approach.

services, befriending schemes and breastfeeding support workers.

3. *Empowerment of the community*. Health needs are identified by the community and people mobilize themselves into action.

These models are based on the belief that when people are engaged in a programme of community development, the result is an empowered community – the product of mutual support and collective action to mobilize resources to make changes within the community. Research Example 11.2 outlines some of the evidence of outcomes that arise from community engagement.

There is a substantial body of evidence on the benefits of community participation and empowerment. Table 11.2 summarizes the possible outcomes and the levels at which they may be evident.

DEFINING COMMUNITY DEVELOPMENT

Community development has been defined as:

Building active and sustainable communities based on social justice and mutual respect. It is about changing power structures to remove the barriers that prevent people from participating in the issues that affect their lives. Community workers support individuals, groups and organisations in this process.

Standing Conference for Community Development (2001)

TABLE 11.2 The Outcomes of Community-Centred Approaches

Individual Outcomes	Community Level Outcomes	Community Process Outcomes	Organizational Outcomes
• Health literacy – increased knowledge, awareness, skills and capabilities • Behaviour change – healthy lifestyles, reduction of risky behaviours • Self-efficacy, self-esteem, confidence • Self-management • Social relationships – social support, reduction of social isolation • Well-being – quality of life, subjective and objective well-being • Health status, physical and mental • Personal development – life skills, employment, education	• Social capital – social networks, community cohesion, sense of belonging, trust • Community resilience • Changes in physical, social and economic environment • Increased community resources – including funding	• Community leadership – collaborative working, community mobilization/ coalitions • Representation and advocacy • Civic engagement – volunteering, voting, civic associations, participation of groups previously at risk of exclusion	• Public health intelligence • Changes in policy • Redesigned services • Increased service use – reach, uptake of screening and preventive services • Improved access to health and care services, appropriate use of services, culturally relevant services

After South, J., 2015. A Guide to Community-Centred Approaches for Health and Wellbeing. Public Health England, London. Available at: https://www.gov.uk/government/uploads/system/uploads/attachment_data/file/402887/A_guide_to_community-centred_approaches_for_health_and_wellbeing.pdf.

Community development is thus both a philosophy and a method. As a philosophy its key features are:

- a commitment to equality, and the challenging of attitudes and practices which discriminate against and marginalize people
- an emphasis on participation and enabling all communities to be heard
- an emphasis on lay knowledge and the valuing of people's own experience
- the collectivizing of experience, seeing problems as shared and working together to identify and implement action
- recognizing the skills, knowledge and expertise that people possess and contribute
- the empowerment of individuals and communities through education, skills development, sharing and joint action.

The community development approach has been influenced by the work of Paulo Freire (1972), a Brazilian educationalist who worked on literacy programmes with poor peasants in Peru and Brazil during the 1970s. Freire saw education as a way to liberate people from cycles of oppression and sought to engage people in critical consciousness-raising or 'conscientization', helping them to understand their circumstances and why they have been oppressed. The process of 'conscientization' begins with problem-posing groups which seek to break down barriers and establish a dialogue between

individuals and between individuals and the facilitator. Eventually a state of praxis is reached, in which there is a common understanding and development of action and practice whereby people collectively can transform their circumstances. The process of conscientization is summarized as:

- reflection on aspects of reality
- search and collective identification of the root causes of that reality
- an examination of their implications
- development of a plan of action to change reality (Freire, 1972).

Community development is a recognized way of working which has given rise to a specific profession – community development workers, who are employed by local authorities to support, facilitate and empower communities. Community development workers have their own training courses, qualifications and professional associations.

COMMUNITY DEVELOPMENT AND HEALTH PROMOTION

Community development is a recurring theme in health promotion, and its role as a strategy reflects a changing political environment. In the 1960s the women's movement emphasized the need for women to reclaim knowledge about their bodies and control over their lives. Shared personal experiences led to a new understanding of health issues as well as providing positive effects and social cohesion for participants. Black and minority ethnic groups also addressed health issues, particularly the effect of racism within the health services. In the 1970s and early 1980s numerous community development projects were set up, prompted by inner city problems and focused on youth work and neighbourhood centres.

Learning Activity 11.2 asks you to consider and discuss why we should prioritize the enabling of communities to take action on their health and express their perspectives in the development of social, economic and environmental policy.

 Learning Activity 11.2 Participation, Involvement and Community Development

Consider the following statements from the World Health Organization on the importance of participation, involvement and community development. What do you think contributed to this emphasis on working with 'the community'?

The people have a right and a duty to participate individually and collectively in the planning and implementation of their health care.
World Health Organization (1978)

Health for all will be achieved by people themselves. A well-informed, well-motivated and actively participating community is a key element for the attainment of the common goal.
World Health Organization (1985, p. 5)

Health promotion works through concrete and effective community action in setting priorities, making decisions, planning strategies and implementing them to achieve better health. At the heart of this process is the empowerment of communities, their ownership and control of their own endeavours and destinies.
World Health Organization (1986)

Community action is central to the fostering of health public policy.
World Health Organization (1988)

Health promotion is carried out by and with people, not on or to people. It improves the ability of individuals to take action, and the capacity of groups, organizations or communities to influence the determinants of health.

Improving the capacity of communities for health promotion requires practical education, leadership training and access to resources.
World Health Organization (1997)

By the 1990s strategies for service delivery were frequently linked to the notion of community. This focus on the community needs to be seen in relation to the developing crisis in the role of welfare state provision and broader debates around accountability. Chapter 7 showed how neoliberal concerns to retreat from welfare have been linked to a focus on individuals as consumers of services. Devolved services and an emphasis on participation and 'consumer involvement' were all strategies designed to achieve these aims. By the turn of the century, the focus was on action aimed to bolster social capital and trust (see Chapter 15 for a discussion of how neighbourhoods and the community became a focus for policy and analysis). In England, a government department of Housing, Communities and Local Government was set up, and there was a new emphasis on civil society – that domain between the state and individuals, households or communities where people volunteer (there are an estimated 3 million volunteers in England), may be carers (there are an estimated 6 million informal carers) or belong to a charity or community group.

The tradition of community development has radical roots and is closely associated with work to challenge the status quo, redistribute resources and address power imbalances across society. Although many have welcomed the adoption of once-radical terms such as empowerment and participation into mainstream policy language, there are those who suggest such mainstreaming has diluted the aims and processes of community development. There have been warnings that such 'state-commissioned' community development results in 'not government by communities but government through communities' (Gilchrist, 2003). The policy focus on communities to bring about change (e.g., in neighbourhood renewal or antisocial behaviour) leads to communities, rather than society, being seen as responsible for the problems they face. This may be viewed as an extension of the 'victim-blaming' principle from individuals to communities. Case Study 11.1 describes an initiative in England, the Troubled Families Programme, that sought to identify and then support those who are most in need. Think about why the programme had such a mixed reception.

CASE STUDY 11.1
The Troubled Families Programme

The Troubled Families Programme was introduced in England in December 2011 as a means to improve outcomes for an estimated 120,000 families identified as having the greatest need, who place a significant burden on public services and are claimed to cost £9 billion a year. According to the government's national criteria, troubled families are defined as those in which there is crime and/or antisocial behaviour, children absent from school or with high levels of truancy, a parent out of work on benefits, domestic violence, 'children who need help' and 'parents and children with a range of health problems'. The programme is based on financial incentives and a payment-by-results scheme, with local councils having to demonstrate successful outcomes to qualify for funding.

There is an active social and political critique of how recent governments have framed these families as 'antisocial' or indeed 'troubling', moving away from a previous discourse which saw people as vulnerable, disadvantaged or having needs (Bond-Taylor, 2014). The 'lumping together' of a number of different problems under the umbrella of 'troubled families' echoes a long-standing discourse from the 1970s that described 'cycles of deprivation' and the 1980s' discourse of the challenging underclass.

WORKING WITH A COMMUNITY-CENTRED APPROACH

The ways in which community-centred approaches are carried out vary enormously. However, there are a number of core principles which overlap and are linked:

- participation
- community empowerment
- community led
- social justice
- asset based.

Participation

Participation, engagement and involvement are frequently used terms in the health sector. While these terms have different meanings, increasing people's involvement in decisions, service design and delivery has been identified as a discrete approach to community engagement (O'Mara-Eves et al., 2013; South, 2015). Participation may be thought of as a ladder which

includes many different activities. The National Institute of Health and Care Excellence (NICE, 2016) guidance describes a range of activities extending from services through to health and social outcomes and demonstrates how the more long-lasting health and social outcomes are only achievable through higher levels of participation. Table 11.3 shows a hierarchical ladder with different levels of power, and what this might imply about ways of working.

There is a distinction between the amount of power sharing and the degree of influence over decisions. At the low or weak end, it may mean consultation to 'rubber stamp' plans already drawn up by official agencies. At the high or strong end of the spectrum, it may mean control over the setting of priorities and implementation of programmes. Learning Activity 11.3 asks you to think about participation and participatory methods and the extent to which they may be empowering.

Learning Activity 11.3   A Ladder of Participation

Consider the following examples of participation. Where would you place them on a ladder of participation?
- A public forum to discuss local health needs.
- The attendance of a mother at a court hearing about the care of her child.
- A service user group to discuss services and give feedback to service providers.

Community Empowerment

Empowerment as a health promotion approach is discussed in Chapter 5, and a distinction is made between empowerment of individuals and empowerment of communities. Empowering communities is a core principle of community development. It has been defined as:

a process by which communities gain more control over the decisions and resources that influence their lives, including the determinants of health. Community empowerment builds from the individual to the group to the wider collective and embodies the intention to bring about social and political change.
Laverack (2007, p. 29)

Community empowerment starts with a process of critical consciousness-raising in which individuals and

TABLE 11.3 Ladder of Participation

Level	Typical Process	Stance
• Supporting local initiatives	• Community development	• 'We can help you achieve what you want, within guidelines'
• Acting together	• Partnership building	• 'We want to carry out joint decisions together'
• Deciding together	• Consensus building	• 'We want to develop options and decide together'
• Consultation	• Communication and feedback	• 'These are the options: what do you think?'
• Information	• Presentation and promotion	• 'Here's what we are going to do…'

Adapted from South, J., 2015. A Guide to Community-Centred Approaches for Health and Wellbeing. Public Health England, London. Available at: https://www.gov.uk/government/uploads/system/uploads/attachment_data/file/402887/A_guide_to_community-centred_approaches_for_health_and_wellbeing.pdf from Wilcox, D., 1994. The Guide to Effective Participation. Partnership Books, Brighton.

RESEARCH EXAMPLE 11.3
Community Mobilization in a Pandemic

Pandemics are invariably managed top down from governments using data science and their own communications. The Ebola outbreak in West Africa in 2015 demonstrated how community engagement and social mobilization can be an effective challenge to distrust of governments and their handling of the disease. In Sierra Leone, the Social Mobilization Action Consortium developed a 'community-led Ebola approach' to trigger local action, using refined messaging and interpersonal contact through thousands of social mobilizers. This approach worked to build a narrative of trust through bottom-up approaches that included a respect for local perspectives. A review of the response (Laverack and Manoncourt, 2016, p. 82) states that:

> The emerging evidence from the current Ebola response suggested that communities have understood what is required and can learn rapidly to change high-risk traditional practices to help to reduce transmission. In particular, community engagement can offer an added value through

the self-management of quarantines, control of crossborder movement, safe and dignified burials, and the siting of Community Care Centers.

Gilmore et al.'s (2020) review restates the importance of community engagement with prevention and control interventions and messaging. During the COVID-19 pandemic around 1 million people in the UK volunteered to check on their neighbours, deliver food parcels and became vaccinators. Similar mutual aid groups started up worldwide. Gilmore et al. (2020) found that almost all examples of community engagement in high-income areas consisted of providing information and support. There were very few examples of groups focusing on equity issues. A study of voluntary groups formed during the pandemic (https://www.volunteerscotland.net/media/1709819/the_role_of_mutual_aid_covid-19.pdf) highlighted some of the tensions explored later in this chapter. These tensions arise from being responsive and flexible within a context of competing interests from formal services and community-led groups.

communities begin to question and challenge the social justice of their situation (Ledwith, 2005) (see the earlier section on defining community development for a more detailed discussion of critical consciousness-raising). Woodall et al. (2012) argue that empowerment has lost its links with its radical origins and is now more closely associated with individual self-empowerment. There is evidence that these approaches can have a positive impact on individuals' self-esteem and sense of control. The evidence that empowerment approaches make a difference to community well-being is less clear cut (Woodall et al., 2011). Research Example 11.3 describes some of the conflicting evidence from recent studies on the nature of the outcomes from community mobilization during pandemics.

Community Led

The term *community led* refers to a commitment to learning from communities and being accountable to, and working with, communities. This is not without its tensions, for example, when needs and priorities identified by communities are not compatible with those identified by statutory and funding bodies. An important aspect of community-centred approaches is legitimizing people's knowledge about health and well-being and giving them a voice. Not only does this pose a challenge to medical dominance, but it is also very different from systematic research into needs (see Chapter 20). Establishing the needs of the community also means a shift towards more participatory and locality-based involvement. Learning Activity 11.4 asks you to consider community development in the context of health promotion. This is followed by Research Example 11.4 which summarizes some recent evidence of the contribution of the arts towards community development.

Learning Activity 11.4   Community Development and Health Promotion

How important do you think community development is as a health promotion strategy?

Social Justice

Inequalities exist within society, and some communities are more privileged and better resourced – and consequently healthier – than others. Community development

> **RESEARCH EXAMPLE 11.4**
> **Arts and Community Development**
>
> There is some evidence that engagement with the arts can lead to prosocial behaviours and enhance social consciousness within communities. Fancourt and Finn (2019) summarize the health benefits of the arts: reaching groups who experience more barriers and are less likely to engage in healthcare; acting as a bridge between different groups, for example, dance, arts classes and theatre have been shown to foster greater social inclusion in people with dementia and disabilities; building social cohesion and supporting conflict resolution through the development of cognitive, emotional and social skills used for constructive engagement with conflict; and among indigenous communities the arts can help to preserve cultural traditions and promote a sense of identity and resilience.

sees these inequalities as having been created by society and therefore amenable to change by society. Community development seeks to strengthen civil society in a democratic and participatory way by giving a voice to communities that are disadvantaged or oppressed. In so doing, it focuses on the determinants of health rather than on individual lifestyles. This may mean:

- working to promote the health of disadvantaged groups
- increasing the accessibility of services
- influencing the commissioning of services
- acting as an advocate and representing the interests of disadvantaged groups
- building a social and health profile of the community.

Asset Based

Asset-based ways of thinking are very different from traditional ways of viewing communities. The asset-based approach is to identify and promote those community characteristics which have the potential to improve and support individuals' health and well-being through self-esteem, coping strategies, resilience skills, relationships, friendships, knowledge and personal resources. This approach is exemplified in a statement in 2009 by Michelle Obama about the Asset Based Community Development Institute at de Paul University:

> *We can't do well serving communities… if we believe that we, the givers, are the only ones that are half-full, and that everybody we're serving is half-empty… there are assets and gifts out there in communities, and our job as good servants and as good leaders… [is] having the ability to recognize those gifts in others, and help them put those gifts into action.*
> **(https://resources.depaul.edu/abcd-institute/news-events/Pages/michelle-obama-mentions-abcd.aspx.)**

An asset is any of the following (Foot and Hopkins, 2011):

- practical skills, capacity and knowledge of local residents
- passions and interests of local residents which energize them for change
- networks and connections – known as 'social capital' – in a community, including friendships and neighbourliness
- effectiveness of local community and voluntary associations

- resources of public, private and third-sector organizations that are available to support a community
- physical and economic resources of a place that enhance well-being.

The concept of asset-based community development is outlined in Case Study 11.2.

TYPES OF ACTIVITIES INVOLVED IN STRENGTHENING COMMUNITY ACTION

A large number of activities may be included as part of a community development approach:

- profiling
- capacity building
- organizing
- networking
- negotiating.

Profiling

Chapter 20 discusses the process of undertaking a community profile and how it differs from a needs assessment. The role of the community worker is to build on initial research and any baseline data and contact with people living and working in the community, so that the needs they identify can be explored and solutions developed (see Chapter 20). Asset mapping is an activity that has gained much importance. Public services have traditionally focused on problems and needs, leading to an absence of information about the wealth of experience, practical skills, knowledge, capacity and passion of local people and associations, and a lack of recognition of the potential of communities to become equal partners.

Capacity Building

Capacity building is working with individuals and groups within communities to recognize and develop the skills and resources they have (their assets) to identify and meet their own needs. This may mean:

- providing opportunities for people to learn through experience – opportunities that would not otherwise be available to them
- involving people in collective effort so that they gain confidence in their ability to influence decisions that affect them.

Case Study 11.3 is about time banking as an example of how communities can develop and share skills and capacities.

Organizing

An important area that community workers are engaged in is helping to organize the community to work together effectively. This may include helping to establish small self-help groups or organizing community events such as health forums.

Networking

Networks are the ties that link people together within a community. Gilchrist (2019) identifies two different types of networks: those linked by strong ties and those linked by weak ties. Networks linked by strong ties are based on bonds of friendship or family relations and

---

CASE STUDY 11.2
Asset-Based Community Development

Asset-based community development has emerged to counter approaches that identify community deficits or needs and then provides services (or not). Asset-based community development uses a salutogenic perspective, identifying the factors that keep people well and resilient within the community. Asset mapping is a process that makes explicit the knowledge, skills and capacities that already exist. This can be 'any factor (or resource) which enhances the ability of individuals, groups, communities and populations to maintain and sustain health and well-being. These assets can operate at the level of the individual, family or community as protective and promoting factors to buffer against life stresses' (Morgan and Ziglio, 2007, p. 18).

CASE STUDY 11.3
Time Banking

Time banking (https://timebanking.org.uk/) works by facilitating the exchange of skills and experience within a community. It aims to build the 'core economy' of family and community by valuing and rewarding both the people (and their skills) and their work. Time banking values everyone's time as equal. For every hour spent helping someone in the community, a person is entitled to an hour of help in return. One of the first time banks in the UK, Rushey Green in south-east London (https://www.rgtb.org.uk/) describes it in very positive terms as 'a chain reaction caused by healthy and productive relationships that bind us together and provide a strong incentive to care for our planet'.

are those we are most likely to turn to for daily support and companionship. Networks based on weak ties link different clusters of networks together. They have been described as the links that operate over the whole network, forming bridges between sections of the community or between organizations. Both types of network are an important asset within a community and an indicator of levels of social capital. Strong networks create opportunities for skills, information and learning to be shared across the community and lead to more effective community action.

Building such networks by making links between individuals, groups and local organizations is therefore an important part of the community development worker's role. As one refugee advocate puts it:

Community development can be quite an invisible job, but the relationships you build with groups over the months or years is vital. By getting to know different groups, you can identify the issues they face and where they can work together. We have strategic bodies at one level, and the communities and grassroots activity at another level, and community development somewhere in the middle. If you take that out, the structures will collapse; the issues which need to be addressed by policy makers just won't reach them… one of the things I have done is to help set up a Refugee Forum. The refugee community organisations now come together in a group and talk about their issues, what action they want to take and how to make a strong voice.

Mani Thapa, community development officer, Refugee Action, quoted in Community Development Exchange (undated)

Negotiating

Community work recognizes the diversity and division that may exist within communities. Communities are not homogeneous entities but include hierarchies, imbalances in power and differences. Such diversity in, for example, prioritizing and meeting needs must be addressed in order to achieve a consensus. As well as negotiating and managing conflict within communities, the community worker must negotiate and advocate on behalf of the community. This may involve negotiating with funding or statutory bodies to ensure that the needs and views of the community are heard and considered.

As we have seen, community development is a challenging form of practice. Learning Activity 11.5 includes a description of this way of working.

Learning Activity 11.5   Community Development in Practice

Community Development Exchange information sheet.

Read the following excerpt. What positive outcomes are attributed to community development working?

Carol Osgerby, community health development worker for West Hull Primary Care Trust, describes community development work.

Question: Please explain your job as simply as possible.

Answer: When people want their community to get more healthy and prevent illness, I help them to set up groups and keep them going, by encouraging them and helping sort out problems.

Question: Please describe a typical week.

Answer:

Monday: Work on an evaluation of the health impact of community groups. Later, I join a local walking group to talk to them about raising funds and developing the group.

Tuesday: Prepare display materials for Thursday's event. Attend a committee meeting of a local community orchard. Discuss insurance, tenancy agreement and annual budget. Agree to work with the secretary to draft a funding application and help them contact other similar groups so they can share information.

Wednesday: Catch up with paperwork and e-mails. Team meeting in the afternoon. We are a team of four community health development workers, covering a city of 250,000 people.

Thursday: More paperwork, and reading the latest news on the reorganization of public health in Hull. Later I attend a health event at a community centre where I run a quiz about food labelling and offer tasters of fruit smoothies. I get into discussion with many of the residents and workers there about nutrition, exercise, slimming and queries about healthcare and illness. My real aim is to publicize community groups and make some links that could lead to new projects. In the evening I attend a neighbourhood management meeting. There is a good turnout of residents and council staff, Community Empowerment Network, youth workers, etc. I help to get residents' ideas recorded in the minutes of the meeting.

Friday: Meet with the community orchard secretary to help draft a budget and fill in a grant application form. We discuss how we can encourage local residents to get involved in winter, when there is less physical work to do. Later, I work on our community group's newsletter.

Question: Please describe what you feel makes your work specifically 'community development'.

Answer: Community development develops and leaves behind structures that were not there before, and which are managed by members of the community. A vital part of community development is to support individuals to develop skills which they can use to develop community groups, organizations and networks. When I'm asked to take on a new piece of work, I ask myself: 'Is there potential to produce a project which is truly led by the community it's meant to serve?' If the answer is no then to me it's not community development work. You have to respect the ability of the communities you work with to make their own decisions.

DILEMMAS AND CHALLENGES IN COMMUNITY-CENTRED PRACTICE

Community-centred practice is challenging. It offers the prospect of improving health and well-being, but there are many practical difficulties to overcome. Table 11.4 illustrates some of the advantages and disadvantages of these approaches.

The question of whether the community worker is engaged in radical practice or supporting the status quo is at the root of much of the ambiguity surrounding practice. Common dilemmas facing the community development worker relate to funding, accountability, acceptability, the role of the professional and evaluation.

Funding

Most community development projects are funded by statutory agencies, such as health and education authorities, sometimes in partnership through joint funding. Other projects which might come under the label 'community development' belong in the voluntary sector and are funded from a variety of sources, including direct government grants and independent fundraising. Most community development work is funded in the short term only. Lack of security and the impossibility of guaranteeing an input in the long term increase the problems of planning and evaluating such work. Insecure funding

TABLE 11.4 Advantages and Disadvantages of a Community-Centred Approach	
Advantages	**Disadvantages**
• Starts with people's concerns, so it is more likely to gain support • Focuses on root causes of ill health, not symptoms • Creates awareness of the social causes of ill health • The process of involvement is enabling and leads to greater confidence • The process includes acquiring skills which are transferable, e.g., communication and lobbying skills • If health promoter and people meet as equals, it extends the principle of democratic accountability	• Time-consuming • Results are often not tangible or quantifiable • Evaluation is difficult • Without evaluation, gaining funding is difficult • Health promoters may find their role contradictory; to whom are they ultimately accountable – employer or community? • Work is usually with small groups of people • Draws attention away from macro issues and may focus on local neighbourhoods

arrangements can also subvert a project's focus, leading workers to spend time fundraising instead of working around defined issues.

Accountability

Community workers have a dual accountability: to their employers and to their communities. This can lead to problems when the priorities of the community and the agency are not the same. Organizational objectives, such as service take-up, may become incorporated into the community worker's role.

Community and worker responses to issues may also differ. For example, both may identify safety as a priority, but whereas the worker may respond by advocating structural changes such as better lighting and common responsibility for shared areas, the community might respond by advocating increased vigilance.

Community development workers may feel themselves trapped in the role of mediator, informing statutory services about community needs and the community about how to access and participate in services.

Acceptability

Employing authorities often view community develop-ment as not quite respectable. Community development and other community-centred approaches may be seen as absorbing unacceptably large amounts of time and resources for dubious results. Community development tends to focus on small numbers of people, whereas employers tend to be responsible for large populations. The long-term nature and diffuse outcomes of commu-nity development and community-centred approaches are at odds with the organizational need to allocate resources on the basis of specific and demonstrable results. Issues raised through a community-centred approach such as institutional racism may be unaccept-able to employing authorities. Community workers may also find that they need to establish and negotiate their role before they are accepted by a community. The role of these workers is ambiguous, with their status and employment setting them apart from the community in which they are working. Relationships of trust may need to be created before any other work can take place.

Role of the Professional

Community-centred work also poses problems for workers whose primary training lies in other areas. Problems may arise from the differences in the client–worker relationship envisaged in professional training and community work. Professional workers are taught a particular area of expertise and tend to assume that they know what is best for their clients. Learning Activity 11.6 asks you to consider and discuss how you would justify working in a community development way.

Learning Activity 11.6   Adopting a Community Development Approach

A health visitor wishes to adopt a community develop-ment approach in her work. She has identified setting up a postnatal mothers' group as an appropriate project.
- What arguments might she use in favour of this kind of work?
- What arguments might her manager use against it?

Community development workers see their role as that of catalyst and facilitator rather than expert. Their task is to enable a community to express its needs and support the community in meeting those needs themselves. This requires a worker–client relationship based on egalitarianism and the sharing of knowledge.

For professionals, trained to be experts, this can be a difficult switch to make.

The skills involved in community work differ from those acquired in professional training and this is the focus of Learning Activity 11.7. Key community work skills concern process rather than content and include:
- organizational skills, for example, developing appro-priate management structures such as management committees or steering groups
- communication skills, for example, consultation and communication with a variety of groups, including community groups, funding agencies and co-workers
- evaluation skills, for example, monitoring the impact of interventions and self-evaluation.

Evaluation

Community development has often been described as difficult to evaluate because it works on so many levels, is a long-term strategy and encompasses many strands of work. The evaluation of community development projects and interventions is an ongoing process of learning for everyone who is involved. Outcomes of community development projects are often hard to mea-sure because they deal with social relationships and the complex functioning of groups and communities rather than easily quantified things.

However, many of the principles used for evaluating health promotion work discussed in Chapter 23, partic-ularly around assessing process, impact and outcomes, are relevant. Barr (2002) provides a useful checklist of questions to consider when evaluating community development work, which reflect the principles and goals of this approach.
- Are we gaining a new understanding of community issues and needs?
- Are we being effective in tackling them?
- Are we being inclusive?
- Are the participants achieving their personal goals?
- Are we building community assets and resources?
- Is our work empowering people?
- Are we building a culture of collaboration, participa-tion and sustainable change?
- Are we learning from our experience?
- Are we contributing to health and well-being?
- Are we making the best possible use of the resources we have?
- Do we have the evidence we need to influence future decisions?

Learning Activity 11.7   Skills in Community Development

The following figure shows aspects of a job role for community-centred working and how this is mapped against the Public Health Skills and Knowledge Framework.

Which, if any, of these aspects are included in your current role?

Which, if any, of these skills were covered in your professional training?

How much time is devoted to these areas compared to other areas in the curriculum?

Do you think your professional training has equipped you to practise community development?

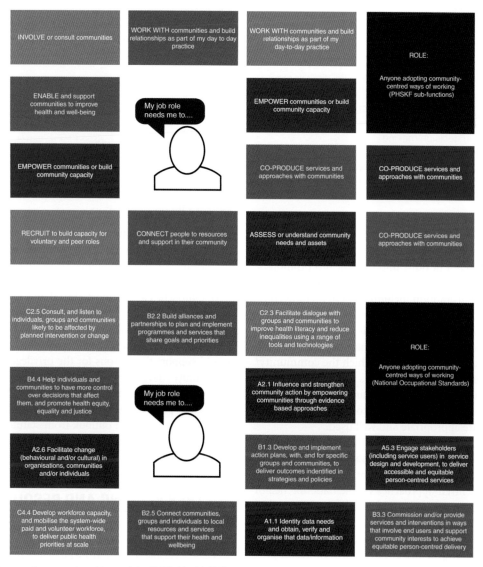

Community-centred working and the Public Health Skills and Knowledge Functions (From Public Health England, 2019. Public Health Skills and Knowledge Framework. Available at https://www.gov.uk/government/publications/public-health-skills-and-knowledge-framework-phskf/public-health-skills-and-knowledge-framework-august-2019-update.)

As we reach the end of this chapter, the last learning activity (Learning Activity 11.8) asks you to reflect on your understanding of community development.

 Learning Activity 11.8   What Is Community Development?

Consider the following statements which describe community development:

- trying to create a 'better' community
- getting the community to do what the authorities want it to do
- promoting equal access to resources
- getting the community to take responsibility for its own problems
- a political process
- controlling social unrest by providing diversionary activities
- helping people to see the root causes of problems
- providing people with opportunities to become involved in decision-making.

Which of these statements would you say were true? What issues or dilemmas were raised when you were thinking about these statements?

CONCLUSION

Community development and community-centred approaches do not fit tidily into most health promoters' working lives although there is an increasing expectation of health promotion including strengthening community action. There are many reasons why community engagement is now seen as desirable. These reasons tend not to be based on a body of evidence but derived from an ideological view of society in which the community/volunteer workforce are the agents of change in creating health and well-being. Service users and people with lived experience of deprivation co-design services to ensure they are appropriate and well used.

Health promotion and community-centred approaches differ in their assumptions about the nature of health and their skills. This can make undertaking community-centred approaches problematic for health promoters. However, practitioners who have espoused community development are enthusiastic about its potential and outcomes. Community development is claimed to be the most ethical and effective form of health promotion, and one which makes a real impact on people's lives. Community-centred approaches appear to address many of the problems inherent in more traditional forms

of health promotion: they avoid victim blaming, address the structural causes of inequalities in health and seek to empower people. This helps explain why community development approaches are so popular with health promoters, and why they are regarded as a central strategy.

REFLECTIONS ON PRACTICE

- Would you consider adopting a community development approach in your work?
- Recent government publications on health systems in England refer to placing communities and citizens at the centre and engaging and empowering communities. What, if any, examples of this have you seen in your practice?
- It is claimed that a higher level of community activity, involving more people, more varied activities and having greater influence on local services, improves health and well-being. What other evidence of its benefits would you put forward for a community-centred approach in your area of work?

SUMMARY

This chapter has examined the history and theoretical underpinnings of community development as an approach to health promotion alongside other community-centred approaches. Workers often view community-centred approaches as the most ethical and effective means of promoting health. However, practising community development poses dilemmas for the health promoter, and evaluation is fraught with problems. However, we would support the reasons for the privileged position of community development. Practical difficulties should not obstruct the continuing development and spread of this health promotion strategy. On the contrary, what is needed is a more open outlook from statutory organizations and a willingness to experiment with community action approaches.

FURTHER READING AND RESOURCES

Chanan, G., Fisher, B., 2018. Commissioning community development for health. Coalition for Collaborative Care. Available at: https://irp-cdn.multiscreensite.com/9163ad55/files/uploaded/0%200%200%200%200%200%200%20Community%20Dev%20for%20Health%20screen%20FINAL%20PUBD%20Dec%2017.pdf.

A practical guide on what local authorities and clinical commissioning groups would look for from community development projects, and how community development can be measured and evaluated.

Gilchrist, A., Taylor, M., 2016. A Short Guide to Community Development, second edn. Policy Press, Bristol.
This book provides an introduction to community development and its origins and current challenges. The book explores how community development can achieve a range of policy objectives.

Laverack, G., 2007. Health Promotion Practice; Building Empowered Communities. Open University Press, Buckingham.
Combines theory with practice in discussing how to build community empowerment using experiences from the UK, Asia and Africa.

New South Wales Service for the Treatment and Rehabilitation of Torture and Trauma Survivors, 2012. Community Development Evaluation Manual. Available at: https://startts.org.au/media/Services-Community-Development-Evaluation-Manual.pdf.
This manual is a guide to planning and evaluating community development projects with refugee communities. It is clear and well laid out and applicable to a range of projects.

NICE, 2016. Community engagement: improving health and wellbeing and reducing health inequalities NG 44. Available at: https://www.nice.org.uk/guidance/ng44.
This guidance shows how community engagement and community development can be used in service design, reaching underserved groups, and developing equity based strategies. The cost effectiveness of such approaches is assessed.

South, J., 2015. A Guide to Community-Centred Approaches for Health and Wellbeing. Public Health England, London. Available at: https://www.gov.uk/government/uploads/system/uploads/attachment_data/file/402887/A_guide_to_community-centred_approaches_for_health_and_wellbeing.pdf.
An invaluable evidence-based guide to place-based approaches that develop local solutions, drawing on all the assets and resources of an area, integrating public services and also building resilience of communities in order to improve health and well-being for all and to reduce health inequalities.

Useful website includes:

Scottish Community Development Centre: www.scdc.org.uk.

FEEDBACK TO LEARNING ACTIVITIES

11.1. You might have identified communities based on geographic location, professional identity, interests, religion or culture. These may or may not be the same communities your parents belonged to. Key characteristics of communities are mutual interests and beliefs, a sense of belonging and identity and a willingness to help in times of need.

11.2. Participation is one of the core principles of health promotion and is a vital component of empowerment. Working with the community helps demarcate health promotion as distinct from healthcare and medicine (where services are provided by medical experts for the community). Working with the community ensures that the right priorities are addressed and builds expertise and knowledge within the community. It is intended that in the long term, this will lead to an empowered, health-promoting community and a reduction in health needs.

11.3. The public meeting involves consultation, but no decisions are made.
The child protection hearing involves information and the parent has little power.
The service user group involves consultation and placation. Service users are invited to be involved but decision-making is likely to be done by the service provider.

11.4. Marking the 25th anniversary of the Ottawa Charter, Laverack and Mohammadi (2011) suggested that strengthening community action has not become part of health promotion's day-to-day work. Actively engaging with communities demands a long-term commitment and dialogue and remains a challenge.

11.5. The outcomes of community development are:
- community members acquiring new knowledge and skills
- building social capital, with people feeling more connected
- networking and bringing together people with common interests
- an increase in the number of people who feel they can influence decisions, and a democratic renewal
- co-production of service design that meets needs.

11.6. The health visitor might argue that such work is important for health because it increases self-esteem, autonomy, confidence and a sense of belonging. She could argue that such work is effective. For example, postnatal networking among mothers could prove effective in reducing mental illness among this client group. The health visitor might also argue that time spent on setting up the group will reduce claims on her time in future and is therefore a cost-effective option.

The health visitor's manager might respond that there is not enough time to carry out such work. Full caseloads and many other priority claims (such as visiting all new mothers and carrying out child development check-ups) mean there is no spare time available for other activities. The manager might also argue that such activities need to be thoroughly evaluated and be of proven effectiveness before resources can be committed.

11.7. Community development is not a core subject within health workers' courses, although specialist community public health nurses may have community development as part of their training. Some postgraduate courses in public health may also include working with communities. As public health is now located within local government, there are increased opportunities for working with local communities.

11.8. Community development is about the community engaging in decision-making and tackling the root causes of problems. As such, it is a political process which empowers people. Community development is not a panacea designed by local authorities to control people or get them to conform to some ideal template. Dilemmas may arise for local authority staff engaged in community development if communities are directly opposed to local authority policies or plans.

REFERENCES

Barr, A., 2002. Learning Evaluation and Planning. A Handbook for Partners in Community Learning. Scottish Community Development Centre. Available at: https://www.webarchive.org.uk/wayback/archive/20150220030253/http://www.gov.scot/Publications/2007/12/05101807/1.

Bond-Taylor, S., 2014. The politics of 'anti-social' behaviour within the 'Troubled Families' programme. In: Pickard, S. (ed.), Anti-Social Behaviour in Britain: Victorian and Contemporary Perspectives. Palgrave, Basingstoke.

Community Development Exchange, undated. CDX Information Sheet: Community Development in Action. CDX, Sheffield.

Fancourt, D., Finn, S., 2019. What is the evidence on the role of the arts in improving health and well-being? A scoping review. World Health Organization, Geneva. Available at: https://www.euro.who.int/en/publications/abstracts/what-is-the-evidence-on-the-role-of-the-arts-in-improving-health-and-well-being-a-scoping-review-2019.

Foot, J., Hopkins, T., 2011. A Glass Half Full: How an Asset Approach Can Improve Community Health and Wellbeing. Improvement and Development Agency, London. Available at: http://janefoot.com/downloads/files/Glass%20half%20full.pdf.

Freire, P., 1972. Pedagogy of the Oppressed. Penguin, Harmondsworth.

Gilchrist, A., 2003. Community development in the UK — possibilities and paradoxes. Comm. Dev. J. 38 (1), 16–25.

Gilchrist, A., 2019. The Well Connected Community. A Networking Approach to Community, third edn. Policy Press, Bristol.

Gilmore, B., Ndejjo, R., Tchetchia, A., de Claro, V., Mago, E., et al., 2020. Community engagement for COVID-19 prevention and control: a rapid evidence synthesis. BMJ Global Health 5 (e003188).

Green, L. W., Raebum, J., 1990. Contemporary developments in health promotion: definitions and challenges. In Bracht, N. (ed.), Health Promotion at the Community Level. Sage, Newbury Park, CA, pp. 29–44.

Laverack, G., 2007. Health Promotion Practice: Building Empowered Communities. Open University Press, Buckingham.

Laverack, G., Manoncourt, E., 2016. Key experiences of community engagement and social mobilization in the Ebola response. Glob. Health Promot. 23 (1), 79–82.

Laverack, G., Mohammadi, N.W., 2011. What remains for the future: strengthening community action to become an integral part of health promotion practice. Health Promot. Int. 26 (Suppl 2), 258–262.

Ledwith, M., 2005. Community Development: A Critical Approach. Policy Press, Bristol.

Lehman, U., Sanders, D., 2007. Community health workers: what do we know about them? the state of the evidence on programmes, activities, costs and impact on health outcomes of using community health workers. World Health Organization, Geneva. Available at: https://www.who.int/hrh/documents/community_health_workers.pdf.

McMillan, D.W., Chavis, D.M., 1986. Sense of community: A definition and theory. Journal of Community Psychology 14 (1), 6–23.

Morgan, A., Ziglio, E., 2007. Revitalising the evidence base for public health: an assets model. Global Health Promotion (Suppl 2), 17–22.

NICE, 2016. Community Engagement: Improving Health and Wellbeing and Reducing Health Inequalities. NICE guidance NG44. Available at: https://www.nice.org.uk/guidance/ng44/resources/community-engagement-improving-health-and-wellbeing-and-reducing-health-inequalities-pdf-1837452829381.

O'Mara-Eves, A., Brunton, G., McDaid, D., Oliver, S., Kavanagh, J., et al., 2013. Community engagement to reduce inequalities in health: a systematic review, meta-analysis and economic analysis. Public Health Res. 1 (4). Available at: http://www.journalslibrary.nihr.ac.uk/phr/volume-1/issue-4#abstract (accessed 19.03.21).

Putnam, R.D., 2000. Bowling Alone: The Collapse and Revival of American Community. Simon and Schuster, New York.

South, J., 2015. A Guide to Community-Centred Approaches for Health and Wellbeing. Public Health England, London. Available at: https://www.gov.uk/government/uploads/system/uploads/attachment_data/file/402887/A_guide_to_community-centred_approaches_for_health_and_wellbeing.pdf.

Standing Conference for Community Development, 2001. Strategic Framework for Community Development. Standing Conference for Community Development, Sheffield.

Woodall, J., Raine, G., South, J., Warwick-Booth, L., 2011. Empowerment and health and wellbeing: evidence review. Available at: www.altogetherbetter.org.uk.

Woodall, J., Warwick-Booth, L., Cross, R., 2012. Has empowerment lost its power? Health Educ. Res. 27 (4), 742–745.

World Health Organization, 1978. Alma Ata 1978: Primary Health Care. WHO, Geneva. Available at: http://www.who.int/publications/almaata_declaration_en.pdf.

World Health Organization, 1985. Targets for Health for All. WHO Regional Office for Europe, Copenhagen. Available at: http://www.euro.who.int/__data/assets/pdf_file/0006/109779/WA_540_GA1_85TA.pdf.

World Health Organization, 1986. The ottawa charter for health promotion. Health Promotion, 1iii–v. Available at: http://www.euro.who.int/en/publications/policy-documents/ottawa-charter-for-health-promotion-1986.

World Health Organization, 1988. Adelaide Recommendation on Health Public Policy. WHO, Adelaide. Available at: http://www.who.int/healthpromotion/conferences/previous/adelaide/en/.

World Health Organization, 1997. New players for a new era: leading health promotion into the 21st century. In: 4th International Conference on Health Promotion, Jakarta, Indonesia, 21–25 July, 1997. Conference Report. World Health Organization, Geneva/Ministry of Health, Indonesia. Available at: http://www.who.int/healthpromotion/conferences/previous/jakarta/declaration/en/index1.html.

12

Developing Healthy Public Policy

LEARNING OUTCOMES

By the end of this chapter you will be able to:
- understand what is meant by healthy public policy
- discuss the development of getting health issues to be considered in all policies and associated challenges
- understand the contribution of health impact assessments to predicting the consequences of a policy or programme
- discuss how to work across sectors so that the policies of all sectors and agencies are health promoting.

KEY CONCEPTS AND DEFINITIONS

Health impact assessment (HIA) A method used to judge the potential effects of a policy or programme on the health of a population.

Health in all policies (HiAP) A commitment since 2006 that all policies across different sectors will systematically take into account the health implications of decisions.

Healthy public policy (HPP) A policy that has a clear concern for health, well-being and equity. The term is also used to describe the role of government in creating conditions that support health.

IMPORTANCE OF THE TOPIC

Health policy is described by Nutbeam (1998, p. 10) as a 'formal statement or procedure within institutions (notably government) which defines priorities and the parameters for action in response to health needs, available resources and other political pressures'. Health policy is often enacted through legislation or other regulations to enable the provision of services. Health policy might also cover issues as wide ranging as the lockdown of populations to prevent the spread of infection, mental health provision for new mothers and organ donation. Many other government actions play a part in improving health, for example, compulsory seat belt wearing and traffic congestion charges in urban areas. Such policies are not within the remit of a Ministry or Department of Health even though air pollution and road safety are crucial determinants of health.

Healthy public policy (HPP) was identified in the Ottawa Charter (World Health Organization, 1986) as one of the five key strategies for promoting health and crucial for the creation of supportive environments for health. HPP focuses on changing the environment in order to make the healthy choice the easier choice. The Adelaide Charter (World Health Organization, 1988, p. 1) describes HPP as 'having an explicit concern for health and equity in all areas of policy and by an accountability for health impact'. Health is affected by many different policy areas:

> *Everyone has the right to a standard of living adequate for the health and well-being of himself and of his family, including food, clothing, housing and medical care and necessary social services, and the right to security in the event of unemployment, sickness, disability, widowhood, old age or other lack of livelihood in circumstances beyond his control*
> ***United Nations Universal Declaration of Human Rights, Article 25(1)***

HPP therefore includes all the major areas of policy that are the responsibility of democratic governments – employment, welfare, education, transport, food, health and social services – and the aim is to embed and implement a concern for health in all policies. Relevant policies may also be instigated by private commercial organizations or devolved government agencies. Promoting HPP across this range of agencies and issues appears to be a daunting task. How to make inroads into this aspect of health promotion is the subject of this chapter, which examines the infrastructure required to facilitate HPP, the role of the practitioner and the potential of this approach to promote health. Understanding the policy process is crucial for health promoters, enabling them to debate what is shaping policy and how it effects change.

DEFINING HPP

Policy is a contested term, with meanings ranging from intentions to decisions and strategies. Milio (2001, p. 622), in a glossary of definitions, describes policy as 'a guide to action to change what would otherwise occur, a decision about amounts and allocations of resources: the overall amount is a statement of commitment to certain areas of concern; the distribution of the amount shows the priorities of decision-makers. Policy sets priorities and guides resource allocation'. We shall adopt a broad definition of policy as a plan of action to guide decisions and actions. Policy can be developed and implemented at many different levels, from organizational to national to international. While policy may be allocated to a specific sphere, such as health, education or transport, in practice its effects are often wide-ranging and extend beyond the sphere originally targeted. Fig. 9.4 in Chapter 9 illustrates the many agencies and organizations that promote health in some way. Although it is based on the structures in England, it is broadly similar in other countries. At government level, the Treasury, for example, tries to influence individual behaviour through taxation of unhealthy products, while the Department of Education tries to do this through school-based health education. Joined-up policymaking is the term used to refer to integrated policymaking across different spheres. The determinants of health are multiple and interconnected, so in order to be effective, policy also needs to be holistic. It is often assumed that policy,

once made and adopted by the relevant agency, translates smoothly into the intended action and anticipated outcomes. However, this is the exception rather than the rule. Policy is (re)interpreted at all levels and its practical application may diverge from the original intention. It is therefore not enough to make policy; it must be followed through, monitored and supported by appropriate training and resources.

The World Health Organization (WHO) defined HPP as 'placing health on the agenda of policy makers in all sectors and at all levels, directing them to be aware of the health consequences of their decisions and to accept their responsibilities for health' (World Health Organization, 1986, p. 2). This is a very broad definition, as is the Ottawa Charter's definition of HPP as a central plank for health promotion (World Health Organization, 1986). The Ottawa Charter cited the following fundamental resources for health: peace, shelter, education, food, income, a stable ecosystem, sustainable resources, social justice and equity. This embraces all governmental activities, except, ironically enough, the provision of health services, although they might be counted as part of the social justice and equity resources. HPP has remained a consistent commitment of the WHO. The second International Conference on Health Promotion in Adelaide, Australia, in 1988 (World Health Organization, 1988) explored HPP. It called for a political commitment to health by all sectors and an explicit accountability for health impacts. The eighth WHO conference in Helsinki in 2013 took the theme of 'health in all policies' (HiAP).

This focus on HPP underpins many governments' commitment to promoting behaviour change. Its importance can be seen in relation to an issue such as the 'obesity crisis' in many countries. While developing personal skills such as dietary know-how (see Chapter 10), and health services to support weight management (see Chapter 9) are important, so too is tackling the obesogenic environment through, for example, transport policy, food policy and food advertising.

UNDERSTANDING THE POLICY PROCESS

Policymaking is the process by which governments translate their political vision into programmes and actions to deliver 'outcomes'. National governments set the fundamental policy direction while local policies develop incrementally. Walt (1994) identifies four phases in policymaking that occur at all levels, whether national or local, and which shape any policy analysis:

1. Problem identification and issue recognition. Why some issues get onto the policy agenda and which issues do not get addressed.
2. Policy formulation. The goals of the policy; different options are identified and analysed; costs and benefits of alternative policies are weighed up; determining who formulates policy; how and where the initiative comes from.
3. Policy implementation. How policies are implemented; what resources are available; how implementation is enforced.
4. Policy evaluation. How progress is reviewed; setting up monitoring systems; how and when adaptations are made.

There is an assumption that policy is the result of rational decision-making in which choices are evaluated and a solution is chosen to achieve objectives. Yet this rational process rarely takes place. As Simon (1947) argued, real-world decision-makers are not 'maximizers' who select the best possible course of action but 'satisfiers' who look for the course of action that is good enough to deal with the problem at hand. Sutton (1999) also refers to other models of policymaking:

• The incrementalist model, where policies which represent the least possible change are preferred, and policy is a series of small steps which do not fundamentally challenge the status quo.
• The mixed-scanning model, which represents a middle position where a broad view of possibilities is considered before focusing on a small number of options for more investigation.

To understand the policy process, it is important to be familiar with the structure of government. There is a complex process for the development of national policy in many countries based on democratic constitutions (e.g., England, Canada, Australia, USA). In England, a new policy is signalled by the publication of a Green Paper for public consultation and discussion. After consultation and amendment, a White Paper, which is the government's plans for legislation, is published. The policy then enters the parliamentary or legislative process, when the bill is scrutinized and amended by the House of Commons and then the House of Lords. If the bill is not thrown out at any stage, it goes on to receive the royal assent, and the bill becomes an Act of Parliament. The policy has now become legislation, which agencies are legally bound to follow.

Numerous factors affect the way in which policy is finally developed and implemented:

• situational: local or timely factors
• cultural: the values and ideologies dominant in the political environment
• structural: the political system and its processes.

Issue Recognition and Framing

For a policy to be approved and enacted, an issue has first to become relevant and identified as a problem. In general, there are three ways in which issues can get onto the agenda:

• following action by community groups leading to a groundswell of public opinion
• initiated by organizations or agencies concerned with the issue
• initiated by key political figures who then mobilize support.

In addition, key incidents may also provide the trigger for gaining support and momentum for a policy, especially if they receive widespread media coverage and spark off a public debate.

Issue recognition, or agenda setting, relies on:

• problem definition
• receptive environment
• policy proposal.

Learning Activity 12.1 asks you to consider the issue of obesity which is a key priority for the health in many nations and yet the issue is defined or framed differently.

 Learning Activity 12.1 Framing the Issue of Obesity

Obesity is identified as a national priority to be addressed in many countries. How is the issue framed?

The public policy environment inevitably involves struggles for power and influence in which politicians, civil servants, the media and pressure groups try to achieve their preferred ends. One problem with public health policy is that it is not usually seen as being newsworthy. Long-term investments in health which prevent illness or disability are not as attractive to the media as topical scandals or 'feelgood' stories focused on high-technology medical services and individual patients. For example, the coverage of the introduction of congestion charging in London, intended as a public health measure to reduce car use, has focused on local objections to the extra 'taxation' and stories of its effect on livelihoods. An exception to this type of coverage is the resurgence of interest in public health protection and hazard management in the wake of the COVID-19 pandemic.

Advocacy is one of the three major strategies for health promotion identified in the Ottawa Charter to gain political commitment, policy support and public acceptance for a particular programme or policy. Nutbeam and Muscat (2021, p. 11) describe advocacy as taking many forms including 'the use of the digital and mass media; more direct political communication, persuasion or lobbying; and community mobilization through, e.g. building coalitions of interest around defined issues'. An example is discussed in Case Study 12.1.

CASE STUDY 12.1
Advocacy

The process of undertaking interventions with the explicit goal of influencing policy is known as advocacy and it is one of the core strategies in the Ottawa Charter. For example, Transport for London's Healthier Food Advertising Policy, which bans the advertising of foods identified as high in fat, sugar or salt, was supported by Sustain, an alliance of organizations campaigning for healthier food and was implemented in February 2019. Such policies attract the attention of several groups with different perspectives, including the commercial food sector. For any policy change to be considered, the issue must be framed in a way that appeals to both policymakers, for example, by piggybacking onto an existing commitment and the public. Cullerton et al. (2018) identify a series of advocacy strategies for influencing government nutrition policy, shown in the figure in this case study.

Understanding the system of governance, particularly with respect to the formal and informal rules of policymaking and who has power over these rules, is crucial to effective advocacy. Practitioners need to understand how power is distributed and exercised between people at different levels. Understanding the positions of these stakeholders and gaining their trust in order to form alliances was found to be more important than arguments using scientific evidence. Policy entrepreneurs who work as lobbyists to make the policy change happen are also central to the process.

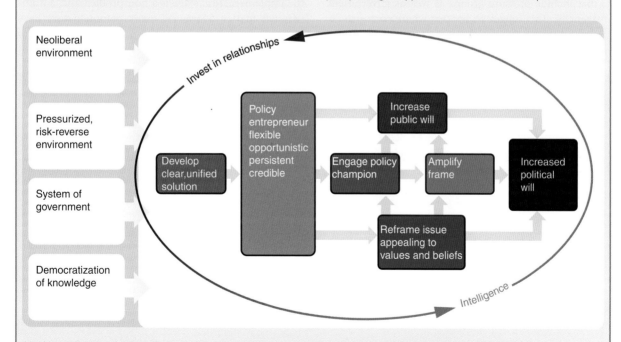

Nutrition policy change (From Cullerton, K., Donnet, T., Lee, A, Gallegos, D., 2018. Effective advocacy strategies for influencing government nutrition policy: a conceptual model. International Journal of Behavioral Nutrition and Physical Activity 15, 83.)

Policy Formulation

Once an issue is on the public agenda, there is an opportunity for stakeholders to influence any resulting policies. Table 12.1 illustrates some of the different views that compete over how to tackle alcohol misuse in the UK. As we saw in Chapter 7, political ideology includes assumptions about, for example, where responsibility lies for health, and how far the state should intervene to regulate behaviour. Such ideological views are important factors in determining how policy is framed and implemented.

Practitioners may be involved in professional, civic or voluntary pressure groups lobbying for particular public health policies. Lobbying may involve individual action (e.g., writing to MPs), collective action (e.g., local demonstrations or petitions), or coordinated and funded media campaigns. Professional associations, such as the Royal College of Nursing, the British Medical Association and the Royal Society of Public Health, have expert views that are often sought and represented to government at the policy consultation stage.

Baggott (2010) identifies three models of stakeholder influence on the policy process:

1. Institutional politics – policy results from the interaction of different institutions and policy networks that include pressure groups as well as government agencies. This suggests a process where consensus is arrived at through negotiation and compromise.

2. Pressure-group politics – policy results from different stakeholders and pressure groups which seek to mobilize public support through the media and direct action. Policy is not a result of consensus but more a product of the most powerful vested interests. For example, the extension of drinking hours in licensed premises has been supported by commercial licensing bodies and alcoholic drinks manufacturers, although many civic groups fear the consequences for public order, and public health practitioners predict an increase in alcohol-related problems.

3. Policy knowledge and policy learning – policy results from the knowledge and experience of experts and interested parties. An example is expert committees which are set up to gather evidence to input into the policy process. This suggests a rational, scientific process driven by a clear evidence base. For example, an independent expert committee, the Scientific Advisory Group for Emergencies (SAGE), advised the British government during the COVID-19 pandemic.

Policy Implementation

Once a policy has been made, it is often assumed that the implementation stage is a non-problematic, administrative matter. However, many commentators have pointed out that implementation is a separate activity

TABLE 12.1   Reducing Alcohol-Related Harm: Strategies Supported by Different Key Stakeholders

Evidence-Based Practitioners	English Government Policies	Alcohol Concern Voluntary Sector Lobbying Group	Portman Group Alcohol Industry Lobbying Group
Blood alcohol concentration laws and minimum legal drinking age	Revision of licensing hours	Alcohol awareness campaign	Information provision
Peer-led prevention programmes	Brief interventions	Education for young people	Education for vulnerable groups
Alcohol screening in hospital accident and emergency departments	Treatment programmes for alcoholics	Resources for counselling	Tighter controls restricting children's access to alcohol
Brief interventions by primary healthcare staff	Control of drinks promotions, e.g., happy hours	Training retailers to prevent sales to under age young people	Inclusion of alcohol education in the national curriculum
Employee assistance programmes	Control of advertising	Ban on glass bottles in pubs Lowering of the blood alcohol driving limit Fewer price promotions	

where policies are reinforced, changed or even sabotaged by frontline workers – the street level bureaucrats identified by Lipsky (1980). Street level bureaucrats are relatively low-level employees who have considerable discretion in how they operate, and who act as an interface between the public and the organization. Examples of street level bureaucrats are teachers, police officers, social workers, environmental health officers and health practitioners. Street level bureaucrats tend to be public service employees working in organizations with the following characteristics:

- demand outstrips supply
- resources are inadequate
- goals are ambiguous, vague or conflicting
- measuring employee performance to meet goals is difficult or impossible
- clients are typically non-voluntary and therefore are not a primary reference group for the organization.

In such situations, 'the decisions of street level bureaucrats, the routines they establish, and the devices they invent to cope with pressure, effectively become the public policy they carry out' (Lipsky, 1980, p. xii). Other potential barriers include practitioners having low levels of commitment to the policy, policy overload and lack of resources.

HEALTH IN ALL POLICIES

By the 21st century, the language and vision of HPP had evolved into 'health in all policies'. This broad strategy focuses on addressing health challenges through an integrated policy response across different sectors of government, such as transport, agriculture, housing, education and public safety. The WHO (2014, p. 1) describes health in all policies as:

An approach to public policies across sectors that systematically takes into account the health implications of decisions, seeks synergies, and avoids harmful health impacts in order to improve population health and Health Equity.

HiAP is difficult to achieve: Governments are divided into departments or ministries responsible for particular areas and with designated budgets. While health is often the biggest ministry, its budget is mostly spent on healthcare rather than the prevention of ill health. HiAP requires intersectoral collaboration, but this rarely happens at government level when each department has its own goals and budget. Electoral cycles, with their focus on short-term demonstrable achievements, are also not conducive to long-term strategies.

No policy would claim to have adverse health effects and most would claim to increase well-being in some way, albeit indirectly. Yet many policies have apparently contradictory effects. For example, it has been argued that the overall economic effect of a reduction in smoking would be negative, due to the loss of tobacco tax revenue to the exchequer and the extra demand on health and social services due to people living longer. Economic policies that increase the income of the wealthiest have been defended on the grounds that there would be a 'trickle-down' effect, despite evidence that increases in relative inequality are detrimental to health (Wilkinson, 1996). The application of stringent animal and environmental welfare regulations in the UK has resulted in an increase in meat imports from other countries where the same regulations do not apply. The consequences of policy programmes therefore need to be thought through in some detail. Health impact assessment (HIA) is an example of this process.

HEALTH IMPACT ASSESSMENT

HIA enables the identification, prediction and evaluation of likely changes to health, both now and in the future, resulting from a policy programme or plan. HIA recognizes that health is affected by a broad range of determinants linked by various pathways. For example, an HIA of a policy to extend pub licensing hours would weigh up the benefits and disadvantages of the proposal's impact on individuals, the local community, the environment and the economy. While the proposal may benefit the local economy, disadvantages for health, law, safety and community cohesion are likely. HIA as an approach is becoming more widespread as various international agreements require an assessment be made of the likely impact of policy. For example, the European Union (EU) requires the establishment of mechanisms to ensure a high level of human health protection in the definition and implementation of all EU policies and activities (Article 152 of the Treaty of Rome). Thailand has made HIA mandatory at all levels of government to identify and address health problems caused by environmental hazards such as pesticides and coal-fired power plants. In the UK, there have been several HIAs that

CASE STUDY 12.2
Health Impact Assessment

Health impact assessments are often used to evaluate the impact of policies that focus on factors other than health. An HIA includes qualitative and quantitative methodologies and collaboration with interested partners, including workers, clients and other stakeholders. This allows for a multidisciplinary definition of health to evolve. Some examples of HIAs may be found at:

- Department of Health (2010) Health Impact Assessment Tools. Available at: https://assets.publishing.service.gov.uk/government/uploads/system/uploads/attachment_data/file/216008/dh_120106.pdf
- Welsh Health Impact Assessment Support Unit network, WHIASU at http://www.wales.nhs.uk/sites3/home.cfm?OrgID=522
- Scottish Health Impact and Inequalities Assessment Network, SHIIAN at http://www.healthscotland.com/resources/networks/shian.aspx.

There are numerous examples of HIAs on topics as varied as building on green space, fast-food outlets and the siting of airports. A rapid HIA of the proposed Olympic Games was conducted for London in 2012, concluding that hosting the Olympics would provide net benefits to local communities due to increased employment, greater physical activity and enhanced community cohesion. In 2020 Public Health Wales conducted an HIA of home working during the COVID-19 pandemic (Green et al., 2020) to identify the differential impacts on the environment, economy and people's mental well-being of such a change.

Conducting an HIA can appear to be a simple matter of collecting epidemiological evidence using models of exposure and outcomes defined primarily in relation to mortality and morbidity. However, HIAs differ from traditional research primarily because they engage with the local community and stakeholders and draw on local knowledge and informed opinion about potential impacts.

There are many different models and guidance, but generally it is agreed that there are several stages to an HIA.

1. Screening: this assesses whether a project or policy is likely to pose significant health questions, and therefore whether it is worth doing an HIA.
2. Scoping: this stage outlines possible hazards and benefits and therefore identifies questions that should be asked in the HIA.
3. Risk assessment: this stage identifies the nature and magnitude of harmful and beneficial factors; how many and which population groups will be affected by them; how they will be affected; and what might enhance or mitigate the factors' impact. This stage includes an evaluation of the level of confidence or certainty in the predicted effects.
4. Decision-making: this stage will be informed by the findings of the previous stages.
5. Implementation and monitoring: ongoing monitoring of the implementation of the project or policy will feed into its evaluation

assess transport plans, housing strategies and the siting of new airports or runways and waste management landfill sites. Case Study 12.2 outlines some of the guidance on conducting an HIA.

THE HISTORY OF HPP

Public policies to promote or protect health have a long history in the UK, dating back to the 19th century and the rise of the sanitary reform movement which was prompted by concerns about the spread of disease in overcrowded slums. Edwin Chadwick's *Report from the Poor Law Commissioners on an Inquiry into the Sanitary Conditions of the Labouring Population of Great Britain* (1842) made it clear that poor people did not have the power to change their living conditions, and that local government was responsible for protecting and

promoting their health. The 19th century saw a plethora of legislation and regulations to protect and promote health – a trend that was carried on into the 20th and 21st centuries.

The inevitably selective list of HPPs in Case Study 12.3 shows how the effects of the physical environment on health dominated the 19th-century view of public health. The 21st-century view of public health, by contrast, is ecological, whereby economic, environmental and social factors interconnect and impact on health, as shown in Table 12.2.

Regulation is just one way in which public policy can support health. Governments may also use fiscal or monetary means, such as taxing unhealthy products or hypothecation (a dedicated tax to support a specific purpose, e.g., funding cycling routes through a congestion charge on motor vehicles). Other examples of

TABLE 12.2   Examples of Policies to Address Obesity Across the Life Course

Type of Policy	Example
Legislation	Restrictions on advertising of unhealthy food and drink to children
Regulation	Front of pack labelling Sugar reduction School meal standards
Fiscal measures	Soft Drinks Industry Levy – as a policy lever to encourage reformulation
Environmental/ context changes	Improving access to active travel Healthy Urban Planning Checklist Removal of confectionary from supermarket checkouts National Child Measurement Programme (NCMP)

hypothecation include the use of the TV licence to fund the BBC in the UK, and the use of tobacco taxation to fund health promotion in some Australian states.

 Learning Activity 12.2 Using Policy to Make the Healthier Choice the Easier Choice

What examples can you think of where the healthier choice has been made the easier choice?

Evidence for the effectiveness of HPP, given the long timescales involved and the complexity of interrelated factors, has proved to be problematic. Policymakers and researchers have long commented on the lack of a robust evidence base for HPP, despite it being adopted as a WHO strategy (Petticrew et al., 2004). The Marmot Review into Health Inequalities (Marmot, 2010) gathered evidence on health inequalities and lobbied to spell out the implications for populations' health. Some of its recommendations were incorporated into subsequent policies, for example early-years education, active transport, sustainable food production and zero-carbon houses.

The focus of HPP can be summarized as follows.

- Health as security: addressing issues that are not global risks but are perceived as security threats, for example, human immunodeficiency virus (HIV)/ acquired immunodeficiency syndrome (AIDS) or avian flu.

- Health as development: policies and programmes that invest in developing the economies and infrastructure of low-income countries.
- Health as a public good: policies that promote collective benefits, for example, tackling climate change.
- Health as a human right: embodied in treaties and covenants.

 Learning Activity 12.3 Global HPP

Globalization is having a huge impact on public health and poses new challenges for public policy. The changes in trade, travel, communication and migration mean that many factors impacting on health operate on a global scale that transcends national boundaries, for example, infectious diseases, poverty and food shortages, war and civil conflict, and climate change. What challenges are posed by addressing global health in public policy?

At the global level, international organizations such as the United Nations (UN), the WHO, the World Trade Organization, the World Bank and the International Monetary Fund (IMF) are all hugely influential in affecting the socio-economic determinants of health (see Chapter 9). Examples of global health promoting policymaking are the WHO's establishment of the Commission on Social Determinants of Health in 2005 and the UN's Sustainable Development Goals (SDGs), which include targets to reduce poverty, hunger, child and maternal mortality, and infectious diseases and to promote universal primary education, gender equality and environmental sustainability. The impact of global players is not always beneficial, however. For example, financial bodies such as the World Trade Organization support free-trade policies which often benefit middle- and high-income countries rather than low-income countries. The IMF has imposed structural adjustment programmes in low-income countries, which has had the effect of reducing their public spending, including spending on health. There is a 'brain drain' of skilled health professionals from low-income countries to middle- and high-income countries, which leads to a spiral of reduced service delivery and further migration of professionals. The outbreak of Ebola in 2015 and COVID-19 in 2019–20 highlighted the fragility of health systems – Liberia, for example, had only 150 doctors for a population of 4 million people.

CASE STUDY 12.3
Some HPP Landmarks in the UK, 1842–2020

1842 Edwin Chadwick's Report from the Poor Law Commissioners on an Inquiry into the Sanitary Conditions of the Labouring Population of Great Britain is published.

1845 Final report from the Royal Commission on the Health of Towns is published.

1848 Public Health Act for England and Wales requires local authorities to provide clean water supplies and hygienic sewage disposal systems, and introduces the appointment of medical officers of health for towns.

1854 John Snow controls a cholera outbreak in London by removing a contaminated local water supply.

1866 The Sanitary Act requires local authorities to inspect their districts.

1868 The Housing Act requires local authorities to ensure owners keep their properties in good repair.

1871 The Local Government Board (which becomes the Ministry of Health in 1919) is established.

1872 The Public Health Act makes medical officers of health mandatory for each district.

1875 The Public Health Act consolidates earlier legislation, and the tone changes from allowing to requiring local authorities to take public health measures.

1906 The Education Act establishes the provision of school dinners.

1907 The Education Act establishes the school medical service. The Notification of Births Act is passed and the development of health visiting is encouraged.

1930 The Housing Act (known as the Greenwood Act after Arthur Greenwood, the Labour Minister of Health) introduces, for the first time, a state subsidy specifically for slum clearance.

1944 The Education Act makes secondary education compulsory until the age of 15 years and the provision of meals, milk and medical services compulsory in every school.

1946 The National Insurance Act provides sickness and unemployment benefits, retirement pensions and widows' and maternity benefits. It is claimed that social provision was made for citizens from the 'cradle to the grave'.

1956 The Clean Air Act to reduce air pollution and respiratory diseases is passed.

1967 The Road Safety Act sets a legal limit of 80 mg of alcohol per 100 mL of blood and imposes a 70 miles per hour maximum speed limit.

1973 The wearing of helmets by motorcyclists becomes compulsory.

1974 The National Health Service (NHS) is reorganized, with community and public health services transferred from local authorities to the NHS.

1974 The Health and Safety at Work Act requires all employers to ensure the health, safety and welfare at work of all employees.

1977 The Housing (Homeless Persons) Act places a duty on local authorities to house homeless people.

1983 Seat-belt legislation. Wearing seat belts in front seats becomes law in 1991. Children are legally required to be restrained in car seats in 2006.

1988 The Water Bill requires privatized water suppliers to conform to health standards.

1989 The tax subsidy on unleaded petrol is introduced.

2000 The Food Standards Agency, an independent body, is established to protect the public's health and consumer interests in relation to food.

2005 Pubs and clubs are able to apply for unlimited extension to their opening hours.

2005 The Civil Partnership Act allows same-sex couples to enter a civil partnership, giving them the same next-of-kin rights in relation to healthcare as married couples.

2006 A smoking ban is introduced in all public places in Scotland.

2006 The Work and Families Act extends maternity and adoption leave from 6 to 9 months paid leave, to be taken by the father or the mother.

2007 A smoking ban in all enclosed workplaces and public places is introduced in England, Northern Ireland and Wales.

2007 Junk-food advertising is banned from television programmes aimed at young children (aged 4–9)

2012 Displays promoting tobacco are banned from supermarkets

2012 Food hygiene rating scheme is displayed in all outlets

2013 Marriage for same-sex couples becomes legal

2014 Free school meals are introduced for children in reception and years 1 and 2 in state-funded schools in England

2015 Displays promoting tobacco are banned from all shops.

2016 Plain packaging for cigarettes is introduced.

2018 The Soft Drinks Industry Levy (SDIL) is introduced, with manufacturers having to pay a charge for drinks containing over 8 g of sugar.

2018 Minimum unit pricing (MUP) is introduced in Scotland for all alcoholic drinks

2018 Fixed-odds betting terminals stake limit is reduced to £2.

2019 A ban of foods high in fats, sugar and salt is introduced across the Transport for London travel network.

2019 Abortion in Northern Ireland is decriminalized.

The role of states is usually emphasized in HPP, but policy is also made at other levels. In Part III, we discuss how settings such as schools and hospitals can be supportive environments for health. Organizational policies, for example, those relating to cultural competence, may have an impact on working practices.

THE STRENGTHS AND LIMITATIONS OF A REGULATORY APPROACH TO IMPROVING HEALTH

HPP is a vehicle for tackling structural and environmental barriers to health by making health improvement choices easier and protecting the public from risks. Learning Activity 12.4 asks you to consider and discuss the policy levers available to tackle an issue which may include legislation, fiscal measures, taxation and organizational change.

 Learning Activity 12.4 The Pros and Cons of HPP

Choose a health topic, for example, obesity, sexual health or drug use. What might be the advantages of a regulatory approach to health promotion? And what might be the disadvantages?

HPP has the potential to make clear inroads into the health of the public. While issues relating to healthcare systems are visible and challenging for governments, HPP requires that all sectors, including those that traditionally do not see health as part of their remit, for example, housing, must appreciate the social determinants of health and see linkages between their policy area and the health and well-being of the public. Attempts to increase cycling in the UK to promote health and reduce carbon emissions have found municipal policies influence individuals' transport choices, by reducing transport costs and making competing modes more expensive (e.g., increasing car-parking costs), and improving infrastructure and safety.

This chapter discusses the elements of HPP and highlights how policy action needs to come from policy sectors other than health. This was emphasized by the Ottawa Charter, and yet there is little evidence of coordinated action that leads to health and social policies that foster greater equity. Learning Activity 12.5 asks you to consider and discuss this.

Learning Activity 12.5 The Use of HPP as a Strategy in Health Improvement and Health Promotion

Why, given the benefits outlined above, has HPP such a low profile?

Opponents of a regulatory approach might argue that it removes personal responsibility and supports a 'nanny state' that dictates to its citizens their opportunities and behaviours. Indeed, Beattie (1993) described legislative action in his model of approaches to health promotion as authoritative and 'top-down' (see Chapter 5). Those who subscribe to conservative and individualistic political beliefs and ideology might be more likely to hold this view. This criticism has been met by the proposal that governments should act as stewards, guiding and protecting the health of the public, but not replacing the need for individual responsibility. Stewardship is about collective responsibility, which requires agreement about what needs to be done. The WHO ranks stewardship as more important than health service delivery or funding, because 'the ultimate responsibility for the overall performance of a country's health system must always lie with government' (World Health Organization, 2000, Section 11, p. 2).

There are certain situations where the public expect the state to act, for example,

- Epidemics and infectious diseases including vaccination, clean water and safe food. Governments have a history of, for example, intervening to establish quarantine or regulating on food safety to keep it free of infection
- Pollution, especially of air and water. Governments have regulated on the burning of fossil fuels and lead in petrol
- Industrial injury and occupational disease
- Industries based on addiction, for example, smoking and alcohol
- Dangerous industries, for example, construction
- Protecting the most vulnerable, for example, safeguarding child and maternal health.

Intervention can be seen as paternalistic, especially when the behaviour (e.g., smoking in one's own space, or the consumption of unhealthy foods) is considered private. Where there are immediate evidence-based risks to health, for example, not wearing seat belts, intervention is often deemed more acceptable. The intervention ladder developed by the Nuffield Council on Bioethics (2007) points to the acceptability and justification for public health policies. All policies, from the least intrusive to the most intrusive, are debated, balancing the size of health effects and the strength of evidence against the potential loss of liberty. Fig. 12.1 shows the ladder of intervention, which has been discussed in relation to numerous issues including food labelling and cutting carbon emissions from cars. Many current governments favour enabling choice following the provision of better information and education or 'nudging' (see Chapter 6).

There are therefore several roles that governments may adopt in order to pursue HPPs. Some, such as the 'nanny state', appear old-fashioned and deeply unpopular. Others, such as stewardship or the 'canny state', appear more contemporary and in tune with a range of current values and ideologies in which people in a civic society determine direction and government 'steers' but does not 'row' (Giddens, 1998). Any form of legislative action requires agreement by the public. Tones (2001) has argued that without health education, HPP would not be possible. Health education can not only set an agenda, such as environmental concern, but can also help 'to create a climate of opinion that will enable government, for example, to institute and claim the credit for change without risking electoral unpopularity' (p. 14). Chapter 5 includes a representation of Tones' model of health promotion which illustrates the importance of agenda setting and consciousness raising in moves towards HPP. Following two case studies (12.4 and 12.5) highlight how the conditions favouring policy implementation are both temporally relative. Case Study 12.4 outlines a legislative policy in workplaces in Japan in relation to obesity, and Case Study 12.5 outlines the globally accepted Framework Convention on Tobacco Control (FCTC).

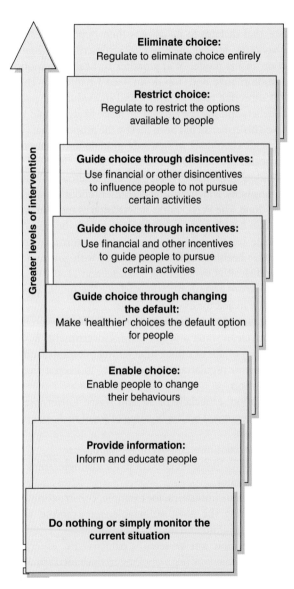

Fig. 12.1 The ladder of intervention (From Nuffield Council on Bioethics, 2007. Public Health: Ethical Issues. Nuffield Council, London. Available at: https://www.nuffieldbioethics.org/publications/public-health.)

THE PRACTITIONER'S ROLE IN HPP

Although many practitioners might not think being a policy advocate is part of their work remit, there are a number of ways in which they might become involved. Depending on the job role and employing organization or service, practitioners may take on various roles in relation to HPP, ranging from leading the process, sharing the vision and promoting the benefits of the HPP approach to active involvement in the process of lobbying, advocacy and partnership working.

 Learning Activity 12.6 HPP in Practice

Identify an example of a policy for health, for example, a smoking ban, food-labelling regulations, transport policy to promote walking and cycling, or a neighbourhood action. What kind of skills and resources are necessary to formulate and implement any change in policy?

CASE STUDY 12.4
The Ethics of Legislating About Obesity

In Japan, the 'Metabo Law' refers to a set of guidelines, officially called the Standards Concerning Implementation of Special Health Examinations and Special Public Health Guidance, which call for local governments and employers to conduct mandatory annual examinations including the measurement of waistlines for people between the ages of 40 and 74 – representing 56 million or 44% of the entire population. Individuals should not exceed a maximum waistline of 33.5 inches (85 cm) for men and 35.4 inches (90 cm) for women. People in the highest measurement category are required to attend counselling sessions over the next 3 months. The individual's insurers and employers can face penalties that will go towards fund elderly care if the person does not lose weight.

In 2011 Denmark passed a 'fat tax' that implemented an across-the-board tax on all foods with saturated-fat content above 2.3%. Instead of leading consumers to make healthier food choices, people bought their fatty foods online or in neighbouring Germany. In 2012 the Danish government announced that it would abolish the tax.

In America, the so-called Safeway Amendment allows employers to offer insurance incentives and discounts to people who take steps towards better health. Employers can increase premiums for all employees by, for example, $500. The employer will pay back $500 if a person meets certain targets, for example, if body mass index is below 25. Those already at a healthy weight get lower premiums, and those who want to change their behaviour may be incentivized; but those for whom the change is difficult get a financial penalty.

CASE STUDY 12.5
The Framework Convention on Tobacco Control

The Framework Convention on Tobacco Control (FCTC) is the first global health treaty and came into force in 2005. The treaty establishes measures to reduce the demand for tobacco through price and tax. The treaty also controls the supply of tobacco, for example, in sales to minors and illicit trade, and agrees measures to control the promotion of tobacco. The FCTC was agreed by the member states of the WHO in 2003, following almost 4 years of negotiation. Lobbying from anti-tobacco pressure groups and the tobacco lobby's persistent manoeuvring from the inside made the creation of the FCTC a difficult task. By 2004 131 countries had signed the treaty and 21 had ratified it. The USA was a notable omission to those ratifying the convention, which illustrates the influence that interest groups can have on HPP.

Based on World Health Organization, 2003. Framework Convention on Tobacco Control. WHO, Geneva, Available at: http://www.who.int/fctc/about/en/.

The Public Health Skills and Knowledge Framework (https://www.gov.uk/government/publications/public-health-skills-and-knowledge-framework-phskf/public-health-skills-and-knowledge-framework-august-2019-update) outlines the standards for those working in public health. The framework identifies a core area in policy and strategy development and expects practitioners to know of methods to assess the impact of policies, to understand the policymaking process and different methods of HIA, to have the ability to compare the health consequences of different policy options and to understand interagency working. These methods have been described elsewhere, and the Ottawa Charter (World Health Organization, 1986) noted three key skills which are necessary for effective action: mediation, advocacy and enablement.

A variety of different skills are needed at each stage of the policymaking process:

Raising the issue and formulation: research, lobbying and advocacy to promote awareness of a particular issue. A force field analysis to identify the enabling and inhibiting factors. Identification of the stakeholders and their relative power and influence. An awareness of different organizational cultures and their interests is vital for partnership working.

Policy development: An HIA can raise awareness of health impacts during the development of a potential policy or policy change. Partnership working and networking are involved. Presenting the case for a policy might mean finding areas of overlap or congruence between the interests of the people you are representing and the key people with influence.

Policy implementation: It cannot be assumed that once a policy has been approved that the implementation stage is straightforward. This stage may be particularly problematic for policies that affect organizational working. Implementation involves getting the agreement of those who are affected by a policy, and their commitment to its operationalization.

Learning Activity 12.7 asks you to reflect on your role, whether and how you might develop skills as a policy advocate or become involved in the policy process.

 Learning Activity 12.7 The Practitioner and the Policy Process

Your local council is proposing a new transport plan to encourage cycling and walking. The plan includes congestion charging, the introduction of cycling lanes and dedicated lanes for cars carrying more than one person. Proponents argue that this will encourage people to integrate exercise into their personal travel plans. Opponents argue that the scheme will lead to more congestion and longer travel times due to reduced road space and more speed restrictions. The council is inviting consultation with all interested parties. What, if anything, would you see as your role as a practitioner? How, if at all, would this differ from your role as a member of the public?

The policy context, process and implementation, as well as specific skills helpful for those engaging with policy, tend to be neglected areas within professional training. This is the current situation despite the fact that practitioners are often crucial in determining whether or not a policy achieves its goals. Policies need to be implemented in order to have an impact. This will usually involve a change in working practices, and there is a tendency to resist change within organizations. Change is often stressful and time-consuming, and unless people are convinced of its merits, there may well be resistance. Inertia or misinterpretation of what is required may also mean policies get no further than the paper they are written on. To be effective, practitioners need to be 'on board' and committed partners in implementing policies. This in turn depends on whether and how their organizations have engaged them in the policymaking process.

Within the health services, there is a long history of continual change and reorganization. This can lead to a degree of cynicism and lack of engagement with the policymaking process. For many, policy implementation in the past has been experienced as increased levels of micro-management, leading to a negative stance towards policy. However, policymaking is a powerful professional tool, and the skills for effective engagement in the policy process need to be embedded in professional training.

 Learning Activity 12.8 Effective Partnership Working

What features or characteristics would lead you to the conclusion that a partnership or collaboration is not working?

EVALUATING AN HPP APPROACH

Evaluating the impact of policies is often difficult, due to the long timescale involved, the lack of controlled comparisons and the complexity of factors and relationships affected by policy changes. The benefits of HiAP are descriptive and rest on assumptions. Areas that are commonly researched to assess the impact of policy changes are:

- knowledge of the policy change
- attitudes towards the policy change – for or against
- self-assessed behaviour change following the policy change
- independently assessed behaviour change, for example, monitoring before and after use of services
- media coverage of the policy change – amount; positive or negative
- economic analysis to determine whether or not the policy change is cost-effective.

More details of the evaluation process are given in Chapter 23.

CONCLUSION

Developing HPP and putting health in all policies is a vital cornerstone of health promotion and at the centre of the Ottawa Charter framework. Despite the strength of evidence and some notable successes, the regulatory approach that this entails remains underused. This is probably due to its complexity and the view that simultaneously addressing the many determinants of health seems too enormous a task. Addressing the social determinants of health calls into question politics, values and ideologies concerning the willingness of governments to intervene and to acknowledge their role in tackling inequalities. The potential of HPP to be an effective and efficient means of promoting health and preventing ill health suggests that the policymaking process should be addressed in professional training. The ability to understand and engage effectively in the policy process should be part of every practitioner's professional skills base.

REFLECTIONS ON PRACTICE

- Think of a policy or policy change with which you are familiar. What were its aims and objectives? What was the action plan (which personnel were involved, what resources)? How was it communicated? How was it monitored and evaluated?
- Think of an issue in relation to your practice about which you feel strongly. How could you have a voice?
- Select a controversial new policy, for example, the implementation of a 'COVID passport' indicating vaccination status, and search the newspapers for coverage about this issue. What issues are highlighted in media coverage about this issue?

■ SUMMARY

This chapter has outlined the history of public policy for health. It has discussed the strategy of attempting to put HiAP in place, and why this poses challenges. HPP is one of the action areas of the Ottawa Charter and, despite political ideologies that have moved away from state intervention, acceptance has grown of the need to legislate and regulate to tackle a range of issues.

The practitioner's role in HPP and the importance of developing an understanding of the policy process are discussed.

FURTHER READING AND RESOURCES

Baggott, R., 2010. Public Health: Policy and Politics, second edn. Palgrave Macmillan, Basingstoke.

Baggott, R., 2015. Understanding Health Policy, second edn. Policy Press, Bristol.
These two books provide a comprehensive account of British, European and international policy and public health and the policymaking process.

Eversley, J., Pitt, B., 2022. Social policy and health. In: Naidoo, J., Wills, J. (eds.), Health Studies: An Introduction, fourth edn. Palgrave Macmillan, Hampshire.
A concise overview of the discipline of social policy, with a focus on health. The chapter includes a historical account and a discussion of methodological issues, including policy analysis and the policy process.

Laverack, G., 2013. Health Activism: Foundations and Strategies. Sage, London.
A short book with numerous examples of practitioners taking action on behalf of a cause. The actions challenge an existing order that contributes to a social injustice or inequality.

FEEDBACK ON LEARNING ACTIVITIES

12.1. Governments frequently frame obesity as a problem for individuals: people eat too much of the wrong kind of food and exercise too little. The government's role is to empower people and help them make better choices (DHSC, 2020). The 2020 obesity strategy (DHSC, 2020) was said to have been introduced because of COVID-19 and evidence that excess weight is a modifiable risk factor. Obesity may also be framed as a disease within a health strategy, or a focus on childhood obesity may be construed as contributing towards future protection. The *Lancet's* Global Syndemic Commission report (Swinburn et al., 2019) locates obesity within the context of global undernutrition, climate change and systemic economic, social and political drivers, rather than as a consequence of individual decisions.

12.2. Making the healthier choice the easier choice can be achieved by legislation or regulation, for example, banning smoking in public places. It can also be achieved by changing the norms of choices and propelling people towards healthier choices, for example, changing the default option in fast-food restaurants from French fries to carrots.

12.3. While the need for global public health policy is acknowledged, it is also seen as challenging. Promoting health can become repressive, for example, when people's movements are restricted to prevent the transmission of disease. Development can be steered by global economic forces. The voice of the WHO is often not heard, while that of the World Trade Organization, where considerations of trade and profit predominate, is usually loud and clear.

12.4. HPP as an approach to health promotion has many strengths. Perhaps most important is its recognition of the multiple socio-economic and environmental determinants of health and the necessity to tackle these determinants to promote health. Alongside this recognition and 'upstream' focus goes a commitment to reducing inequalities in health and promoting equity. An upstream approach also has economic benefits. A positive impact on the determinants of health will prevent much ill health and disease, thus saving money on services and treatment. Prevention is typically far more cost-effective than treatment.

12.5. There are many barriers to achieving HPP, including the tendency of both government and the public to focus on health services instead of public health, and the silo mentality of government departments which means cross-departmental working to promote public health remains an aspiration rather than a reality.

12.6. Influencing, planning for and operationalizing HPP calls for a variety of skills including health education, partnership working, lobbying, advocacy, management, leadership and public relations.

12.7. As a practitioner faced with a proposed new policy affecting your clients, you would probably consider it your duty to assess the policy in terms of its likely impact on the health of your clients. This might include initiating discussions and forums with clients to gauge their reaction to the proposal or a more *ad hoc* process of sounding things out with individuals as and when you deem it appropriate. You might take it upon yourself to translate research findings into plain English or to spell out the likely effects of the proposed policy. You might propose that a rapid HIA is undertaken, which would ensure the views of community groups are heard. You might also discuss the topic with your professional association and oversee its active involvement in the issues.

As a member of the public, you might be involved in the same spectrum of activities (apart from working with professional associations). However, your role and expertise would be different, and you would engage with the issues as an interested member of the public rather than as a practitioner with a duty of care. This might give you more freedom to voice your opinions and make your principles and values known.

12.8. A partnership or collaboration that is not working well may exhibit the following:
- Leadership and vision: Lack of agreed vision; competing targets; divergent organizational priorities; differing perspectives (e.g., medical versus social models of health)
- Organisation and involvement: Key agencies missing from the table; lack of clarity about the relative roles of partners; unrealistic expectations of partners' capabilities and capacity (e.g., voluntary sector)
- Development and co-ordination: Lack of agreement in relation to needs; no clear agreed plans; no sense of co-ordinated joint endeavour
- Learning and development: Unwilling to share knowledge and skills; organizational or professional defensiveness; unwilling to take risks and be innovative
- Resources: Unwilling to share human, financial, technical and information resources
- Evaluation and review: No clarity or consensus about the criteria used to define a 'good' output or outcome; no process review; no agreed measures of success.

REFERENCES

Baggott, R., 2010. Public Health: Policy and Practice, second edn. Palgrave Macmillan, Basingstoke.

Beattie, A., 1993. The changing boundaries of health. In: Beattie, A., Gott, M., Jones, L. (eds.), Health and Wellbeing: A Reader. Macmillan/Open University, London, pp. 260–272.

Chadwick, E., 1842. Report from the Poor Law Commissioners on an Inquiry into the Sanitary Conditions of the Labouring Population of Great Britain. Poor Law Commission, Home Office, London.

Cullerton, K., Donnet, T., Lee, A., Gallegos, D., 2018. Effective advocacy strategies for influencing government nutrition policy: a conceptual model. Int. J. Behav. Nutr. Phys. Act. 15, 83.

DHSC (Department of Health and Social Care), 2020. Tackling obesity: empowering adults and children to live healthier lives. Policy Paper 27 July. Available at: https://www.gov.uk/government/publications/tackling-obesity-government-strategy/tackling-obesity-empowering-adults-and-children-to-live-healthier-lives.

Giddens, A., 1998. The Third Way The Renewal of Social Democracy. Polity Press, Cambridge.

Green, L., Lewis, R., Evans, L., Morgan, L., Parry-Williams, L., Azam, S., et al., 2020. A COVID-19 Pandemic World and Beyond: the Public Health Impact of Home and Agile Working in Wales. Summary Report. Public Health Wales NHS Trust, Cardiff. Available at: https://phw.nhs.wales/news/home-working-can-enhance-mental-well-being-but-also-increases-risk-of-stress/the-public-health-impact-of-home-and-agile-working-in-wales-supporting-information-report/.

Lipsky, M., 1980. Street Level Bureaucracy. Russell Sage, New York.

Marmot, M., 2010. Fair Society, Healthy Lives. Institute of Health Equity, London. Available at: http://www.instituteofhealthequity.org/resources-reports/fair-society-healthy-lives-the-marmot-review.

Milio, N., 2001. Glossary: healthy public policy. J. Epidemiol. Community Health 55, 622–623.

Nuffield Council on Bioethics, 2007. Public Health: Ethical Issues. Nuffield Council, London. Available at: http://nuffieldbioethics.org/project/public-health/.

Nutbeam, D., 1998. Health Promotion Glossary. WHO. Available at: https://www.who.int/healthpromotion/about/HPR%20Glossary%201998.pdf.

Nutbeam, D., Muscat, D., 2021. Health Promotion Glossary 2021. Health Promotion International. Available at: https://academic.oup.com/heapro/advance-article-abstract/doi/10.1093/heapro/daaa157/6211341.

Petticrew, M., Whitehead, M., Macintyre, S.J., Graham, H., Egan, M., 2004. Evidence for public health policy on inequalities: 1: the reality according to policymakers. J. Epidemiol. Community Health 58, 811–816.

Simon, H., 1947. Administrative Behaviour: A Study of Decision Making Processes in Administrative Organization. Macmillan, New York.

Sutton, R., 1999. The Policy Process: An Overview. Overseas Development Institute, London. Available at: https://odi.org/en/publications/the-policy-process/.

Swinburn, B., Kraak, V., Allender, S., Atkins, V.J., Baker, P.I., et al., 2019. The global syndemic of obesity, undernutrition, and climate change: The Lancet Commission report. Lancet 393 (10173), 791–846.

Tones, K., 2001. Health promotion: the empowerment imperative. In: Scriven, A., Orme, J. (eds.), Health Promotion Professional Perspectives, second edn. Palgrave Macmillan, Hampshire, pp. 3–18.

United Nations. Universal Declaration of Human Rights, Article 25(1). United Nations, Geneva. Available at: https://www.un.org/en/about-us/universal-declaration-of-human-rights (accessed 16.04.21).

Walt, G., 1994. Health Policy: An Introduction to Process and Power. Zed Books, London.

Wilkinson, R., 1996. Unhealthy Societies: The Afflictions of Inequality. Routledge, London.

World Health Organization, 1986. Ottawa Charter for Health Promotion: An International Conference on Health Promotion. November 17–21. WHO, Copenhagen. Available at: http://www.who.int/healthpromotion/conferences/previous/ottawa/en/.

World Health Organization, 1988. Second International Conference on Health Promotion. WHO, Adelaide, Australia. Available at: https://www.who.int/teams/health-promotion/enhanced-wellbeing/second-conference.

World Health Organization, 2000. The World Health Report 2000: Health Systems; Improving Performance. WHO, Geneva. Available at: https://www.who.int/whr/2000/en/whr00_en.pdf.

World Health Organization, 2014. Health in All Policies (HiAP) Framework for Country Action. Available at: https://www.who.int/healthpromotion/hiapframework.pdf.

13

Communicating About Health

LEARNING OUTCOMES

By the end of this chapter you will be able to:
- understand how information is used to promote behaviour change
- discuss the contribution of mass media and public information to behaviour change
- consider the potential contribution of different communication strategies (interpersonal, digital and other media)

- critically assess health communication to determine how credible, understandable and actionable it is for its intended audience.

KEY CONCEPTS AND DEFINITIONS

Behaviour change communication Communication strategies designed to promote positive behaviours. Strategies follow a systematic process from formative research to planning, implementation and evaluation.

Health literacy The ability of individuals to access and critically assess information. Health literacy includes the ability to interact and express personal and societal needs for promoting health.

Medium/media Channels of communication e.g., television, social media.

Media advocacy The use of media to promote a policy change.

Message The content or what is being communicated.

Social marketing An approach aimed at changing people's behaviour, borrowing ideas from commercial marketing.

IMPORTANCE OF THE TOPIC

Communication of information and advice about health is central to health promotion strategies. A knowledge of how communication takes place between the sender and receiver of messages, and an understanding of the medium through which communication occurs, are therefore important tools for the health promoter. Giving health-related information is a key task for most practitioners involved in health education, which typically involves conveying a message about reducing health risks, compliance with advice and the effective use of services. Communication is top down, with the

health promoter as the holder of the scientific knowledge, which is transmitted to the public. As we have seen throughout this book, information alone is not enough to enable people to take control over their health. A key challenge is making communication relevant and provided in ways that are empowering. To do this effectively, a practitioner needs to understand the audience and the best means of reaching them and to foresee how information will be received. Marshall McLuhan's famous dictum from 1964 that 'the medium is the message' tells us that the method and channel of communication is as important as the message. A wide range of methods are used to communicate about health, ranging from interpersonal to digital, online and mass media. In addition to the traditional media (radio, television, press), social media, most notably the internet, have changed communication patterns with the capacity to reach large numbers of people and the ability to be accessed individually as and when people choose.

INTRODUCTION

Communicating about health may seek to:

- provide health information and raise awareness about an issue, for example, the risks of smoking during pregnancy
- change opinions on an issue through advocacy, for example, the importance of vaccination
- influence behaviours, for example, wearing a helmet when cycling
- demonstrate a skill or practice, for example, handwashing.

Communication may do this through different channels and be below-the-line, targeting specific groups, or above-the-line, targeting a wider audience through the use of billboards or television. Communication channels include:

- web, including targeted search engine marketing and websites
- broadcast media (radio and television)
- social media (e.g., Facebook)
- print (leaflets, posters)
- billboards
- interpersonal communication.

Good communication is a vital health promotion skill. Most practitioners in most settings communicate health messages as part of their daily work. Health messages may be about a health condition or treatment; a desirable lifestyle change; or advice on how to manage a situation that may be impacting on a person's health. A practitioner may be giving information, teaching or educating or counselling, and may use a variety of communication tools.

Beattie et al. (1993) describe the use of media as 'health persuasion', by which they mean a top-down conservative method designed to infuse an audience with information (see Chapter 5). Many public health issues, for example, human immunodeficiency virus/acquired immunodeficiency syndrome (HIV/AIDS), alcohol misuse, smoking and, more recently, COVID-19, have been the subject of extensive mass-media campaigns.

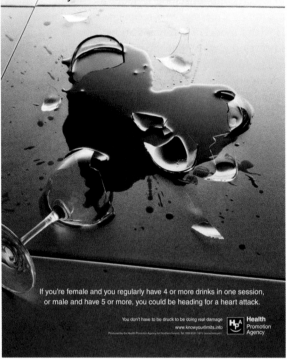

Fig. 13.1 Alcohol poster from Health Promotion Agency Northern Ireland (Reproduced with permission from the Health Promotion Agency for Northern Ireland: photography, David Gill.)

The aim of such campaigns is usually to raise awareness or present a message advocating healthy lifestyles, as shown in the example in Fig. 13.1.

The media may also be an unhealthy influence, advertising unhealthy products (e.g., alcohol), or transmitting unhealthy messages (e.g., that drinking excessively is fun and fashionable). The media also play a major role in constructing society's views on health issues and services. What health issues are covered, and the slant the reporting takes, are powerful forces in public discourse around health. Social media have emerged in the last couple of decades, and Twitter, Facebook and YouTube have enabled rapid and widespread sharing of information and opinions.

UNDERSTANDING HEALTH COMMUNICATION

There are many process models of communication, all of which adopt a mechanistic and linear orientation, in which communication is about the transfer of information or a message to a recipient. The American Yale-Hovland model of communication, which was designed to develop ways of influencing public attitudes, is shown in Fig. 13.2. This model suggests that the process of mass communication entails five variables: source, message, channel, receiver and destination. The effectiveness of the communication, which may aim to change opinions or attitudes, or influence a behaviour change, depends on:

- the extent to which the source of the communication is credible and trustworthy
- the way the message is constructed and distributed
- the receiver's receptiveness and readiness to accept the message.

Communication is concerned with the transmission of messages from a sender to a receiver. Messages are coded into signs and symbols that have meaning within specific codes. The message is encoded by the sender and decoded by the receiver (as shown in Fig. 13.2). The aim is that messages should be decoded and understood according to the intentions of the sender, but this can be problematic when using mass media. This is because mass media target large audiences simultaneously and, unlike direct personal communication, there is typically no feedback loop from the receiver back to the sender of the message. This means messages may be interpreted in ways that were not anticipated or intended by the sender. For example, the commonly used term 'healthy eating' may be variously understood as a diet for weight loss, eating particular foods or a balanced diet (Buckton et al., 2015). Later in this chapter we discuss the role of social marketing and how this strategy is based on research on the views and reception of audiences to targeted messages.

Mass media may be important in raising awareness, communicating basic information and disseminating new ideas. Mass communication influences key opinion leaders who are active members of the mass-media audience. These opinion leaders then spread ideas to other people through interpersonal means of communication (Katz and Lazarsfeld, 1955). The process of diffusing innovative or new ideas through a population is based on the finding that the adoption of new behaviours typically follows an S-shaped trajectory (Rogers and Scott, 1997). There is usually a slow initial uptake followed by rapid acceptance, as opinion leaders or early adopters (who are

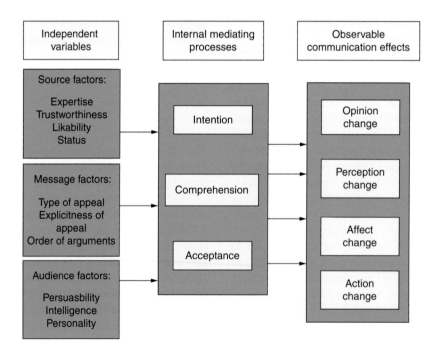

Fig. 13.2 Model of communication (With permission from Peter Bearman, INCITE/TAA, Columbia University.)

usually from higher socio-economic groups) communicate the benefits of the behaviour, and then a final slowing as a minority (who tend to be from isolated traditional communities) resist acceptance or change. Social media can accelerate this process and new ideas can get adopted very quickly, which is illustrated in Case Study 13.1.

The media also play a key role in creating beliefs and values about health, medicine, disease and illness. The ways in which these are presented, from the kindly doctor in soap operas to news bulletins on miracle cures and high-tech interventions, all contribute to people's understanding of health (Lupton, 2012). Many studies use discourse analysis to reveal the underlying values, concepts and messages implicit in media portrayals of health and ill health. Public health's long timescale and basis in numerical data make it unattractive to the mass media. Instead, 'shock-horror' stories of crisis within the National Health Service (NHS) or the appearance of rare diseases tend to dominate the news headlines. Learning

Activities 13.1 and 13.2 ask you to consider and discuss the influence of media representations.

 Learning Activity 13.1   The Portrayal of Drinking Alcohol in Television Programmes

Some people argue that representations of people drinking alcohol in television programmes encourage viewers to do the same. What do you think? Why?

 Learning Activity 13.2   Media Coverage of Public Health

Monitor media coverage on television, in magazines, on radio and in broadsheet and tabloid newspapers for items about health over a 1-week period. Use the following categories to allocate coverage:

- medical dominance, for example, medical breakthroughs, high-technology interventions
- crisis or scare stories, for example, failures in services or outbreaks of unusual diseases or illnesses
- individual consumerism and lifestyles, for example, stories about how to choose and access healthier lifestyles and health services
- celebrities illustrating how health or anti-health behaviours can be perceived as attractive
- social, economic or political health determinants, for example, policy changes and how these might affect health
- environmental or global determinants of health, for example, the loss of agriculture and the ability to grow food due to climate change.

Does the media coverage you monitored fit into these categories?

Which categories were the least and most common? What are the implications of this?

How much of the coverage was in entertainment programmes?

Think about and find some examples of how the following are represented in popular media culture:

- doctors
- hospitals and healthcare services
- chronic illnesses, for example, coronary heart disease, cancer
- acute illnesses, for example, flu
- social and environmental health
- individual state of positive health and well-being
- prevention of ill health
- protection of health.

 CASE STUDY 13.1

South Africa's Brothers for Life Tackles Men's Involvement in HIV Prevention

Brothers for Life (BFL) is a South African health communication programme that promotes HIV testing, voluntary medical male circumcision (VMMC), male involvement in the prevention of mother-to-child transmission (PMTCT) of HIV and prevention of gender-based violence. BFL uses a variety of innovative approaches to diffuse the principles of positive behaviour among South African males. BFL promoted positive HIV testing behaviour by creating 1000 Twitter accounts for World AIDS Day 2011 and recruiting HIV-positive volunteers to tweet about HIV stigma and promote HIV testing using the hashtag #HIVarmy. Within hours, the #HIVarmy hashtag was 'trending' (i.e., a Twitter hashtag tagged at a greater rate than other tags) in South Africa and then globally. Local celebrities picked up the hashtag and joined the conversation. At midnight all 1000 accounts were terminated with the word 'deceased' displayed in the avatar. The last tweet warned South Africans that 1000 of their fellow citizens needlessly die from AIDS-related causes daily. This innovative Twitter campaign created a virtual social network, recruited opinion leaders and used a new communication channel to achieve diffusion of HIV testing and awareness messages (Communication Initiative Network at https://www.comminit.com/global/category/sites/global).

COMMUNICATING ABOUT HEALTH

Practitioners communicate about health to:
1. Provide or give information.
2. Explain risk.
3. Encourage a behaviour change with a specific message through a planned campaign or social marketing.

GIVING INFORMATION

The conveying of information is, as we saw earlier, a two way process in which the information needs to be in a form likely to be accepted and understood. Practitioners often underestimate a person's need for information, and overestimate their own ability to convey information effectively (Britten et al., 2000). Studies have shown that up to 80% of the medical information patients are told during a medical visit is forgotten immediately, and nearly half of the information retained is incorrect (Kessels, 2003).

As most people cannot concentrate for longer than 15 minutes, any structured activity to give information needs to be planned:
- What does the person already know? People learn better if any information is linked to their experiences.
- What is to be learned or understood? Is it factual information? Practical skills?
- How could the information be presented in a logical, sequenced way?
- Are there complex points, terms or concepts? Will a visual aid be helpful?
- How will the person's understanding and interest be checked?

Case Study 13.2 describes the technique of Teach-Back, which has become widely adopted in practitioner–patient consultations.

CASE STUDY 13.2
Teach-Back

Teach-back is a method of ensuring that patients/clients understand what you have told them. During teach-back, you ask patients/clients to explain in their own words what they need to know or do to take care of their health. The practitioner asks the person to teach back to them what they have been told. If a person is asked whether they have any questions, they will usually say they do not, even if they do not really understand what you have told them.

They may be embarrassed or intimidated, or they may think they understand. Using teach-back helps a practitioner more accurately determine a person's level of understanding. The figure in this case study shows how this simple technique might enable the practitioner to adapt their communication (from https://www.ahrq.gov/sites/default/files/wysiwyg/professionals/quality-patient-safety/patient-family-engagement/pfeprimarycare/teachback-module.pdf).

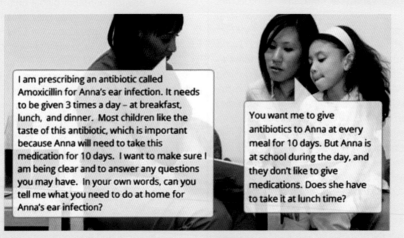

I am prescribing an antibiotic called Amoxicillin for Anna's ear infection. It needs to be given 3 times a day – at breakfast, lunch, and dinner. Most children like the taste of this antibiotic, which is important because Anna will need to take this medication for 10 days. I want to make sure I am being clear and to answer any questions you may have. In your own words, can you tell me what you need to do at home for Anna's ear infection?

You want me to give antibiotics to Anna at every meal for 10 days. But Anna is at school during the day, and they don't like to give medications. Does she have to take it at lunch time?

Agency for Healthcare Research and Quality. *Teach-back.* Agency for Healthcare Research and Quality, US Department of Health and Human Services. (Available at https://www.ahrq.gov/sites/default/files/wysiwyg/professionals/quality-patient-safety/patient-family-engagement/pfeprimarycare/teachback-module.pdf.)

A person's health literacy needs to be taken into account when providing information. Health literacy is a term that encompasses many of the skills necessary to access, assess and use information in making life choices. Health literacy has been defined in many different ways. A broad definition is provided by Zarcadoolas et al. (2005, p. 196): 'the wide range of skills and competencies that people develop to seek out, comprehend, evaluate, and use health information and concepts to make informed choices, reduce health risks, and increase quality of life'.

Functional health literacy is being able to read and understand information about health risks and health services, which facilitates the appropriate and effective use of services. This is very similar to the general lay definition of literacy as the ability to read and write. Interactive health literacy includes the ability to develop skills in a supportive environment, leading to increased self-confidence and independent action to improve health, including being able to actively engage in health care communications. Critical health literacy includes the ability to assess information on the wider socio-economic determinants of health, and to use this information to improve health and tackle health inequalities.

Even though 70%–90% of people in high-income countries are connected online, many people prefer to use traditional media (such as books, brochures, magazines) or healthcare professionals as their primary source of health information. Trust, confidence in the information source and access are the main reasons for choosing one source over another (Coulter et al., 2006). Leaflets and pamphlets have been used to educate the public since the beginning of the twentieth century. When the Central Council for Health Education was established in 1927 it listed the provision of better and cheaper leaflets as its main aim. The greatest use of written material is to support one-to-one interactions with clients and patients. As only 50% of information can be recalled by patients 5 minutes after a consultation (Kessels, 2003), this seems an effective use of leaflets. There is some evidence that written information can not only improve patients' understanding and recall, but also provide reassurance. Learning Activity 13.3 asks you to think about when and with whom you might use written communication in order to promote health.

 Learning Activity 13.3 Health Communication

What would be the key considerations for using written information as part of health communication?

EXPLAINING RISK

The COVID-19 pandemic has highlighted the importance of presenting information about risk clearly so that people can take informed decisions to protect themselves and their families. Risks are generally seen as being more worrying (and less acceptable) to the public if they are perceived to be:

- involuntary (such as exposure to pollution) rather than voluntary (dangerous sports or smoking)
- inequitably distributed (some benefit while others suffer the consequences)
- inescapable and uncontrollable through taking personal precautions
- arise from an unfamiliar or novel source
- result from man-made, rather than natural, sources
- cause hidden and irreversible damage, such as through the onset of illness many years after exposure
- pose some particular danger to small children or pregnant women or, more generally, to future generations
- threaten a form of death (or illness/injury) arousing particular dread
- damage identifiable rather than anonymous victims
- poorly understood by science
- subject to contradictory statements from responsible sources (or, even worse, from the same source).

The development of the COVID-19 pandemic led to a vast amount of information being communicated quickly from a huge range of sources and when so much scientific knowledge is uncertain. Fig. 13.3 shows an example of guidance from WHO to counter one of the many examples of misinformation that circulated on the internet.

Vraga and Jacobsen (2020) suggest that communication about risk, for example, during a pandemic should:
- Address information overload
  - Identify the core message and communicate one simple point
  - Communicate the most important information first
  - Make the target population clear
  - Promote concrete actions that encourage healthy behaviours.
- Address information on certainty
  - Avoid sharing incomplete information
  - Tailor messages depending on whether audiences are likely to be sceptical
  - Describe the strength of evidence

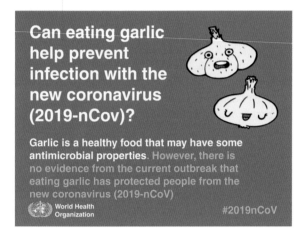

Fig. 13.3 Combatting misinformation about COVID-19 (From World Health Organization, 2021. Coronavirus Disease (COVID-19) Advice for the Public: Mythbusters. World Health Organization, Geneva. Available at https://www.who.int/emergencies/diseases/novel-coronavirus-2019/advice-for-public/myth-busters.)

- Acknowledge uncertainty.
- Address misinformation
  - Disseminate accurate information
  - Actively seek to minimize inaccurate information.

❓ Learning Activity
13.4   Communicating Risk

If you were trying to explain the risk, chance or probability that a person will develop cancer from smoking cigarettes, which of the following statements might have the greater effect?

- 'Cigarette smokers are 12 times more likely to die of lung cancer than non-smokers.'
- 'The number per 100,000 smokers who will develop lung cancer' (actual number depends on factors such as their age and how many years they have been smoking).
- 'You will live longer and healthier if you quit smoking.'
- 'Smoking causes cancer, heart attacks, and lung disease.'

COMMUNICATING BEHAVIOUR CHANGE

Campaigns have been used by national health promotion agencies in the UK and worldwide to promote various health messages. Different media, including billboards, press advertisements and radio announcements, have been used, but television is the principal medium because, although it is expensive, it reaches much larger audiences and achieves better recall. The end goal of most media campaigns is to achieve a specific behaviour change, although their ability to do so is disputed. Fig. 13.4 is an example of a poster to promote the wearing of helmets, targeted especially at young people, as over 40% of road traffic deaths involve people aged 0 to 25 years.

The examples given here of mass-media campaigns suggest that, on their own, they are unreliable in achieving behaviour change. However, used in combination with other strategies, such as personal reinforcement from trusted peers or experts, or policy changes affecting the environment, mass-media campaigns can be effective.

Campaigns adopt a variety of tactics to communicate their message, including emotional appeals, shock tactics and reassurance. The evidence on whether or not fear is an effective strategy is inconclusive. Early studies showed that people may attend to, comprehend and retain information when shocked, but may also

---

👥 RESEARCH EXAMPLE 13.1
The Effectiveness of Mass-Media Campaigns for Smoking Cessation

Mass-media campaigns have been shown to increase smoking cessation and reduce smoking prevalence and uptake among adults, but have been less successful in preventing smoking uptake among young people. Campaigns tend to convey messages about the negative health consequences of smoking, or information about how to quit (e.g., Bala et al., 2008; Brinn et al., 2010; Durkin et al., 2012), although a counter-marketing campaign in Florida called 'Truth' was very successful. This campaign used the techniques of traditional marketing satirically. One poster promoted a spoof cigarette called 'True' (Hicks, 2001), with the strapline 'No other cigarette can make this statement: US government tests show True is lowest in both tar and nicotine of the 20 best selling cigarettes.'

In England, a new approach has been adopted termed Stoptober, reframing the usual call to action from 'quit now', which might feel an unsurmountable challenge, to 'join the 28-day quitting challenge'. It also aimed at creating a social movement around quitting smoking for 28 days as in 'dry January'. An evaluation of the 2019 Stoptober campaign (Public Health England, 2019) showed that the campaign generated high levels of brand recognition (82%) and quit attempts among 25% of all smokers and recent ex-smokers, the majority using a form of support (quit aid, behavioural support or digital tool).

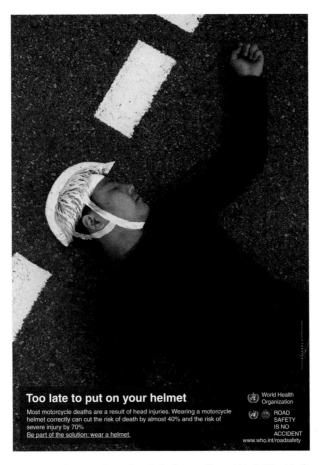

Too late to put on your helmet

Most motorcycle deaths are a result of head injuries. Wearing a motorcycle helmet correctly can cut the risk of death by almost 40% and the risk of severe injury by 70%
Be part of the solution: wear a helmet.

World Health Organization

ROAD SAFETY IS NO ACCIDENT
www.who.int/roadsafety

Fig. 13.4 A poster to promote the wearing of cycle helmets (From World Health Organization. Available at: www.who.int/roadsafety (accessed 30.09.21).)

RESEARCH EXAMPLE 13.2

Evaluation of Mass-Media Campaigns

1. Sun safety – evaluation of repeated campaigns in Australia using the mass media to promote sun protection measures among children concluded that using the message 'slip, slap, slop' was linked to a decrease in the incidence of melanoma in young people since the 1990s. However, health promotion campaigns are competing against a range of commercial messages, for example, about the safety of sunscreens and vitamin D deficiency (www.sunsmart.com.au).

2. Change for Life – a social marketing campaign to reframe childhood obesity as a health issue. Mass media were effective in raising awareness in the targeted group, but there was little impact on behaviour (Croker et al., 2012).

3. Weight gain – a repeated campaign aimed at preventing weight gain in the Netherlands resulted, after the final campaign wave, in high awareness (88%) and message recall (68%), and positive attitudes and motivation. However, the campaign had mixed effects on self-efficacy and negative effects on risk perception (Wammes et al., 2007).

---

become resistant or deny the relevance of the message (Montazeri et al., 1998). The use of fear appeals in social marketing has been criticized (Hastings et al., 2004) for its relative ineffectiveness and its unintended negative consequences (e.g., anxiety, complacency and increased social inequity). Case Study 13.3 gives examples of public information campaigns and how the presentation of key messages has changed over time.

CASE STUDY 13.3

The Changing Face of Health in Social Marketing

The following posters about substance use from the archives of Public Health England (https://publichealthengland.exposure.co/100-years-of-public-health-marketing) show the changing impetus for health marketing and the acceptability of messages according to the social and cultural context.

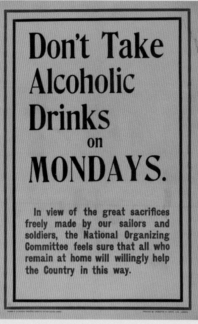

1916: During the First World War it was important to maintain a workforce in factories and on farms. Beer was watered down, pub hours were restricted and it was against the law to buy a round of drinks.

1974: Consumption of alcohol and deaths from cirrhosis doubled from 1950 to the mid 1970s. A series of poster campaigns aimed to get people to drink in moderation.

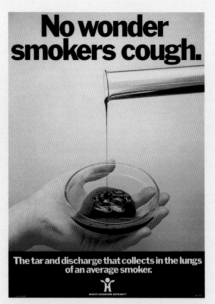

1988: Increasing evidence about the harmful effects of smoking and of secondhand smoke led to a stronger and darker tone in campaigns. A dramatic rise in the use of heroin in the 1980s led to a series of shock campaigns.

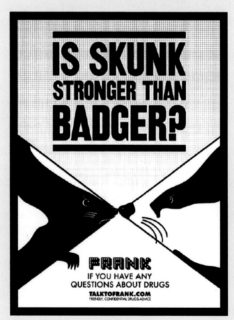

2003: Digital technology transforms the ways that people access and share information. More emphasis is given to personalised messaging, practical tools and enabling people to be active participants. The FRANK service is a website and telephone line set up in 2003 to provide information and advice about drugs for young people and their parents www.talktofrank.com.

All figures in this case study are from Public Health England. (Available at: https://publichealthengland.exposure.co/100-years-of-public-health-marketing (accessed 01.08.21).)

Extensive reviews of media campaigns now conclude that they may be successful if their goals are reasonable and there is no expectation of immediate results. Simple awareness or market penetration is relatively easy to achieve; to inform or reinforce attitudes is more difficult; and to have any effect on behaviour is even more difficult. There are certain preconditions for success:

- favourable public opinion, which is most likely when there has been extensive market research at the design stage
- emotional appeal, for example, a child death arising from drink driving
- time available for the presentation of complex information, for example, nutritional information
- a clear action which individuals feel confident that they can take, for example, putting a baby to sleep on its back
- support through interpersonal communication.

As we have seen public information campaigns about health remain a key strategy and yet the evidence for their effectiveness is equivocal. Learning Activity 13.5 asks you to consider and discuss what should be taken into account in an evaluation of such campaigns.

 Learning Activity 13.5   Evaluating Mass-Media Campaigns

How would you evaluate a mass-media campaign to reduce drink-driving?

Evaluations of mass-media campaigns take many forms:

- coverage (the percentage of the target population who were exposed to the message)
- recall (the percentage of the population who could accurately recall the message)
- impact of the campaign on behaviour
- cost-effectiveness.

Campaigns are unlikely to be successful when they seek to:

- convey complex information, for example, the relative risks of different kinds of fat in the diet
- teach skills, for example, how to negotiate safer sex
- shift people's attitudes or beliefs – if messages are presented which challenge basic beliefs, it is more likely that the message will be ignored, dismissed or interpreted to mean something else

- change behaviour in the absence of other enabling factors.

Another way of gaining awareness is having health events. Most countries have a calendar of health awareness weeks or months designed to raise awareness of particular conditions, for example, Mental Health Awareness Week or Breast Cancer Awareness Month. Very few comprehensive evaluations of these events have been conducted. Public awareness of some events, which are supported by coloured ribbons, is high, for example, breast cancer and HIV/AIDS. The effect of such events on health behaviours is less clear, and unlikely to be significant if the desired health behaviour is not yet a social norm.

Most health communications treat audiences as consumers, targeting them with information so they can reduce their risk of illness or injury, or top-down messages exhorting healthier behaviour. Media advocacy is less about delivering a message and more about using the media to raise voices and apply pressure for policy change. Its objectives are:

- to get an issue discussed
- to get an issue discussed in different ways
- to discredit opponents
- to bring in new voices
- to introduce new facts or perspectives
- to shift perceptions of risk.

An example of successful media advocacy involving international cooperation was the Nestlé boycott of the 1970s and 1980s, which led to the World Health Organization's International Code of Marketing for Breast Milk Substitutes (McKee et al., 2005). Direct action can also be successful, as evidenced by Billboard Utilising Graffitists Against Unhealthy Promotions (BUGA-UP), an Australian group which targeted tobacco advertising (Fig. 13.5).

More recently, the Manchester United footballer Marcus Rashford used his extensive profile to lead an eventually successful campaign for the UK government to provide free meals in the holidays for schoolchildren during the pandemic.

Just as commercial companies are able to get the public to buy products (even those they may not really need), so health promoters should be able to get people to choose healthy behaviours. Some of the techniques of marketing are widely used in health promotion to influence the acceptability of healthy lifestyles so that they appear desirable and easy to adopt.

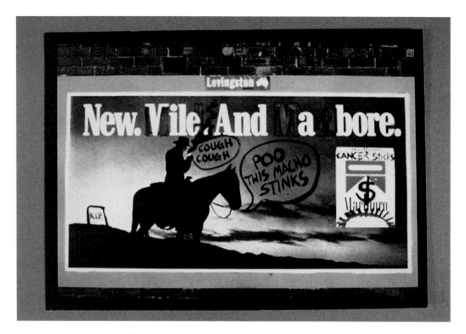

Fig. 13.5 Defaced billboard (Courtesy of Cecilia Farren.)

Learning Activity 13.6   Public Health Campaigns About COVID-19

Here are three examples of public health campaigns about the COVID-19 pandemic from the UK, New Zealand and Oregon, the USA. Which do you think is most effective at conveying a protective message and why?

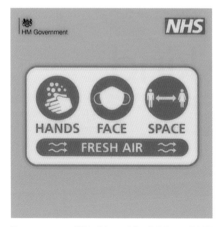

From Department of Health and Social Care, 2020. 'New campaign to prevent spread of coronavirus indoors this winter'. UK government. Available at: https://www.gov.uk/government/news/new-campaign-to-prevent-spread-of-coronavirus-indoors-this-winter.

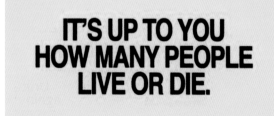

From Office of the Governor, 2020. Oregon. Available at: https://www.campaignlive.co.uk/article/dont-accidentally-kill-someone-says-oregon-coronavirus-public-service-spot/1678630.

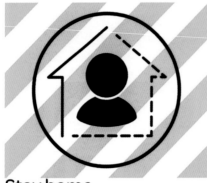

Stay home if you are sick

Call your GP or Pharmacy before visiting them.
Or call Healthline on 0800 358 5453.

Find out more at
Covid19.govt.nz

New Zealand Government

Unite against COVID-19

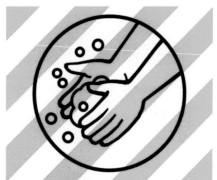

Washing and drying your hands kills the virus

Wash often. Use soap. 20 seconds. Then dry.
This kills the virus by bursting its protective bubble.

Find out more at
Covid19.govt.nz

New Zealand Government

Unite against COVID-19

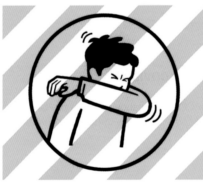

Cough or sneeze into your elbow

It keeps the virus off your hands, so you won't spread it
to other people and make them sick too.

Find out more at
Covid19.govt.nz

New Zealand Government

Unite against COVID-19

Be kind

Please be patient with our staff and others,
while we deliver this service for you.

Thank you for your support.

New Zealand Government

Unite against COVID-19

From Unite Against COVID-19, New Zealand Government. Available at https://covid19.govt.nz/posters (accessed 01.08.21).

Marketing segments the population into different subgroups based on attitudes and behaviour, as well as cruder socio-economic and demographic variables. Psychographic segmentation helps to reveal patterns or differences between groups of people who may be similar in age, gender or socio-economic status. Knowledge about the target audience's demographic, social and psychographic variables will help to identify their priorities, values, beliefs and lifestyles. This will enable the practitioner to 'package' information in ways that will appeal to them. Table 13.1 shows some ways in which segmentation has been used in recent studies of health behaviour.

Commercial marketing is based on the idea of 'exchange' – that the marketer tries to offer something the consumer wants at an acceptable price. Health promoters are beginning to recognize the importance of formative research, which identifies what people see as the benefits of particular health behaviours, so that these can be incorporated into the campaign message. In a sense this is merely an application of the health belief model (see Chapter 10), which suggests that for people to make a change in their health behaviour they need to see the benefits outweighing the costs (such as time and effort). For example, the marketing of condom use involves acknowledgement of the costs (money, embarrassment and less pleasure) and an emphasis on the benefits (protection against pregnancy and

sexually transmitted infections, a sense of control and less anxiety).

Communicating to the public during the pandemic about simple behavioural protective actions posed enormous challenges and was approached very differently as shown in Learning Activity 13.6. The message needs to be perceived as relevant and credible (credibility may be enhanced by the use of people who are perceived to be experts, for example, medical doctors, or conversely 'people like me'). There also needs to be an appeal to desired values or attributes in order to convince people to act on the information. Commonly used motivating values are youth, energy and attractiveness. The behaviour change also needs to seem possible. This might mean acknowledging that implementing changes to behaviour is not

TABLE 13.1   Psychographic Segmentation and Health Behaviours

Segmentation Type	Used By	Description	Sample Segment
Geodemographic	Mosaic – UK profiling tool[a]	Classifications identify neighbourhood household types and person types based on demographic data (e.g., age, sex, socio-economic status, property characteristics, location) and financial measures indicating behaviour	*Bright Young Things:* well-educated young singles paying high rents to live in smart inner-city apartments
Psychographic	Sport England market segmentation[b]	Used results from the Active People survey to identify 19 sporting segments and better understand the nation's attitudes to sports and motivations for action	*Sports Team Lads:* young blokes enjoying football, pints and pool
Life course	Healthy Foundations[c]	Classification based on life stages which can encourage healthy or unhealthy behaviours; nine life stages were identified	*Young Settlers:* people aged 16–44 who have a partner, no children in the household, no caring responsibilities and are not retired
Pen portraits	Maximizing the appeal of weight management services[d]	Based on interviews and focus groups, this study identified nine people segments based on motivations, barriers and ideal services	*Younger Women:* aspiring to 'body beautiful'; desire a youthful and glamorous service that is active and energizing

From Wills, J., Crichton, N., Lorenc, A., Kelly, M., 2014. Using Population Segment to Inform Local Obesity Strategy in England. Health Promotion International. Available at: https://academic.oup.com/heapro/article/30/3/658/625358. Based on
[a] Experian, 2004. MOSAIC United Kingdom: The Consumer Classification for the UK Experian. Nottingham. Available at: www.experian.co.uk/assets/business.
[b] Sport England, 2009. Market Segmentation. Available at: http://segments.sportengland.org.
[c] Department of Health, 2010a. Ambitions for Health: A Strategic Framework for Maximizing the Potential of Social Marketing and Health Related Behaviour. Department of Health, London.
[d] Department of Health, 2010b. Maximising the Appeal of Weight Management Services. Department of Health, London, Available at: http://webarchive.nationalarchives. gov.uk/20130107105354/http://www.dh.gov.uk/prod_consum_dh/groups/dh_digitalassets/documents/ digitalasset/dh_114723.pdf.

straightforward, and including information on negotiating barriers to change. This section has discussed some of the considerations in developing a message to promote a health behaviour or action and Learning Activity 13.7 asks you to apply this learning to an example.

? Learning Activity 13.7   Social Marketing

How would you go about social marketing to raise awareness of a 'taboo' issue such as incontinence?

Marketing a commercial product is very different from trying to sell health. Advertising typically mobilizes existing predispositions, whereas health promotion typically tries to counter them. For example, advertising associates the product (beer, crisps) with something people desire, such as fun. All too often, health promotion messages are about not indulging, and therefore by implication not having fun (e.g., don't drink and drive, eat less fat). Advertising is selling things in the here and now, to be consumed and enjoyed immediately. By contrast, health promotion messages are often about forgoing present enjoyment for future benefits.

Branding plays a major part in selling commercial products. People buy things not just to satisfy a functional need but also to be seen to identify with a group. A very successful example of the development of a tangible product that indicates support of a cause is the Red Ribbon first used by a small charity in New York in 1991 as a symbol to unite the various groups working to get the AIDS epidemic acknowledged. Its success has led to the wearing of a coloured ribbon being adopted by other groups, for example, those working for awareness of breast cancer use a pink ribbon. Learning Activity 13.8 asks you to reflect on several messages that have been developed to promote organ donation.

? Learning Activity 13.8   Promoting Organ Donation: What's the Message?

Consider the following messages designed to promote organ donation. What is each message? Which do you find most persuasive?

- 'Every day thousands of people who see this page decide to register.'
- 'Three people die every day because there are not enough organ donors.'
- 'You could save or transform up to nine lives as an organ donor.'
- 'If you needed an organ transplant, would you have one? If so, please help others.'

- 'If you support organ donation, please turn your support into action.'

Social Media and Web-Based Technologies

Multimedia tools and other new technologies offer many new opportunities for the dissemination of information. The worldwide web offers the possibility of interactive dialogue and for the public to select the information they require at a time convenient for them. The Pew Internet Project in the USA (www.pewinternet.org and www.pewglobal.org) found that:

- 87% of US adults use the internet
- 90% of US adults own a cell (mobile) phone and 58% own a smartphone
- 95% of adults in China own a cellphone
- 59% of adults in Uganda own a cellphone and 12% own a smartphone
- 28% of people in Nigeria and 30% in Venezuela say they get information about health and medicines from the internet.

The definition of 'social media' is broad, generally referring to internet-based tools that allow individuals and communities to gather and communicate; to share information, ideas, personal messages, images and other content; and, in some cases, to collaborate with other users in real time. Digital technology has progressed from Web 1.0, one way, read only; to Web 2.0, two way and interactive; to the third generation of the internet where communication relies on artificial intelligence and machine learning. The accessibility and immediacy of digital technology allows users to create, collaborate and share information in networks and virtual environments. Social networking sites such as Facebook, YouTube, Instagram and Twitter allow for virtual communication and are settings for health communication. Research Example 13.3 summarizes some of the evidence on digital literacy about health.

Case Study 13.4 outlines a successful initiative to capitalize on the ubiquity of mobile phones and use them to promote maternal health.

Personal wearables, such as the Fitbit, can help to increase physical activity levels as well as helping people set goals and motivate change, although their effectiveness may not be sustained over time (Stephenson et al., 2017). Telemedicine, including the helpline NHS 111, offers a two-way dialogue allowing people who are unable to access primary care to ask questions and get feedback about their symptoms. These new technologies

RESEARCH EXAMPLE 13.3
Digital or eHealth Literacy

Digital or eHealth literacy is the ability to seek, find, understand and appraise health information from electronic sources, and to apply the knowledge gained to addressing or solving a health problem. Individuals may be motivated to go online to obtain health information, find out about health services, prepare for and understand a health consultation, get help in decision-making and find others for emotional support. It is often not a one-way process as individuals can become purveyors of information and engage in conversational platforms in online communities. The figure in this research example shows the ways in which individuals may seek information and support in relation to infertility (Sykes et al., 2020).

Mobile phones are a cheap and accessible tool for health communication. They can be used for text messaging to, for example, improve self-management of long-term conditions, or apps to promote goal setting.

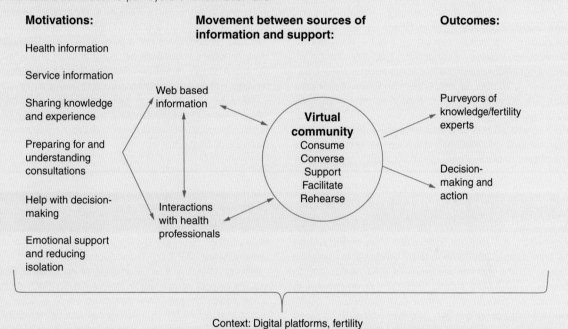

New conceptualization of eHealth literacy in the context of infertility (From Sykes S., Wills J., Frings D., Church S., Wood K., 2020. Multidimensional eHealth literacy for infertility. International Journal of Environmental Research and Public Health 17 (3), 966.)

offer a simulation of human interaction – conversations, the café, support groups – all of which can be harnessed to link health information with the important element of sociability. Telehealth and telecare are platforms to support the self-management of long-term conditions and allow the remote monitoring of patients at home as data can be exchanged from the home to a healthcare professional. Some of the evidence of the effectiveness is provided in Research Example 13.4.

The proliferation of avenues of communication does not necessarily mean that people are better informed about health issues today. Quality control is often absent (e.g., in much of the worldwide web), and even when it exists, the criteria used are often not explicit. A review by Ventola (2014) highlights the potential dangers for practitioners pertaining to the quality of information and reputational damage potentially arising from social media use. Practitioners need to evaluate the quality of any website or social media that they share or advise the public to use. Digital technologies can increase accessibility and enhance health services provision but they can also exacerbate inequalities and emphasize that individuals should be able to manage their health online.

CASE STUDY 13.4
Mobile Midwife in Ghana and Nigeria

In Ghana the need to reduce infant and maternal mortality is acute. In 2008:

- the mortality rate for children under the age of 5 years was 79 per 1000
- the maternal mortality rate was 350 per 100,000
- the percentage of births attended by skilled staff was 57% (the world average was 65% in 2009)
- the adolescent (ages 15–19) fertility rate was 69 per 1000 births.

Mobile Technology for Community Health (Motech) was launched in July 2010 in Ghana by the Grameen Foundation and initially funded by a grant from the Bill & Melinda Gates Foundation (http://www.who.int/woman_child_accountability/ierg/reports/2012_08S_improving_access_to_maternal_child_health_service.pdf). The scheme involves pregnant women registering by providing their phone number, area in which they live, their estimated due date and language preference. They then receive information and advice via text and voice messages, including general information – such as the location of the closest health facility and treatments that they should receive – and messages tailored to their antenatal history.

After each appointment, the nurse updates medical records electronically using a mobile phone. By reviewing a digitally generated monthly report, she can, for example, see who has had the correct vaccinations. This system also means that the health service can gather centralized data on maternal health. A desk-top nurse application has been developed to make it easier to enter large amounts of data, as well as an app for android smartphones.

Mobile technology is not a quick fix – many Ghanaians claim to have a mobile phone, but it is often shared with an entire family, drastically limiting access. Healthcare workers can regard automation such as this as extra work.

The scheme has since being extended to Nigeria (https://www.gsma.com/mobilefordevelopment/wp-content/uploads/2015/06/Connected-Women-Grameen-Case-Study-final.pdf).

RESEARCH EXAMPLE 13.4
Telehealth

Telehealth and telecare involve the use of technology to help people with a long-term condition to maintain independence and feel in control of their health, and to promote health and safety. Telehealth is equipment to monitor people's health in their own homes, for example, a small device that can take readings such as blood pressure, oxygen levels, weight and temperature via a telephone line to a monitoring centre. Telecare includes a system of alarms, sensors and other equipment around the home that detects risks, for example, falls.

A study of the effects of telehealth on people with long-term conditions found that there was a small decrease in admissions to hospital compared with a control group. Other measures of hospital use (elective admissions, out-patient attendances and emergency department visits) were not significantly different between the groups, nor were the differences in notional hospital costs (Steventon et al., 2012). A review by the Centre for Reviews and Dissemination (2013, p. 11) concluded that:

although there is a large amount of evidence evaluating the effects of telehealth interventions, much of it is weak and/or contradictory. However, there is good evidence that telehealth monitoring can reduce mortality in patients with heart failure, particularly those recently discharged from hospital.

The COVID-19 pandemic precipitated a more widespread use of telehealth as healthcare providers sought to minimize the risk of disease transmission whilst maintaining access to care (Monaghesh and Hajizadeh, 2020). Telehealth took the form of live video conferencing or a simple mobile call and allowed for the triaging for consultations and for the collection of routine information in the home about, for example, blood pressure and oxygen levels.

CONCLUSION

Communication tools are a significant resource for health, but one that needs to be understood and used according to priorities. For example, expecting a mass-media campaign to produce large shifts in behaviour and contribute directly to reduced morbidity and mortality is unrealistic. But campaigns can work for health by supporting individual and social change, although effects are often small and generally information seems to have more impact on knowledge and beliefs than on actual behaviour. Some messages that provoke changes in social norms have been effective but, as Robertson (2008) states, it is not clear exactly which messages do this and how.

On an individual level, communication tools such as leaflets and posters can supplement, but not substitute for, one-to-one education and advice. Even with sophisticated marketing and audience research, media remain a fairly blunt instrument with little opportunity for feedback or clarification. However, different media can raise awareness, provide information and motivate people to change if their environment is supportive. The mass media can also be used to advocate for public health by shifting public opinion and encouraging the formation of healthy public policies.

SUMMARY

This chapter has looked at the ways in which health promoters and practitioners communicate about health and the tools they use. It has discussed different strategies, including information giving, advertising as part of a planned campaign, media advocacy and the marketing of health messages. There is now greater awareness of how to use the mass media more effectively, and the chapter looked at how media coverage can be generated and used to influence public opinion. It has reviewed evaluation studies that demonstrate how effective communication combines information with the key element of interaction.

FURTHER READING AND RESOURCES

Atkin, C.K., Rice, R.E., 2014. Theory and principles of media health campaigns. In: Rice, R.E., Atkin, C.K. (eds.), Public Communication Campaigns, fourth edn. Sage, London. An American textbook on designing campaigns that discusses principles such as persuasion and using fear. The book includes examples such as being sun smart, condom use and organ donation.

Corcoran, N. (ed.), 2013. Communicating Health: Strategies for Health Promotion, second edn. Sage, London. Chapter 4 examines the role of mass media in health promotion and engages with practical issues of how to design mass-media campaigns. Social marketing and media advocacy are also discussed.

French, J. (ed.), 2017. Social Marketing and Public Health: Theory and Practice, second edn. Oxford University Press, Oxford. An analysis and case studies of social marketing applied to public health.

O'Neil, I., 2019. Digital Health Promotion: A Critical Introduction. Polity, Bristol. A thoughtful discussion of the positive benefits of modern technologies to health services provision and their challenges in the focus on the individual and neglect of social, environmental and economic determinants of health.

World Health Organization, 2020. Communicating for Health: WHO Strategic Framework for Effective Communications. Available at: https://www.who.int/about/communications.

REFLECTIONS ON PRACTICE

- Think about the last time you used a communication tool with a patient, client or member of the public. How effective do you think it was in supporting your interaction?
- Pick up a commonly used leaflet about a topic of your choice – are its main points clear? Is it attractive and visually appealing? Are the images appropriate, for example, are they representative of a diverse population and non-stereotypical? Is it easy to read with technical terms explained? Is it accurate and up to date in its information and evidence? Is it sponsored, for example, by a commercial company?
- Look at a display in a health facility or other public building. Is it attractive? Is it at eye level? Is it readable from distance? Are the elements in good condition? Are they well positioned?
- Look back at Learning Activity 13.2 and think about what and how those you work with as patients, clients or members of the public learn from the mass media about the health issues that concern them.

FEEDBACK TO LEARNING ACTIVITIES

13.1. Studies of media representations show that alcohol consumption is both frequent and presented as normal and unproblematic, with the portrayal of negative consequences being rare (e.g., Coyne and Ahmed, 2009; Van Hoof et al., 2009). Assumptions that media affects an audience's drinking behaviour are explained by social cognitive theory (Bandura, 1977). This theory suggests that a vicarious learning effect can be induced by media exposure, whereby the observation of a character experiencing a reward or punishment for a specific behaviour, such as drinking, will help viewers build attitudes toward this action and model their own behaviour after it. Views on the effects of the mass media shifted from an early belief that they could produce dramatic changes in attitudes and behaviour to the opposite view, that the media have negligible effects (Gatherer et al., 1979). Today there is a more tempered view, which regards the media as influential in certain circumstances and in specific ways.

13.2. It is likely that the greatest representation of health items, in both factual and entertainment programmes, will be about medicine. As the COVID-19 pandemic has raged across the world perhaps for the first time, public health and health promotion received much media coverage about how they communicate health messages, how they persuade people to adopt behaviour change, and how they test and screen individuals. The tendency to sensationalize means that it is the emotional, the dramatic or the tragic that gets coverage and space. Stories tend to relate to individuals, and issues that concern population groups such as older people, or the determinants of health, tend to be ignored. The emphasis on behavioural journalism means that personalities or real-life case studies are also prominent. Newsworthiness depends less on the importance of an issue than on its immediate impact, which is often heightened by being linked to celebrities in emotive ways. For example, the involvement of celebrity chef Jamie Oliver led to a dramatic increase in media coverage of children's diets and healthy school meals.

13.3. Any information should:
- be suitable for the target audience, for example, culturally sensitive and representative of the intended audience
- be available in different formats, for example, in different languages and in Braille
- be pitched at an appropriate literacy level
- have an effective design and structure
- have accurate and up-to-date content.

13.4. The communication of risk is complex and there are numerous studies assessing understanding. Naik et al. (2012) conclude that loss-framed messages, that is, you are more likely to develop cancer, are more effective than gain-framed messages about living a longer life. They show that people have great difficulty in processing mathematical expressions of probability (e.g., 1:1000), and numeracy is low even among highly educated people, so verbal presentation of risk with use of words such as 'likely' and 'rare' is easier and more effective to use.

13.5. Evaluation of a mass-media campaign to reduce drink-driving could take many forms, for example:
- coverage (the percentage of the target population who were exposed to the message)
- recall (the percentage of the population who could accurately recall the message)
- behaviour (changes in behaviour, such as statistics relating to the incidence of drink-driving)
- incidence of alcohol-related car accidents (this is the main cause for concern and is likely to be better monitored than drink-driving).
- cost-effectiveness of such a campaign.

13.6. 'Hands, face, space' was the public communication campaign from the UK government in September 2020. The order of actions stresses handwashing and mask wearing over physical distancing which has been identified as the critical factor in airborne virus protection. The New Zealand campaign has been praised for presenting a brand – attention-grabbing yellow and white stripes and national solidarity in 'Unite against COVID-19' and the 'Be kind' message (see a critique in the Guardian newspaper https://www.theguardian.com/world/2021/feb/26/words-matter-how-new-zealands-clear-messaging-helped-beat-covid). The central message of the Oregon campaign is 'Don't accidentally kill someone' with the key message being to stay home.

13.7. Social marketing can seek to raise awareness or prompt a behaviour change. For an issue that is rarely discussed in public, the message must be made to seem relevant. It should identify a clear action the audience could take or some form of engagement, and make clear the benefits.

13.8. The first message:
- is intended to act as a social norm – people like themselves are taking the action.
- is framed as a loss
- is framed as a gain
- is that fairness and reciprocity should prompt action
- (e) is addressing the intention-behaviour gap, that people may intend to act and put themselves on an organ donation register or carry a donation card but not get round to it.

REFERENCES

Bala, M., Strzeszynski, L., Cahill, K., 2008. Mass media interventions for smoking cessation in adults. Cochrane Database Syst. Rev. (1), CD004704. Available at: http://onlinelibrary.wiley.com/doi/10.1002/14651858.CD004704.pub3/full.

Bandura, A., 1977. Social Learning Theory. Prentice Hall, Englewood Cliffs, New Jersey.

Beattie, A., 1993. The changing boundaries of health. In: Beattie, A., Gott, M., Jones, L., Sidell, M., (eds.), Health and Wellbeing: A Reader. Macmillan/Open University, Basingstoke.

Brinn, M., Carson, K., Esterman, A., 2010. Mass media interventions for preventing smoking in young people. Cochrane Database Syst. Rev. 11, CD001006.

Britten, N., Stevenson, F.A., Barry, C.A., Barber, N., Bradley, C.P., 2000. Misunderstandings in prescribing decisions in general practice: qualitative study. BMJ 320 (7233), 484–488.

Buckton, C.H., Lean, M.E.J., Combet, E., 2015. 'Language is the source of misunderstandings'–impact of terminology on public perceptions of health promotion messages. BMC Public. Health 15, 579. https://doi.org/10.1186/s12889-015-1884-1.

Centre for Reviews and Dissemination, 2013. Telehealth for People with Long-term Conditions. CRD, York. Available at: https://www.york.ac.uk/media/crd/Telehealth.pdf.

Coulter, A., Ellins, J., Swain, D., Clarke, A., Heron, P., et al., 2006. Assessing the Quality of Information to Support People in Making Decisions about Their Health and Healthcare, Picker Institute. Oxford, Available at: http://www.pickereurope.org/wp-content/uploads/2014/10/Assessing-the-quality-of-information-to-support-people-in-makin.pdf.

Coyne, S.M., Ahmed, T., 2009. Fancy a pint? Alcohol use and smoking in soap operas. Addic. Res. Theory 17, 345–359.

Croker, H., Lucas, R., Wardle, J., 2012. Cluster randomized trial to evaluate the 'Changing for Life' mass media/social marketing campaign in the UJK. BMC Public. Health 12, 404. Available at: http://www.biomedcentral.com/content/pdf/1471-2458-12-404.pdf.

Durkin, S., Brennan, E., Wakefield, M., 2012. Mass media campaigns to promote smoking cessation among adults: an integrative review. Tob. Control. 21, 127–138. Available at: http://m.tobaccocontrol.bmj.com/content/21/2/127.full.pdf.

Gatherer, A., Parfit, J., Porter, E., Vessey, M., 1979. Is Health Education Effective? Health Education Council, London.

Hastings, G., Stead, M., Webb, J., 2004. Fear appeals in social marketing: strategic and ethical reasons for concern. Psychol. Mark. 21, 961–986.

Hicks, J., 2001. The strategy behind Florida's "truth" campaign. Tob. Control. 10, 3–5. Available at: http://m.tobaccocontrol.bmj.com/content/10/1/3.full.pdf.

Katz, E., Lazarsfeld, P., 1955. Personal Influence: The Part Played by People in the Flow of Mass Communication. Free Press, Glencoe, Illinois.

Kessels, R.P., 2003. Patients' memory for medical information. J. R. Soc. Med. 96 (5), 219–222. https://doi.org/10.1258/jrsm.96.5.219. Available at https://www.ncbi.nlm.nih.gov/pmc/articles/PMC539473/pdf/0960219.pdf.

Lupton, D., 2012. Medicine As Culture: Illness, Disease and the Body, third edn. Sage, London.

McLuhan, M., 1964. Understanding media: the extensions of man. Routledge, London.

McKee, M., Gilmore, A.B., Schwalbe, N., 2005. International co-operation and health: part two: making a difference. J. Epidemiol. Community Health 59, 737–739. Available at: http://m.jech.bmj.com/content/59/8/628.full.pdf.

Monaghesh, E., Hajizadeh, A., 2020. The role of telehealth during COVID-19 outbreak: a systematic review based on current evidence. BMC Public. Health 20, 1193. https://doi.org/10.1186/s12889-020-09301-4.

Montazeri, A., McGhee, S., McEwan, J., 1998. Fear inducing and positive image strategies in health education campaigns. Int. J. Health Promotion Educ. 36, 68–75.

Naik, G., Ahmed, H., Edwards, A.G., 2012. Communicating risk to patients and the public. Br. J. Gen. practice: J. R. Coll. Gen. Practitioners 62 (597), 213–216. Available at: https://bjgp.org/content/bjgp/62/597/213.full.pdf.

Public Health England (2019) Stoptober 2019 Campaign evaluation. Available at: https://assets.publishing.service.gov.uk/government/uploads/system/uploads/attachment_data/file/924685/Stoptober_2019_Evaluation__1_.pdf.

Robertson, R., 2008. Using Information to Promote Healthy Behaviours. Kings Fund, London, Available at: http://www.kingsfund.org.uk/sites/files/kf/field/field_document/information-promote-healthy-behaviours-kicking-bad-habits-supporting-paper-ruth-robertson.pdf.

Rogers, E.M., Scott, K.L., 1997. The Diffusion of Innovations Model and Outreach from the National Network of Libraries of Medicine to Native American Communities. Available at: https://communitas.co.za/the-diffusion-of-innovations-model-and-outreach-from-the-national-network-of-libraries-of-medicine-to-native-american-communities-2/.

Stephenson, A., McDonough, S.M., Murphy, M.H., Nugent, C.D., Mair, J.L., 2017. Using computer, mobile and wearable technology enhanced interventions to reduce sedentary behaviour: a systematic review and meta-analysis. Int. J. Behav. Nutr. Phys. Act. 14, 105. https://doi.org/10.1186/s12966-017-0561-4.

Steventon, A., Bardsley, M., Billings, J., Dixon, J., Doll, H., et al., 2012. Effect of telehealth on use of secondary care and mortality: findings from the Whole System Demonstrator cluster randomised trial. BMJ 344, e3874. Available at: http://www.bmj.com/content/344/bmj.e3874.

Sykes, S., Wills, J., Frings, D., Church, S., Wood, K., 2020. Multidimensional ehealth literacy for infertility. Int. J. Env. Res. Public. Health 17 (3), 966.

Van Hoof, J.J., De Jong, M.D., Fennis, B.M., Gosselt, J.F., 2009. There's alcohol in my soap: Portrayal and effects of alcohol use in a popular television series. Health Educ. Res. 24, 421–429. Available at: https://pubmed.ncbi.nlm.nih.gov/18640968/.

Ventola, C.L., 2014. Social media and health care professionals: benefits, risks, and best practices. P T. 39 (7), 491–520. Available at: https://www.ncbi.nlm.nih.gov/pmc/articles/PMC4103576/.

Wammes, B., Oenema, A., Brug, J., 2007. The evaluation of a mass media campaign aimed at weight gain prevention among young Dutch adults. Obesity, 152780–2789. Available at: http://onlinelibrary.wiley.com/doi/10.1038/oby.2007.330/epdf.

Wills, J., Crichton, N., Lorenc, A., Kelly, M., 2014. Using population segment to inform local obesity strategy in England. Health Promot. Int. Available at: https://academic.oup.com/heapro/article/30/3/658/625358.

Vraga, E.K., Jacobsen, K.H., 2020. Strategies for effective health communication during the Coronavirus pandemic and future emerging infectious disease events. World Med. Health Policy 12, 233–241. Available at: https://onlinelibrary.wiley.com/doi/full/10.1002/wmh3.359.

Zarcadoolas, C., Pleasant, A., Greer, D., 2005. Understanding health literacy: an expanded model. Health Promotion Int. 20, 195–203. Available at: https://academic.oup.com/heapro/article/20/2/195/827483.

Settings and Supportive Environments for Health Promotion

Part III focuses on the settings and environments that have the potential to promote health. Our lives are spent in different settings – at school, at work, in neighbourhoods, in our contact with health services and, for some, in prisons. The Ottawa Charter (World Health Organization, 1986, p. 3) stated that 'health is created and lived by people within the settings of their everyday life: where they learn, work, play and love'. One of the five key action areas identified in the Ottawa Charter was creating supportive environments. As we have seen in this book, the focus of health promotion activity is moving away from identifying the diseases and conditions contributing to ill health and the groups at risk and towards identifying the complex interplay of factors which create health. It is in settings – at school or university, at work, in our neighbourhood, in hospital or in prison – that we live our lives, and these settings need to be made more supportive for health.

Health promotion has been carried out in particular settings for many years. Workplaces and schools, for example, have provided established channels to reach defined populations. The COVID-19 pandemic placed an emphasis on online settings to promote health rather than physical settings. The concept of a settings approach to health promotion, however, is quite distinct and first emerged in the 1980s. The settings approach seeks to make systemic changes to the whole environment. This contrasts with using the setting as a convenient route to access individuals and provide traditional health education messages.

The aim of the settings approach is to move beyond individual behavioural change towards changing organizational processes and structures that have an impact on their members' health.

A concern for health is built into the fabric of the system and ensures that the routine activities of the system take account of, and seek to promote, health whenever possible. Adopting a healthy settings approach is fundamentally different to carrying out a one-off short-term health promotion project within a particular setting. This section of the book focuses on approaches to create health promoting settings. Nutbeam (1998) describes a setting as:

> *where people actively use and shape the environment and thus create, or solve problems relating to, health. Settings can normally be identified as having physical boundaries, a range of people with defined roles, and an organizational structure.*

The settings approach is long-term. In most cases it is implemented through defined projects which are designed to:
- introduce specific interventions to create healthy working and living environments
- develop health policies
- integrate health into quality, audit and evaluation procedures in order to build evidence of how health can make the system perform better.

The first and most well-known example of settings-based health promotion is the Healthy Cities project. Originally this was a small project initiated by the World Health Organization in 1986 to put the 'Health for All' and 'Ottawa Charter' principles into practice (World Health Organization 1985; 1986). The Healthy Cities project subsequently expanded to become a worldwide movement incorporating over 1200 cities in more than 30 countries in the European region (https://www.euro.who.int/en/health-topics/environment-and-health/urban-health/who-european-healthy-cities-network). Parallel initiatives have been developed and are coordinated by international networks in schools, hospitals, workplaces, prisons and universities.

The settings approach is complex and characterized by several unique factors (Dooris, 2005):
- an ecological model of health promotion that conceptualizes health as determined by a range of socio-economic, organizational, environmental and personal factors
- a focus on health and well-being rather than illness
- a focus on populations rather than individuals
- a holistic, salutogenic view of health that focuses on how health is created
- a systems perspective that sees settings as complex systems interacting dynamically with their environment and other settings

- a whole-organization focus that seeks change from within the organization.

A key factor behind the interest in the settings approach has been the ecological perspective of health promotion which has expanded beyond the psychological perspectives evident in social marketing, behaviour change and health education. This demands that individuals are not to be treated in isolation from the larger social units in which they live, work and play and the contributions of both behaviour and the environment must be considered in the creation and maintenance of health and well-being, and points to the duality of structure and agency (Dooris et al., 2014).

Implementing health promotion in settings requires the setting itself to change, and Poland et al. (2009) list a series of questions to guide practitioners in their understanding of a setting's features. These include thinking about how the setting (e.g., hospitals) is different from (or similar to) other settings (e.g., schools, workplaces), and how the setting interacts with other related settings and systems as well as the local environment to accomplish its goals. Poland et al. (2009) draw attention to not only the physical and built environment that may be causing ill health in this setting (e.g., through ergonomics, noxious hazards, physical and social isolation or lack of opportunities for access to green space, etc.), but also the psychosocial environment that has a bearing on health and the possibilities for intervention in this setting, for example, the workload and decision latitude, control over pace, status hierarchies and the quality of human relations (trust, reciprocity, local social capital and social cohesion, bullying). As we will see in the following chapters, it is important to consider different stakeholder perspectives on the meaning of health in the setting, and its salience to them.

The benefits of such an approach are hard to quantify but appear to be significant. They include encouraging partnership working and collaboration, embedding health in organizational structures and systems, and taking account of broader determinants of health. Perhaps not surprisingly, given the complexity of this approach, evaluation and evidence of the effectiveness of the settings approach is scanty:

> *The settings approach has been legitimated more through an act of faith than through rigorous research and evaluation studies... much more attention needs to be given to building the evidence and learning from it.*
>
> ***St Leger (1997, p. 100)***

Indeed, if the approach is successful then health would be part of the core business and 'the way things are done round here', so unpicking the contribution of the settings approach is a challenge. The premise of the settings approach is that health is produced outside of health services, where health is not the primary remit. Within organizations there are difficulties in translating the healthy settings philosophy into tangible activities, and barriers to such activities exist regarding structures and finance (Whitelaw et al., 2001).

Each setting is addressed in a separate chapter, but it is important to remember that the settings are not discrete but coexist as part of a wider independent network. Schools, universities, workplaces and hospitals are all sited in neighbourhoods, and there is a constant flow of people within and between the different settings. Prisons, although more separated from their neighbourhoods, are sited in a specific locality and impact upon that locality in terms of employment and transport. There are many other settings where health promotion interventions may be delivered, for example, barber shops and hairdressers, airports (Crimeen et al., 2018), sports clubs (Kokko, 2014) and libraries (Whitelaw et al., 2017).

Each of the following chapters examines why the setting is appropriate for health promotion, identifying how the setting affects health and giving examples of health promoting initiatives, which have been developed in that setting.

REFERENCES

Crimeen, A., de Leeuw, E., Freestone, R., 2018. Towards a health promotion paradigm for airport development. Cities Health 2, 134–144.

Dooris, M., 2005. Healthy settings: challenges to generating evidence of effectiveness. Health Promot. Int. 21, 55–65.

Dooris, M., Wills, J., Newton, J., 2014. Theorising healthy settings: a critical discussion with reference to healthy universities. Scand. J. Public Health 42 (Suppl. 15), 7–16.

Kokko, S., 2014. Sports clubs as settings for health promotion: fundamentals and an overview to research. Scand. J. Public Health 42 (15 Suppl), 60–65.

Nutbeam, D., 1998. Health Promotion Glossary. WHO, Geneva. Available at. http://www.who.int/healthpromotion/about/HPR%20Glossary%201998.pdf?ua=1.

Poland, B., Krupa, G., McCall, D., 2009. Settings for health promotion: an analytic framework to guide intervention design and implementation. Health Promot. Pract. 10 (4), 505–516.

St Leger, L., 1997. Health promoting settings: from Ottawa to Jakarta. Health Promot. Int. 12, 99–101.

Whitelaw, S., Baxendale, A., Bryce, C., MacHardy, L., Young, I., et al., 2001. 'Settings' based health promotion: a review. Health Promot. Int. 16 (4), 339–353.

Whitelaw, S., Coburn, J., Lacey, M., McKee, M.J., Hill, C., 2017. Libraries as 'everyday' settings: the Glasgow *MCISS* project. Health Promot. Int. 32 (5), 891–900.

World Health Organization, 1985. Targets for Health for All. WHO Regional Office for Europe, Copenhagen.

World Health Organization, 1986. Ottawa Charter for Health Promotion. Geneva. Available at: http://www.who.int/healthpromotion/conferences/previous/ottawa/en/.

World Health Organization, Europe. Healthy Cities. Available at: https://www.euro.who.int/en/health-topics/environment-and-health/urban-health/who-european-healthy-cities-network.

Health Promoting Schools

LEARNING OUTCOMES

By the end of this chapter you will be able to:
- understand how health promotion can be incorporated into the school setting
- understand how schools can enhance or inhibit health
- describe the elements of a health promoting school.

KEY CONCEPTS AND DEFINITIONS

Curriculum The lessons and academic content taught in a school or in a specific course or programme.

Health promoting school A health promoting school is one that constantly strengthens its capacity as a healthy setting for living, learning and working. A health promoting school seeks to provide a healthy environment that engages all parties (children, parents, teachers and communities).

PSHE Personal, social, and health education (PSHE) was introduced as part of UK schools' national curriculum in 2000. In 2008 the subject was renamed as personal, social, health and economic education. It includes relationships and sex education (RSE). PSHE promotes healthy living by providing young people with appropriate knowledge, understanding, attitudes and practical skills.

School-based health promotion Health promotion activities that take place within a school setting, for example sex education, traffic awareness education and physical activity sessions.

IMPORTANCE OF THE TOPIC

The view that schools can promote the health and welfare of children and young people has a long history. The development of a school health service, the requirement for school boards to provide meals and, more recently, the inclusion of physical education in the national curriculum and the setting of nutritional standards for school meals are examples of how the school was, and is, seen as a key setting in which a captive audience could be encouraged to adopt lifestyles conducive to good health.

The World Health Organization (WHO) defines a health promoting school (HPS) as one that fosters health and learning; strives to provide a healthy environment; and implements policies and practices that respect well-being and dignity (https://www.who.int/health-topics/health-promoting-schools#tab=tab_1). The school is seen as a total environment in which many of its aspects affect the health of its pupils and staff. Such aspects include its organization, ethos, culture and layout as well as teaching about health issues and the provision of medical and nursing services. Schools also act as referral agencies, signposting children and parents to other health, welfare and voluntary services when appropriate. This chapter looks at how schools, using the curriculum and everyday practices, can be powerful agents in the promotion of young people's physical, mental and social health and well-being.

WHY SCHOOLS ARE A KEY SETTING FOR HEALTH PROMOTION

Education is a resource for health. This is recognized by the WHO, and the United Nations included 'quality education' as one of its 17 Sustainable Development Goals. Health is also a prerequisite for education: 'Children who face violence, hunger, substance abuse, and despair cannot possibly focus on academic excellence. There is no curriculum brilliant enough to compensate for a hungry stomach or distracted mind' (National Action Plan for Comprehensive School Health Education, 1993).

Schools are seen as an important context for health promotion, principally because they reach a large proportion of the population for many years. Most children spend a large proportion of their time in school. Learning health-related knowledge, attitudes and behaviour begins at an early age and is crucial for a healthy life course. As observed by Gugglberger (2021, p. 297) 'turning schools into health promoting settings can therefore be considered as a significantly positive social investment'. Learning Activity 14.1 in this chapter asks you to consider what is the purpose of health promotion in the school setting.

Research Example 14.1 pulls out some of the key findings from a cross-national study of adolescent health and well-being that is now undertaken in over 50 countries.

 Learning Activity 14.1 The Aims of Health Promotion in Schools

Consider each of the following statements about the aims for health promotion for young people, and indicate how important you would rate each aim.

Health promotion should:	Very Important	Important	Not Very Important	Not at all Important
1. Provide information about how the body works				
2. Foster positive personal and social relationships				
3. Teach young people to keep fit and feel good				
4. Equip young people with the skills to make informed and responsible decisions				
5. Inform young people about local services and how to get help				
6. Teach young people about the dangers of certain behaviours, such as taking drugs				
7. Help young people to express their feelings and emotions				
8. Teach young people how to say 'no'				
9. Show young people the wonders of the human body, so they do not damage it				
10. Put young people off unhealthy behaviour by emphasizing the risks to their health				
11. Prepare young people for parenthood				
12. Provide information about human sexuality, puberty and contraception				
13. Teach young people how to reduce their risk from drug taking or sexual activity (i.e., safer sex and safer drug-taking)				
14. Prepare young people to be active citizens				
15. Show young people how to cope with stress				
16. Equip young people with the skills to negotiate, and be assertive in, relationships				
17. Help to build young people's self-esteem				

RESEARCH EXAMPLE 14.1
The Health Behaviour of School-Aged Children Study

The WHO study on health behaviour in school-aged children (HBSC) looks at patterns of health in 43 countries in Europe and North America. The HBSC findings show that those who perceive their school as supportive are more likely to engage in positive health behaviours and have better health outcomes, including lower smoking prevalence.

The latest report in 2020 (https://www.euro.who.int/en/health-topics/Life-stages/child-and-adolescent-health/health-behaviour-in-school-aged-children-hbsc) reveals a rise in adolescents feeling pressured by schoolwork and a decline in young people reporting that they like school. Adolescent mental well-being declines with age, and girls are at particular risk of poor mental health outcomes. Other key findings from this latest study include:

• Risky sexual behaviour remains a concern: one in four adolescents who have sex are having unprotected sex. At age 15, one in four boys (24%) and one in seven girls (14%) report having had sexual intercourse.
• Drinking and smoking have continued to decline among adolescents, but the number of current alcohol and tobacco users remains high among 15-year-olds, with alcohol the most commonly used substance. One in five 15-year-olds (20%) has been drunk twice or more in their lifetime, and almost one in seven (15%) has been drunk in the last 30 days.
• Fewer than one in five adolescents meet the WHO recommendations for physical activity – levels have declined in around one-third of countries since 2014, especially among boys. Participation in physical activity remains particularly low for girls and older adolescents.
• Most adolescents are failing to meet current nutritional recommendations, undermining their capacity for healthy development. Around two out of three adolescents do not eat enough nutrient-rich foods, with one in four eating sweets, and one in six consuming sugary drinks, every day.
• Levels of overweight and obesity have risen since 2014, and now affect one in five young people, with higher levels among boys and younger adolescents. One in four adolescents (predominantly girls) perceive themself to be too fat.

Childhood and adolescence are times of great change, when young people often acquire lifetime habits and attitudes. One function of a healthy school environment is to enable children to develop healthy behaviours. While adolescence is characterized by powerful peer-group attachments, the school setting provides an opportunity to communicate with young people and gives learning opportunities and a safe environment to practise new skills. Learning Activity 14.2 asks you to consider whether and in what circumstances might there be an association between a child's health and their educational development.

 Learning Activity 14.2   The Relationship Between Health and Learning

In what ways might a child's educational potential and achievement be influenced by their health?

HEALTH PROMOTION IN SCHOOLS

The development of health education and promotion in schools has reflected many approaches to health promotion. The medical view of health has dominated health education, which in many countries is almost exclusively concerned with hygiene, nutrition and fitness. Education in the 1960s became more child-centred, and educational methods sought to develop autonomy and responsibility through discovery learning. Health education emerged as a complex theme of well-being and fulfilment of maximum potential. Health promotion in schools is now closely linked to personal and social development, and delivered in the curriculum as personal, social health and economic education (PSHE). The aim is for young people to be in charge of their own lives, and the role of the school is to develop self-esteem and self-awareness. Emphasis is placed on the *process* of education, and finding teaching and learning strategies which encourage reflection and personal awareness. The direction and organization of the health promotion programme also aims to reflect the needs of the children and young people. The provision of PSHE in schools remains patchy, and often focuses on knowledge rather than skills and attitudes. There are many reasons for this, including the lack of training in this subject for teachers, and mixed messages from government regarding the importance of PSHE within the curriculum, for example, PSHE is not a statutory requirement in the UK but is strongly encouraged.

Alongside these attempts to promote autonomy and decision-making skills are more traditional information-giving approaches. Behind such an approach lies the assumption that people are rational decision-makers whose behaviour will change once they have information about how to live more healthily. Much health promotion in schools therefore focuses on the provision of information about the health-damaging effects of certain behaviours, such as smoking and taking drugs.

The provision of sex education in schools reflects these views of health promotion. Sex education is now commonly referred to as 'relationships and sex education' (RSE), in recognition of the need to move away from a focus on biology to a focus on emotional health, values and life skills. RSE is a contentious area and a recent consultation prior to the latest guidance received over 23,000 responses. The Department for Education's latest guidance (DofE, 2019) states that:

- Relationships Education is compulsory in primary schools and Relationships and Sex Education (RSE) is compulsory from age 11 onwards.
- In primary schools, children are taught about respectful relationships with family and friends and online.
- In secondary schools RSE involves teaching about risks such as drugs and alcohol, as well as knowledge about intimate relationships and sex.
- All schools must have a written policy on sex education, which they must make freely available to parents.

The distinction between schools that offer health education and those that are health promoting was made by Young and Williams (1989), and is shown in Table 14.1.

THE HEALTH PROMOTING SCHOOL

Schools are organizations whose core business concerns teaching and learning, the curriculum and students' performance, not the promotion of health. To be health promoting, the school has to be seen as a whole system and its key processes have to be addressed. If education for the health of young people is to focus on more than individual behaviour and be health *promoting*, it needs to acknowledge the influence of the school itself as a health promoting environment and as part of a wider community.

The whole-school context, as illustrated in Fig. 14.1, includes its:

- ethos
- organization and family and community partnerships
- management structures
- relationships and social environment
- physical environment
- taught curriculum.

In the HPS all these aspects will reinforce and support each other, leading to a synergistic effect. In reality, different aspects of the school may give conflicting messages. Many aspects of a school can be health promoting or health inhibiting. Educationalists have long talked of a 'hidden curriculum', and the way in which messages can be transmitted through children's daily experience of their surroundings and relationships at school. For example, the state of many school toilets might suggest that hygiene is not valued, or that pupils do not require (or deserve) cleanliness or care. Knowing that someone (e.g., personal tutor, school nurse) is always available to talk to about any personal concerns, or incidents at

TABLE 14.1 Health Education in School Versus the Health Promoting School	
Traditional Health Education	**The Health Promoting School**
• Health education is delivered in the classroom only	• The whole school and all its activities are considered health promoting
• Emphasizes physical health and hygiene	• Sees health as the interaction of physical, mental, social, emotional and environmental dimensions
• Uses didactic and instructional methods	• Uses participatory methods that seek to empower students
• Tends to respond to perceived problems or crises, for example drug use or violence, on a one-off basis	• Recognizes that skills and processes are common to all health issues and should be incorporated into the curriculum
• Takes little account of psychosocial aspects of health	• Sees the development of positive self-image and self-efficacy as important
• Does not involve parents	• Considers parental support as central
• Views school health services only in relation to disease prevention and screening	• Helps to integrate services within the curriculum and enables students to be consumers of health services

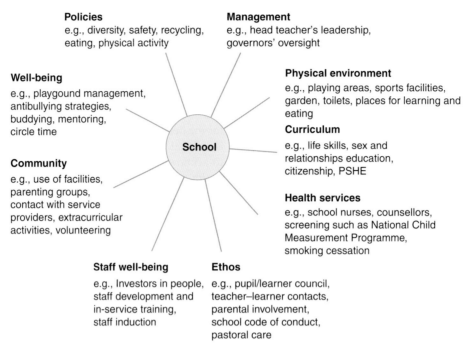

Policies
e.g., diversity, safety, recycling, eating, physical activity

Management
e.g., head teacher's leadership, governors' oversight

Well-being
e.g., playgound management, antibullying strategies, buddying, mentoring, circle time

Physical environment
e.g., playing areas, sports facilities, garden, toilets, places for learning and eating

Curriculum
e.g., life skills, sex and relationships education, citizenship, PSHE

School

Community
e.g., use of facilities, parenting groups, contact with service providers, extracurricular activities, volunteering

Health services
e.g., school nurses, counsellors, screening such as National Child Measurement Programme, smoking cessation

Staff well-being
e.g., Investors in people, staff development and in-service training, staff induction

Ethos
e.g., pupil/learner council, teacher–learner contacts, parental involvement, school code of conduct, pastoral care

Fig. 14.1 The whole-school approach to health promotion

school such as bullying or teasing, is important for children's mental health and well-being.

The International Union of Health Promotion and Education guidelines for HPSs (www.iuhpe.org/images/PUBLICATIONS/THEMATIC/HPS/HPSGuidelines_ENG.pdf) include the following principles:

- promote the health and well-being of students
- uphold social justice and equity concepts
- involve student participation and empowerment
- provide a safe and supportive environment
- link health and education issues and systems
- address the health and well-being issues of staff
- collaborate with the local community
- integrate into the school's ongoing activities
- set realistic goals
- engage parents and families in health promotion.

In common with other settings, effective health promotion in schools depends on it being coordinated and taking place within structured frameworks. Many countries have HPS networks. In England the Healthy Schools rating scheme (https://assets.publishing.service.gov.uk/government/uploads/system/uploads/attachment_data/file/906875/Healthy_schools_rating_scheme.pdf) is a voluntary scheme that recognizes schools' contribution

to supporting children's health and well-being. As with other award schemes for hospitals and workplaces, the Healthy Schools rating scheme encourages institutions to work towards specific targets.

POLICIES AND PRACTICES

The policies that a school develops represent its values. Schools may have policies on equal opportunities, discipline and rewards, health and safety, child protection and safeguarding, bullying, healthy food and various curriculum issues, including sex education. Policies may be merely 'paper exercises' unless they have been influenced by consultation within the school and the community, have been clearly written and disseminated, and are consistently applied. The practices of a school can be evidenced in its daily life and the ways in which decisions are taken. Democratic participation by pupils is a key element in an HPS and Learning Activity 14.3 asks you to consider student participation.

Social Environment

The quality of social interactions among pupils, between staff and pupils and among the staff contributes to the

Learning Activity 14.3   Student Participation in Schools

The Ottawa Charter describes health promotion as a process of 'enabling people to take more control over and improve their health' (WHO, 1986). How can pupils in schools be enabled to make decisions about their education and their health?

ethos or climate in a school. Increasingly, schools are recognizing that healthy schools which value positive relationships, prioritize learning and build self-esteem may also drive up educational standards.

Curriculum

The formal curriculum includes knowledge and understanding of health-related topics (e.g., biology and nutrition) at a level appropriate for pupils' ages and social and cognitive development. The informal curriculum refers to areas not formally taught or examined, including pastoral care and extracurricular activities, in areas such as sports and arts. In England and many other countries there is no statutory provision for health promotion, and its integration into the curriculum is patchy.

Physical Environment

The physical environment and layout of a school may be stimulating or depressing. Learning Activity 14.4 focuses on the playground area of schools. Schools should provide a clean and safe environment with no litter or graffiti, clean toilets and a welcoming but secure entrance. There should be areas for play, for social interaction and for quiet study or reading, including a library. In many countries the provision of basic amenities such as sanitation, water and air cleanliness may be priorities.

Learning Activity 14.4   Health Promoting Playgrounds

Think back to your primary school and try to picture the playground area. Was it a health promoting environment? What would constitute a health promoting playground?

Links With the Community

How well the school communicates and connects with its local community, where its pupils and their families live, is an important criterion for the HPS. Partnerships with parents may vary from information about school events, fundraising requests and consultation about uniform or meals' provision to the active involvement of all parents in decision-making about the curriculum, pastoral care and resource issues. Parents may also become involved in school life through reading schemes, practical parenting classes and breakfast clubs. Learning Activity 14.5 asks you to consider and discuss what a HPS would be doing in relation to healthy eating. Schools are part of a wider community and should be open to that community. Many agencies and services can provide support to schools. For example, the police and emergency services often provide educational sessions concerning accident prevention.

Learning Activity 14.5   School Healthy-Eating Policies

In the broad areas of policy, curriculum, social and physical environment and community links, what would demonstrate that the school was health promoting in its approach to healthy eating?

Effective Interventions

Health promotion interventions in schools differ substantially in their nature, ranging from programmes providing physiological information and life skills to abstinence-oriented programmes, in addition to the comprehensive whole-school approaches outlined above. Many curriculum programmes aim to have outcomes relevant to risk reduction, such as increased knowledge or changes in behaviour. They may have a focus on building resilience and improving mental health. Programmes may thus be specific to a particular health issue (e.g., smoking education) or more generic life-skills programmes, aiming to develop self-esteem and social and communication skills. They may target pupils only, or extend their reach to include teachers, parents and the wider community.

Schools are dynamic communities, and there are many varied influences on young people both within and outside the school setting, so demonstrating the particular effect of health promotion programmes is extremely difficult. The majority of interventions aim to develop health-enhancing behaviours. These health outcomes will not be apparent until later in life. For example, the Australian 'no hat – no play' policy will not demonstrate an effect on skin cancer rates until well into adulthood. Evidence shows that increasing children's knowledge is feasible, but changing their attitudes and behaviour, even in the short term, is far more difficult (Lister-Sharp et al., 1999).

A Cochrane review of HPSs (Langford et al., 2015) found that the settings approach was effective for certain outcomes related to fruit and vegetable intake, tobacco use, physical activity and bullying. An earlier review (Stewart-Brown, 2006) found that mental health promotion programmes were among the most effective. Factors associated with increased effectiveness included long duration, high intensity, involvement of the whole school, a focus on the school environment, multifactorial interventions and peer-led health promotion (Stewart-Brown, 2006). There is evidence that integrated, holistic and strategic programmes are more effective than classroom education programmes (St Leger, 2005).

Reviews do show that the implementation of HPS varies and often includes only some elements. There are many practical difficulties associated with implementing a whole school approach, and for many teachers and school staff, health promotion is just one of many issues that need to be considered within the school's remit as a provider of education (Mannix-McNamara and Simovska, 2015).

CONCLUSION

Schools are widely seen as playing a key role in health promotion. Young people are seen as a key target group for the provision of information and encouragement of responsible and health promoting attitudes and behaviour. The habits acquired in childhood and adolescence may prove influential for the rest of one's life course. Research suggests that narrow information-based programmes are less effective than broader programmes that address the school as a whole. This is the direction taken by the HPS initiative, which seeks to promote a whole-school approach, encompassing not just the formal curriculum but also the informal curriculum, the school's physical and social environment, and its links with its community. The evolving evidence base suggests that the HPS approach is effective and contributes to children and young people's health, education and welfare.

REFLECTIONS ON PRACTICE

- You are asked to produce a strategy to make your old school, or a school you are working with, an HPS. How would you go about this task? What areas would you prioritize, and why? How would you integrate the following health promotion principles within school structures:
  - equity
  - empowerment
  - collaboration
  - participation.

SUMMARY

This chapter has examined why schools are a key setting for health promotion. Health and education have a reciprocal relationship, so enhancing either one will impact favourably on the other. The holistic HPS approach has been identified as providing the most promising strategy. There is an accumulating evidence base to support the whole-school integrated approach.

FURTHER READING AND RESOURCES

Green, J., Cross, R., Woodall, J., Tones, K., 2019. Health Promotion: Planning and Strategies, fourth edn. Sage, London. *Chapter 10, pp. 497–526 focuses on settings.*

Langford, R., Bonell, C.P., Jones, H.E., Pouliou, T., Murphy, S.M., et al., 2015. The WHO Health Promoting School Framework: A Cochrane Systematic Review and Meta-analysis. Cochrane Collaboration. Wiley. Available at: https://bmcpublichealth.biomedcentral.com/articles/10.1186/s12889-015-1360-y. *A systematic review of studies of health promoting schools.*

Samdal, O., Rowling, L. (eds.), 2012. The Implementation of Health Promoting Schools. Routledge, London. *Developing a 'healthy school' has been a key aim for many schools across the globe. This edited book shows how guidelines can best be implemented by building upon scientific knowledge of 'implementation theory', as well as empirically-based practice from health promoting school initiatives.*

Whitman, C., Aldinger, C., 2009. Case Studies in Global School Health Promotion. Springer, USA. *A review of case examples from over 20 developing and developed countries.*

The Schools for Health in Europe network supports the development of school health promotion: www.schools-for-health.eu/she-network.

Many countries have networks and/or guidance to provide information and good practice, for example

Scotland: https://www.gov.scot/policies/schools/wellbeing-in-schools/.

New Zealand: hps.tki.org.nz/.

Australia: https://www.achper.org.au/advocacy/australian-health-promoting-schools.

Canada: https://phecanada.ca/activate/healthy-school-communities.

South Africa: https://www.afro.who.int/sites/default/files/2018-02/2014-03-06-the-healthy-schools-programme-in-south-africa.pdf.

FEEDBACK ON LEARNING ACTIVITIES

14.1. Children spend a large proportion of their waking lives in school, so it is an important setting for them. Schools can create a healthy environment, for example by providing healthy lunches and snacks and encouraging children to walk to school. The school curriculum can also foster health, for example by teaching children about healthy lifestyles. The school ethos is important in fostering self-respect and helping children to be happy and healthy.

14.2. There is a relationship between health and education and the ability to learn. Young people's experiences in school influence the development of their self-esteem, self-perception and health behaviours. Pupils with low school performance and educational aspirations and high levels of absence from school are more likely to engage in earlier risk-taking behaviour such as drug use. School attendance is particularly important, and provision of food at school, for example through breakfast clubs, can improve attendance rates. Equally, health can impact on educational performance

(e.g., https://www.gov.uk/government/publications/breakfast-clubs-in-high-deprivation-schools)

14.3. Participation is recognized as a desirable feature in school inspections. Participation can range from supporting children to express their views to enabling them to share decision-making through school councils.

14.4. Health promoting playgrounds seek to encourage children to be active. Strategies include playground markings for games; child 'buddies' to discourage bullying; areas for reflection; and protection from the sun (e.g., Australia has a 'no hat – no play' policy).

14.5. Indicators of a school healthy-eating policy might include:
- a whole-school food policy
- a welcoming eating environment
- consultation with children about food choices
- a breakfast club
- water fountains to promote hydration and reduce plastic waste
- healthy school lunches with fruit and vegetables and low levels of salt, sugar and fat.

REFERENCES

Department for Education, 2019. Relationships Education, Relationships and Sex Education (RSE) and Health. HMSO, London. Available at: https://assets.publishing.service.gov.uk/government/uploads/system/uploads/attachment_data/file/908013/Relationships_Education__Relationships_and_Sex_Education__RSE__and_Health_Education.pdf.

Gugglberger, L., 2021. A brief overview of a wide framework—Health promoting schools: a curated collection. Health Promotion Int. 36 (2), 297–302.

Langford, R., Bonell, C.P., Jones, H.E., Pouliou, T., Murphy, S.M., et al., 2015. The WHO Health Promoting School Framework: A Cochrane Systematic Review and Meta-analysis. Cochrane Collaboration. Wiley. Available at: https://bmcpublichealth.biomedcentral.com/articles/10.1186/s12889-015-1360-y.

Lister-Sharp, D., Chapman, S., Stewart-Brown, S., Sowden, A., 1999. Health promoting schools and health promotion in schools: two systematic reviews. Health Technol. Assess. 3 (22).

Available at: http://www.journalslibrary.nihr.ac.uk/__data/assets/pdf_file/0010/64657/FullReport-hta3220.pdf.

Mannix-McNamara, P., Simovska, V., 2015. Schools for health and sustainability: Insights from the past, present and for the future. In: Mannix-McNamara, Simovska V. (ed.), Schools for Health and Sustainability. Springer, pp. 3–17.

National Action Plan for Comprehensive School Health Education, 1993. Working together for the future: 1992 comprehensive school health education workshop. J. Sch. Health 63, 46–66.

Stewart-Brown, S., 2006. What Is the Evidence on School Health Promotion in Improving Health or Preventing Disease and, Specifically, What Is the Effectiveness of the Health Promoting School Approach. WHO, Copenhagen.

St Leger, L., 2005. Protocols and guidelines for health promoting schools. Promotion Educ. 12 (3–4), 145–146.

World Health Organization, 1986. Ottawa Charter for Health Promotion. WHO, Geneva. Available at: http://www.who.int/healthpromotion/conferences/previous/ottawa/en/.

Young, I., Williams, T., 1989. The Healthy School. Scottish Health Education Group, Edinburgh.

Health Promoting Universities

By the end of this chapter you will be able to:
- understand how health promotion can be incorporated into the university setting
- understand how universities can enhance or inhibit health
- understand a whole system approach to health promoting universities.

Health promoting university (HPU) An HPU aims to create a learning environment and organizational culture that enhances health, well-being and sustainability. Some authors make a distinction between an HPU and a healthy university, which refers to a state of health and well-being for everyone at a university.

Whole systems approach A whole systems approach encourages individuals and organizations to understand the complex relationships and contexts surrounding social and health issues in order to best influence and navigate the system.

IMPORTANCE OF THE TOPIC

The rationale for seeking to improve health through the settings within which people live their lives is based on an ecological model of health, where health is determined by many interacting social and environmental factors. The university setting defines the population targeted for intervention – students, staff, all university workers and the local community. The channels for predisposing, enabling and reinforcing positive health behaviours of these targeted populations are shown in the PRECEDE model of implementation outlined in Chapter 22. The setting will 'define the position of health promotion relative to the core business of the setting in question, which shapes the incentives required to assure the cooperation of the setting' (Kokko et al., 2014, p. 495). A systems perspective and whole system focus recognizes that investment for health can contribute positively to a setting's performance and to the delivery of its core goals. A systems perspective demands a focus not only on the learning environment of the university, but also on its organizational culture.

Higher education institutions (HEIs) have often served as settings for projects and interventions on topical issues, such as drugs, alcohol, sexual health, student mental well-being and workplace health. Universities are, like many other communities and organizations, influenced by a range of factors including norms, social networks, patterns of leadership and physical, economic and cultural environments.

This whole university approach embraced by Healthy Universities has three overarching aims (https://healthyuniversities.ac.uk/healthy-universities/):
- to create healthy, supportive and sustainable learning, working and living environments for students, staff and visitors

- to increase the profile of health and sustainability in the university's core business – its learning, research and knowledge exchange
- to connect with, and contribute to, the health, well-being and sustainability of the wider community.

Several documents have been developed to guide universities towards becoming an HPU. In 1998, the European Regional Office of World Health Organization (WHO) published the experiences of English universities to inspire other universities in Europe to implement HPUs (Tsouros et al., 1998). In 2005, the Edmonton Charter reinforced the definition and principles of an HPU and proposed objectives to be pursued by HPUs (WHO, 2006). Ten years later, the Okanagan Charter consolidated the key principles of an HPU. The Okanagan Charter (2015; https://open.library.ubc.ca/cIRcle/collections/53926/items/1.0132754) is an international guide for HPUs and campuses, which defines them as 'infusing health into everyday operations, business practises and academic mandates'. HPUs enhance the success of our institutions; create campus cultures of compassion, well-being, equity and social justice; improve the health of the people who live, learn, work, play and love on our campuses; and strengthen the ecological, social and economic sustainability of our communities and wider society.

WHY THE UNIVERSITY IS A KEY SETTING

There are 167 HEIs in the UK, with almost 2.5 million students from increasingly diverse backgrounds and more than 400,000 staff (https://www.hesa.ac.uk/). There are 39 universities in Australia with over 1.3 million enrolled students and 100,000 employees. The higher education sector therefore offers enormous potential for the promotion of health and well-being.

Universities are large complex settings within which people learn, work and live. There are four main reasons why universities should aim to be health promoting settings:

1. **Enhancing learning**: Evidence from settings such as schools and workplaces suggests that having healthy learners and staff increases levels of achievement, performance, productivity and reputation – thereby helping universities conduct their core business more effectively.

2. **Health improvement**: Through their roles in education, research, knowledge exchange and community engagement, universities have the potential to make a significant contribution to the long-term health improvement of the population.

3. **Social and civic responsibility** Universities can also act as a wider 'generator' of health and well-being in society – through acting as socially and environmentally responsible corporate citizens; and through helping shape the views, values, aspirations and priorities of future decision-makers and community leaders.

4. **Building citizenship:** University provides the opportunity to explore and experiment with new experiences, build life skills, clarify values and develop potential for individuals, many of whom may be living away from home for the first time and transitioning from childhood to adulthood without the close support of family. The move towards widening access to higher education has also resulted in an increasingly diverse student profile with a corresponding focus on the student experience.

In Chapter 14 you were asked to consider the aims of health promotion in that setting and so Learning Activity 15.1 asks you to consider and discuss what would be the aims of a health promoting university.

THE HEALTH PROMOTING UNIVERSITY

As with schools, there are several aspects of the university that can enhance or inhibit health, as shown in Fig. 15.1. Universities are much larger organizations than schools, with academic and administrative staff and students at different stages of their higher education. Universities have strong associations with a place and will have links with other organizations within the setting, such as hospitals and health services, colleges and employing organizations.

The activities of any organization take place at three levels: macro, meso and micro. For a university, the macro level encompasses the overall policies and orientation of activities. The meso level relates to the activities managed by the university, for example facilities and services, and also its research and knowledge exchange activities. The micro level refers to activities conducted by staff (academic, administrative and those responsible for health and well-being),

Learning Activity 15.1   The Aims of a Health Promoting University

Consider each of the following statements about the aims of a health promoting university and indicate how important you would rate each.

A Healthy University Should:	Very Important	Important	Not Very Important	Not Important At All
1. Provide a mental well-being service with counsellors for students				
2. Have nutritional standards and labelling for its catering services				
3. Have student representation on all executive boards				
4. Have an active travel policy providing healthy routes to campus				
5. Have green space				
6. Hold health days/fairs, e.g., mental health day				
7. Have clean toilets				
8. Have accessible and supportive staff				
9. Have protected working time for staff and tenured posts				
10. Have a health theme across the curricula				
11. Have a policy to deal with drunkenness on campus				
12. Have an on-site sexual-health service				
13. Have a safe and secure campus with CCTV, patrols and lighting				
14. Have swift and transparent systems for investigation into allegations of sexual harassment or bullying				

 Learning Activity 15.2   The Characteristics of a Health Promoting University

Think about your own university or college. To what extent and in what ways is it a healthy university?

 Learning Activity 15.3   Similarities and Differences Between a Health Promoting School and a Health Promoting University

Look back at Fig. 14.1 that shows the whole school approach to health promotion. What are the similarities and differences to Fig. 15.1 on the healthy university?

which guide and support the education and health of students.

1. *Policies*

Universities may have policies on numerous issues that affect health and well-being, for example equality and diversity, harassment and bullying,

as well as the regulation of unhealthy products and the encouragement of healthy lifestyles including physical activity. A whole-system approach is one where health is an integral part of all the university's activities. The promotion of health should be visible and identifiable in the university's mission statement and all its processes. Research Example 15.1 focuses on actions taken in UK HEIs towards alcohol and Case Study 15.1 describes a university's actions to promote healthy eating.

2. *Physical environment*

Four aspects are cited in reviews of healthy universities (Suárez-Reyes and Van den Broucke, 2016): green spaces, cafeterias, places to study and rest and opportunities for physical activity. Additionally, to promote sustainability, there is more emphasis on safer travel and the encouragement of cycling where feasible. How healthy food and drink is procured, cooked and served, considering environmental and social issues, and how students and staff are enabled to make informed choices, are all aspects of a healthy university. Case Study 15.1

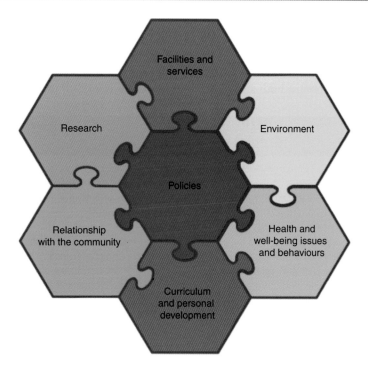

◆ Facilities and services, e.g., on-site gym, fruit truck, water stations, on-site health service

◇ Health and well-being issues, e.g., student representation, staff working practices

◇ Research, e.g., interdisciplinary and focused on the grand challenges of health and well-being

◇ Environment, e.g., green space, gardening opportunities, sustainable, building design incorporating study and rest space

◆ Curriculum, e.g., health across all fields

◇ Community, e.g., having a civic responsibility, providing services, sharing facilities

◆ Policies, e.g., equality and diversity, alcohol

Fig. 15.1 The health promoting university

RESEARCH EXAMPLE 15.1
Alcohol and Universities

A review of actions at UK higher education institutions (HEIs) (Orme and Coghill, 2014) found that:

- Six HEIs reported having a policy specifically related to alcohol. A further three had documented procedures for dealing with excess consumption of alcohol amongst their students.
- Several discouraged alcohol-promotion type activities, such as drinking games and 'happy hour'.
- Three HEIs offered non-alcohol-focused social events.

Initiatives aimed at promoting sensible drinking included:

1. Promotional material relating to sensible drinking and alcohol-free areas mailed out to all freshers from the students' union
2. Alcohol-free events and soft drinks promotions.

3. Working with local police and retailers to reduce alcohol-related antisocial behaviour
4. Protocols to report alcohol-related antisocial behaviour
5. Training sport and social committee members in sensible drinking strategies to discourage irresponsible drinking
6. Training on-campus bar staff in the responsible retailing of alcohol, management techniques and how to deal with intoxicated customers.

Orme and Coghill (2014, p. 199) argue that 'university students are future leaders and policy-makers, and their learning and experiences will inform future policies which in turn will impact on future populations. For these reasons, higher education is a key setting in which to explore how sensible drinking patterns can be facilitated and embedded in people's lifestyles.'

outlines how one campus-based university attempted to improve its catering and food provision.

3. *Health and well-being issues and ethos*

A university can contribute to a sense of powerlessness and a feeling of neglect amongst both staff and students. A key finding of Newton et al.'s (2016) case study was that both staff and students understood the characteristics of a healthy university to include management processes relating to communication and a respectful organizational ethos. This

---

CASE STUDY 15.1
Healthy University and Food

This case study about one campus-based university – the University of the West of England (UWE) – was collected by the healthy universities network in the UK (https://healthyuniversities.ac.uk/wp-content/uploads/2016/10/food_and_health_at_uwe_case_study.pdf):

- Access to fresh fruit and vegetables is enhanced by the market stalls on campus every day at some sites.
- New catering partners encourage staff and students to take proper breaks from work and study. Improving access to a wider choice of healthy food and drinks is a continual process.
- UWE is a Fairtrade university and its catering services provide Fairtrade tea and coffee in all outlets.
- Staff can order locally sourced menus.
- Support for students to improve their cooking skills is available through cookery demonstrations and taster sessions.

- Disposable cup usage is reduced by encouraging staff and students to 'use their mug for the environment' and rewarding those who recycle their cups with a reduced tariff.
- The availability of filtered still and sparkling bottled water has reduced the use of plastic water bottles in all meetings and conferences.
- The research agenda in the area of food and health is strong and includes externally funded multidisciplinary research projects involving public health, environmental health, the built environment and psychology. The integration of different perspectives of this work within multiple curricula can enhance student learning.

The figure in this case study shows some of the ways in which food and its provision would need to be addressed across all the layers of the university setting.

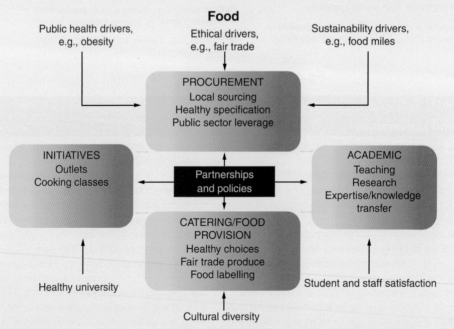

Addressing food and health in a health-promoting university (From Dooris, M., Powell, S., Parkin, D., Farrier, A., 2021. Health promoting universities: effective leadership for health, well-being and sustainability. Health Education 121(3), 295–310. Available at: https://doi.org/10.1108/HE-12-2020-0121.)

was described by students as feeling valued, being listened to, having their concerns addressed and having access to formal mechanisms for complaints.

4. *Community*

Universities can be seen as anchor institutions in their communities and cities. This term was also used in Chapter 9 to describe the NHS. The term 'anchor institutions' is used to refer to organizations which:

- Have an important presence in a place. Universities are large-scale employers, often the largest purchasers of goods and services in the locality and have control over large areas of land and buildings.
- Are tied to a particular place by their mission, histories, physical assets and local relationships. Universities that adopt a place-based approach can improve social mobility, making higher education as accessible as possible to those in the area. It can help develop strong partnerships between the university and local and regional organizations that can help set up student placements and nurture links to local employers.

5. *Facilities and services*

Providing services, especially health services, specifically for students has challenges. As students move between a family doctor or GP and university services, information about their condition and treatment may not travel with them. This means that students either need to repeat their situation several times, acting as their own case co-ordinators, and access treatment and support with incomplete information or not access it at all. Young people at university are adults, and parents and carers may be frustrated in their efforts to support a young person (e.g., in mental health support), by issues of data protection and consent.

EFFECTIVENESS OF THE HEALTH PROMOTING UNIVERSITY

Newton et al. (2016) offer several explanations as to why the HPU approach has been slow to be taken up, especially by comparison to healthy schools. One explanation is the paucity of evidence for the effectiveness of the settings approach, both generally and with regard to healthy universities in particular (Dooris, 2005). Another explanation is that although universities have enormous potential to increase staff, student and community well-being, it is a challenge to demonstrate the added value of the whole-system healthy universities

approach, both for health and for the 'core business' of higher education. A key driver for the healthy schools movement was to be publicly acknowledged as such and awarded for the achievement of standards, and this has been slow to take off in relation to universities, although the Green Gown awards recognize sustainability initiatives in universities and colleges (https://www.greengownawards.org/about and https://www.greengownawards.org/green-gown-awards-australasia). By contrast, the Okanagan Charter is largely unknown in the UK and is not widely used as a lever for action (Dooris et al., 2021).

? Learning Activity 15.4 Universities and the COVID-19 Pandemic

In what ways have universities been impacted by the COVID-19 pandemic? How might the legacy of the pandemic contribute to universities becoming more health promoting?

IMPLEMENTING THE HEALTHY UNIVERSITY

To implement the HPU framework, several key elements must be addressed:

- The context, for example, size of university, its culture, its mission
- Leadership, for example, structure of senior management, nature of senior roles
- Funding and coordination
- The 'business model' and how health aligns with other strategic objectives.

The application of the whole-systems approach as a key element of a successful HPU implementation reinforces the idea that health is everyone's responsibility, and that the initiative targets all members of the university community. For health and well-being to become a strategic priority means finding 'appropriate entry points and windows of opportunity for agenda-setting; engaging with strategic planning cycles; utilizing the potential offered by organizational change; advocating for health to be within a senior leader's role and embedded in multiple roles across the university and learning to navigate the large-scale and complex nature of universities' (Dooris et al., 2021, p. 304).

Routes to implementing a whole university and whole system approach are shown in Fig. 15.2

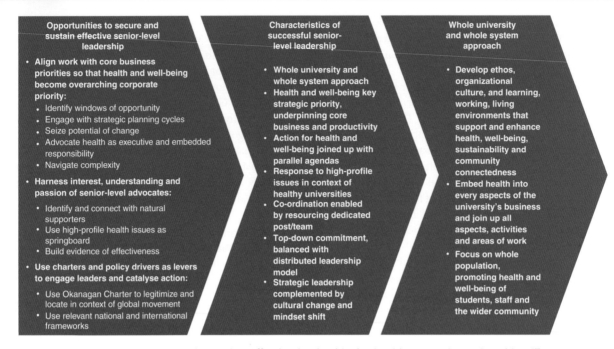

Fig. 15.2 Developing and securing effective leadership for health promoting universities (From Dooris, M., Powell, S., Parkin, D., Farrier, A., 2021. Health promoting universities: effective leadership for health, wellbeing and sustainability. Health Education 121 (3), 299.)

CONCLUSIONS

It is often concluded that universities provide an ideal health promoting environment as students are in a learning environment with numerous facilities and many are of an age when behaviours that impact on health in later life can be improved (see e.g., Plotnikoff et al., 2015). Many initiatives are included under the settings label, even when they might be focussed on individual-based health promotion activities, such as awareness campaigns about HIV/AIDS or mental health, which are delivered in the university as the channel or portal (Suárez-Reyes and Van den Broucke, 2016). A settings approach emphasizes the health determinants and decision-making processes of the university (e.g., active participation).

Universities operate within constantly changing economic contexts and policy environments and what constitutes success spans their research, teaching, enterprise, civic engagement and internationalization. A recent article (Dooris et al., 2021, p. 305) emphasizes the importance of

knitting together agendas in a positive way ...... with effective leadership involving a recognition that more can be achieved by connecting health with parallel agendas such as sustainability, resilience, equality and diversity – and by taking a proactive, integrated and even sometimes "opportunistic" approach to high-profile concerns such as student mental well-being.

Dooris et al. (2021) argue that a health promoting university can bridge core and aspirational values, and unite under one strategy the pressing agendas of climate emergency commitments and student mental health.

REFLECTION ON PRACTICE

Think about the university in which you last studied – was there attention to the health of students (and/or staff)? Where was this evident?

SUMMARY

This chapter has described the characteristics of an HPU and why it is a challenging approach to implement in large and complex organizations with many agendas. The whole-university approach is characterized as building a broad understanding and framing of health, developing a supportive ethos and culture, embedding health within the university and joining up areas of work on for example, sustainability and mental health. In common with other settings that aim to be health promoting, key questions are asked about how health is or could be created in the university and how health promotion can be introduced and embedded into the setting (Dooris et al., 2014).

FURTHER READING AND RESOURCES

Healthy university networks have a number of guides and resources:
https://healthyuniversities.ac.uk/wp-content/uploads/2016/10/HU-Final_Report-FINAL_v21.pdf
https://www.healthpromotingcampuses.org/okanagan-charter-2/

FEEDBACK TO LEARNING ACTIVITIES

15.1. Health promoting university initiatives are often directed at the most common health problems of young people – mental health, sexual health and alcohol misuse.

15.2. A review by Holt et al. (2015) found that students had a focused expectation of what a healthy university should be like, with an emphasis on healthy catering, the provision of water and a green and clean environment. By contrast, a study by Newton et al. (2016) found that staff and students placed a much greater emphasis on the social environment and feelings of being valued.

15.3. As a setting relates to its context you might expect the educational settings of schools and universities to share elements. A review by Kokko et al. (2014) of settings-based practices in cities, schools, universities, hospitals, workplaces and prisons mapped out some shared characteristics and setting-specific factors. First, the Ottawa Charter (1986) and its five action areas have provided the frame for all the settings-based models. Second, in all the cases the settings are broad and complex entities, which emphasizes a need for multi-level actions. Third, the focus is primarily on organizational change and settings-based factors that can generate this change.

15.4. During the COVID-19 pandemic most universities offer blended learning, trying to maintain a high quality student experience at a distance. In addition to prioritizing the long-term mental health and the safety of staff and students, many universities become centres in the wider community as testing facilities. There are however significant sustainability benefits as universities reduce their energy use and commuting and business travel, and experiment with new ways of educating and communicating.

REFERENCES

Dooris, M., 2005. Healthy settings: challenges to generating evidence of effectiveness. Health Promot. Int. 21 (1), 55–65.

Dooris, M., Wills, J., Newton, J., 2014. Theorising healthy settings: a critical discussion with reference to healthy universities. Scand. J. Public. Health 42 (Suppl 15), 7–16.

Dooris, M., Powell, S., Parkin, D., Farrier, A., 2021. Health promoting universities: effective leadership for health, wellbeing and sustainability. Health Educ. 121 (3), 295–310.

Holt, M., Monk, R., Powell, S., Dooris, M., 2015. Student perceptions of a healthy university. Public. Health. 129, 674–683.

Kokko, S., Green, L.W., Kannas, L., 2014. A review of settings-based health promotion with applications to sports clubs. Health Promot. Int. 29 (3), 494–509.

Newton, J., Dooris, M., Wills, J., 2016. Healthy universities: an example of a whole-system health-promoting setting. Glob. Health Promot. 23 (Suppl. 1), 57–65.

Orme, J., Coghill, N., 2014. Wasted potential: the role of higher education institutions in supporting safe, sensible and social drinking among students. Health Educ. J. 73 (2), 192–200.

Plotnikoff, R.C., Costigan, S.A., Williams, R.L., Hutchesson, M.J., Kennedy, S.G., et al., 2015. Effectiveness of interventions targeting physical activity, nutrition and healthy weight for university and college students: a systematic review and meta-analysis. Int. J. Behav. Nutr. Phys. Act. 12, 45.

Suárez-Reyes, M., Van den Broucke, S., 2016 Marr. Implementing the Health Promoting University approach in culturally different contexts: a systematic review. Glob. Health Promot. 23 (1 Suppl), 46–56.

Tsouros, A., Dowding, G., Thomson, J., Dooris, M. (eds.), 1998. Health Promoting Universities. WHO Regional Office for Europe, Copenhagen. Available at: http://www.euro.who.int/document/e60163.pdf.

WHO, 2006. The Edmonton Charter for Health Promoting Universities and Institutes for Higher Education. Available at: http://www.gesundheitsfoerdernde-hochschulen.de/Inhalte/E_Gefoe_HS_internat/2005_Edmonton_Charter_HPU.pdf (accessed 04-05-21).

Health Promoting Workplaces

LEARNING OUTCOMES

By the end of this chapter you will be able to:
- describe the relationship between work and health
- understand how the workplace can enhance or inhibit health
- describe the elements of a health promoting workplace.

KEY CONCEPTS AND DEFINITIONS

Employer A person or business that employs one or more people and pays that person or people wages or a salary.

SME A small- or medium-sized enterprise. Definitions vary but in the UK this means less than 50 employees.

Work A job or paid employment. It may include unpaid or voluntary work, education and training, and caring.

Worker A person employed to carry out specific functions, usually in return for a wage or salary.

Workplace The physical environment where work takes place.

IMPORTANCE OF THE TOPIC

A comprehensive review found that work is good for health (Black, 2008). A key recommendation of the review was to encourage people to remain in work and those who were off sick to return to work. The workplace is significant both in affecting people's health and as a context in which to promote health. At the same time, many people are trapped in low-quality and poorly paid jobs, which have been shown to be bad for health (Institute of Health Equity, 2015).

Office of National Statistics data for the UK for the first quarter of 2021 show that 75.1% of people aged 16 to 64 were in work, 1.4 percentage points lower than the previous year. Promoting health in the workplace will therefore reach a large percentage of the adult population, and will impact on a setting where many adults spend a considerable amount of their time.

This chapter looks at the workplace as a social system and explores how it can contribute to health or ill health. The chapter reviews how health promotion has been implemented in the workplace. Most health promotion interventions have tended to focus on individual lifestyle risk factors and employers' legal responsibilities to provide a safe working environment. Interventions that address the workplace organization and culture as a whole are less common, but evaluation shows they are more effective. The different partners and stakeholders involved in workplace health promotion are identified, and their contribution to interventions discussed.

WHY IS THE WORKPLACE A KEY SETTING FOR HEALTH PROMOTION?

A global survey of workplace health promotion strategies (www.ncbi.nlm.nih.gov/pubmed/18173386) found that improving productivity and reducing staff absence rates were the main priorities. There are five main reasons for prioritizing the workplace:

1. The workplace gives access to a target group – healthy adults, especially men – who are often difficult to reach in other ways. Employees in the workplace are a captive audience. It is easy to follow up interventions in the workplace and encourage participation in health programmes because there are established modes of communication. The cohesion of the working community also provides peer pressure and support.

2. Promoting health in the workplace may acts as a counter to some of the harmful effects on health caused by some jobs.

3. There are economic benefits associated with healthy workplaces (Wanless, 2004). American research studies provide evidence that workplace health promotion programmes are associated with lower medical and insurance costs, decreased absenteeism and enhanced performance, productivity and morale (https://www.cdc.gov/workplacehealthpromotion/health-strategies/index.html). Some of this evidence are shown in Research Example 16.1.

   The Health and Safety Executive (HSE) identifies the costs of work-related ill health, which include sick pay, damage from injuries, and compensation, insurance costs and recruitment costs. Some of the statistics from the HSE about the scale and type of work-related injuries and illness are outlined in Case Study 16.1. Research has shown that employees who have three or more risk factors (e.g., smoking, overweight, excessive alcohol intake, physical inactivity) are likely to have 50% more sickness absence from work than employees with no risk factors (Shain and Kramer, 2004). Investing in health and preventing ill health increases productivity and staff retention, so adopting a healthy workplaces approach makes sound business sense.

4. The workplace provides a resource for health that is relevant to a large percentage of the adult population. Creating a healthy environment at work will benefit employees' health and have positive spin-offs for their families and communities as well as their workplaces. The traditional workplace focus has been on hazards and illnesses, but a health promoting approach has great potential.

5. Enabling people to work, to stay in work and safeguard their health at work is beneficial for them. Presenteeism (when people go to work but are not

---

CASE STUDY 16.1
Work-Related Ill Health

HSE statistics for the UK for 2019–2020 (https://www.hse.gov.uk/statistics) showed that:

- 111 workers were killed at work (the majority in the construction industry)
- 168,000 employees suffered serious injuries at work
- 1.6 million workers suffered from work-related ill health (new or long-standing)
- 12,000 deaths from lung disease were estimated to be linked to past exposures to harmful substances whilst at work
- 30% of work-related conditions were musculoskeletal disorders (MSDs), leading to an average of 18.4 days off work,
- 51% of work-related conditions were stress, depression or anxiety, leading to an average of 21.6 days off work
- 38.8 million working days were lost due to sickness absence in 2019.

---

productive) due to poor mental health is an invisible but substantial cost.

This chapter considers what a health promoting workplace is. In earlier chapters we have discussed the difference between health promotion activities that take place in a setting and whole-system approaches. Research Example 16.1 provides some evidence that promoting health of workers is beneficial for the employer.

THE RELATIONSHIP BETWEEN WORK AND HEALTH

The relationship between work and health is complex. In general, attention has focused on the effects of work on health, although it is also acknowledged that poor health will have negative effects on the capacity for paid employment. There is evidence that paid work is good for health and that unemployment can be linked to ill health (Waddell and Burton, 2006). Some of this evidence are cited in Research Example 16.2. Work is beneficial for health because it provides an income, a sense of self-worth and social networks of colleagues and friends. However, work may also harm health, and most research has concentrated on this. Learning Activity 16.1 asks you to reflect on your most recent work and how it affected your health and well-being.

RESEARCH EXAMPLE 16.1

Economic Benefits of Workplace Health Promotion Programmes

Many evaluations of workplace health promotion programmes have reported positive results, including the following cited by ERS (2016):

- British Gas introduced back-care workshops for employees engaged in physically demanding activities. Almost 300 employees participated, and the company saw a 43% reduction in back pain-related absence, valued at £1,660 per participating employee. The company received a return of £31 for every £1 invested in the workshop.
- A manufacturer with 20,000 employees made cost savings of £11m over 3 years due to savings of 1% in absenteeism reduction. For every £1 pound invested in health policy development and management training, almost £53 was saved.
- A manufacturer with 200 employees funded occupational health services and activities alongside counselling and annual health screenings at a total cost of £7,150. For every £1 invested, £11 was saved on injury claims from employees.
- A public sector transport organization with approximately 400 employees introduced a sickness absence management plan alongside support and return-to-work interviews. The occupational health services provided cost £16,000 per annum and resulted in a 70% reduction in absenteeism between 1999 and 2003. Long-term sickness leave fell from 16 to 3 days at any one time.

 Learning Activity 16.1 The Impact of Work on Health

Think of a recent work experience.

In what ways, if at all, do you think work contributed to your health?

In what ways, if at all, do you think work had a negative impact on your health?

The workplace can affect health in many different ways. Fig. 16.1 provides a means of classifying these different kinds of relationship.

In addition, the Marmot Review ten years on (Marmot et al., 2020, section 3C) identifies good-quality work as providing:

- job security
- adequate pay

- strong relationships and social support
- provision of health, safety and well-being
- support for the employee voice and representation
- varied and interesting work
- the promotion and development of skills
- effort–reward balance
- autonomy, control and task discretion.

Hazards tend to be what people think of first when health in the workplace is mentioned. Most legislation is directed towards the containment of hazards, and safety legislation has been enshrined in numerous Factory Acts in the UK dating back to the mid-19th century. Work that involves handling hazardous or toxic materials may have a direct negative effect on health (e.g., occupational asthma or cancers caused by asbestos). Work that provides easy access to hazardous substances is also linked to associated ill health (e.g., doctors and pharmacists have high rates of suicide caused by drug overdose). There is a downward trend in fatal and non-fatal injuries at work, probably due to automation and fewer physical jobs that present hazards. Almost one-third of deaths occur in the construction sector, with high death rates in agriculture and waste and recycling industries.

The workplace is characterized by fragmented information collected by different bodies (including the HSE and occupational health services). This poses obvious difficulties when trying to plan and implement a health promotion intervention. Health is often affected by risky behaviour or changed routines. Risky behaviour is the preferred explanation for most official accounts of accidents and injuries sustained in the workplace. There are extensive regulations to cover manual handling, which require employers to provide training and equipment. Nevertheless, employees are expected to, according to the Health and Safety at Work Act, 'take reasonable care for the health and safety of themselves and any others who may be affected by their acts and omissions'. This approach extends the victim-blaming ideology of some brands of health promotion to the workplace. Behaviour that carries health risks may be an integral part of the job or the work culture. For example, bartenders have high rates of alcohol-related ill health because drinking heavily is associated with work (Wilhelm et al., 2004).

The general work environment and its effects on health are the most neglected aspects of the work–health relationship. This is due in part to ideological or political reasons, and in part to the fact that such a generalized relationship is hard to research or prove. Because

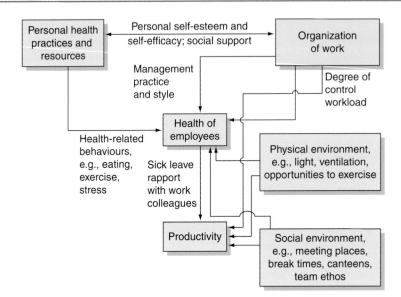

Fig. 16.1 The relationship between health and productivity in the workplace (Adapted from Shain, M., Kramer, D.M., 2004. Health promotion in the workplace: framing the concept; reviewing the evidence. Occupational and Environmental Medicine 61, 643–648.)

the relationship between work and health is to a large extent indirect, it is often difficult to trace ill health to what happens in the workplace. This in turn leads to the true impact of work on health being underestimated. Focusing on the work environment instead of individual workers' behaviour shifts responsibility onto the employer and has resource implications.

Although the relationship is difficult to quantify, strong evidence implicating the importance to health of the general work environment is becoming available. Work-related aspects that have a positive impact on health include adequate pay, protection from hazards, job security and opportunities for progression, and a good work–life balance (Marmot, 2010). Research demonstrates that factors associated with some types of work, such as repetitive tasks, lack of autonomy and pressures to meet deadlines, have harmful effects on health. In particular, a lack of control by workers over what they do and how they do it is associated with an increased risk of ill health (Marmot and Wilkinson, 2003). Health-adverse work conditions are concentrated among more disadvantaged social groups, reinforcing existing inequalities. There is also evidence that adverse work conditions are more common among ethnic minority groups and disabled people. For example, low pay is more common among Pakistani and Bangladeshi groups, and people with a longstanding illness or disability are more likely to earn a below-average income (Institute of Health Equity, 2015).

The concept of well-being at work is also receiving attention. Key components of well-being relate to being valued, having opportunities to engage in decision-making, and being able to work productively and creatively (Foresight, 2008). Working environments may also pose risks for mental well-being. For example, an imbalance between the effort required at work and the rewards received can lead to stress. Long-term exposure to stress results in poor health and may also lead to less healthy lifestyle choices, such as smoking. There is a growing acknowledgement of the impact of workplace stress on health:

- work-related stress accounts for nearly half of all new incidents of ill health and this is a rising trend
- 17.9 million working days were lost due to stress, depression and anxiety in 2019/2020
- there is some evidence that working long hours can lead to stress, depression or mental ill health
- the occupations reporting the highest rates of work-related stress were health professionals (especially nurses), teaching and education professionals, and social care professionals (https://www.hse.gov.uk/statistics/causdis/stress.pdf).

There are two main ways in which workplace stress is being addressed. The traditional approach has been to see the individual as unable to cope with the demands and pressures, and therefore in need of support. Many large workplaces offer stress management courses, counselling services and employee assistance programmes to help people adjust to new demands. Organizational approaches to stress reduction are still rare despite a growing literature linking stress with organizational factors, such as lack of control or lack of consultation over changes. These approaches start from the view that illness and stressed behaviour are responses to workplace factors which individuals may not even be aware of. As the Department of Health (2004, Chapter 7, para. 16) points out:

A focus on individual stress can be counterproductive, leading to a failure to tackle the underlying causes of problems in the workplace. Evidence has shown that poor working arrangements, such as lack of job control or discretion, consistently high work demands and low social support, can lead to increased risks of CHD [coronary heart disease], musculoskeletal disorders, mental illness and sickness absence. The real task is to improve the quality of jobs by reducing monotony, increasing job control, and applying appropriate HR [human resources] practices and policies – organizations need to ensure they adopt approaches that support the overall health and well being of their employees.

The HSE identifies six areas, listed later, that contribute to stress in the workplace. In addition, the report by the Institute of Health Equity (2015) on addressing inequalities cites structural factors including low pay, insufficient hours, job insecurity and temporary work. Learning Activity 16.2 asks you to consider your work and workplace and how it contributes to stress and how it could mitigate that stress.

Stress-related factors in the workplace (https://www.hse.gov.uk/stress/causes.htm#:~:text=us%20improve%20it.-,Causes%20of%20stress%20at%20work,the%20demands%20of%20their%20jobs):

1. Demands – workloads, work patterns.
2. Control – how much of a say employees have over things that affect them.
3. Support – encouragement, appreciation, sponsorship, resources.
4. Relationships at work – managing conflict or unacceptable behaviour.

5. Role – understanding of work role and no conflicting roles.
6. Change – how it is managed and communicated.
7. Culture – management commitment, and open and fair procedures.

 Learning Activity 16.2 Stress at Work

What could your organization do to reduce stress at work?

Research Example 16.2 takes the idea that work is good for health by considering some of the evidence in relation to unemployment. Although this data is now quite old, trends are still similar.

RESPONSIBILITY FOR WORKPLACE HEALTH

The relationship between work and health may appear substantial, but it is viewed in different ways by different groups of people. One of the defining characteristics of the workplace setting is that it brings together a variety of groups who have different agendas with regard to work and health. The key parties are workers or employees and their trade unions or staff associations, employers and managers, occupational health staff, health and safety officers, public health specialists and environmental health officers.

Workers

It has always been a priority for workers' organizations to ensure that employees are working in safe and healthy conditions. Membership of trade unions is now just over a quarter of the working population in the UK (https://www.gov.uk/government/statistics/trade-union-statistics-2019). Changing patterns of employment also mean that part-time (mainly female) workers make up a significant percentage of the working population. So, although consultation with unions is an important means of reaching workers, it does not reach everyone. As the key target group, workers need to be fully involved as partners in decision-making processes. This is recognized by the European Network for Workplace Health Promotion (ENWHP), which states that effective workplace health promotion involves employees in decision-making processes and develops a working culture based on partnership (www.enwhp.org).

RESEARCH EXAMPLE 16.2
Unemployment and Health

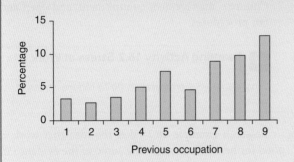

1. Management and senior officials
2. Professional
3. Associate professional and technical
4. Administrative and secretarial
5. Skilled trades
6. Personal service
7. Sales and customer service
8. Process, plan and machine operatives
9. Elementary

Unemployment and Health (Office for National Statistics, 2009. Economic and Labour Market Review: Further Labour Market Statistics, Unemployment Rates by Previous Occupation (cited in Marmot 2010, p. 68); licensed under the Open Government Licence v.3.0)

This figure charts unemployment rates from 2013 by previous occupation and shows that unemployment is unevenly distributed across society, with those in lower socio-economic positions more likely to be without work. Unemployed people have higher rates of long-term illness, mental illness and cardiovascular disease. Unemployment has also been linked to increased suicide rates, although research shows that countries with strong systems of social protection, including active labour market programmes, were able to maintain long-term declines in suicide rates despite rapid increases in unemployment (Stuckler et al., 2009). Unemployment affects mortality and morbidity rates in three ways:

1. Unemployment leads to increased financial problems, which lowers living standards and may reduce social integration.
2. Unemployment can be a trigger for distress, anxiety and depression.
3. Unemployment can trigger unhealthy behaviours, such as smoking and drinking alcohol.

A summary of this evidence can be found in the Marmot Review (2010), section 2.6.3.

Employers and Managers

Employers and managers have as their first priority the viability of the organization. Health is relevant in so far as it can be shown to be linked to organizational goals. Examples of 'hard' benefits are improvements in productivity due to lower rates of sickness, absenteeism and staff turnover, and improved recruitment and retention of trained staff. 'Soft' benefits, such as enhanced corporate image, are also influential.

The Health and Safety at Work Act (1974) states that employers are responsible for the health, safety and welfare of their employees. There is evidence of a recent shift in attitudes to, and awareness of, health and safety issues in the workplace. The Investors in People standard, which has been widely adopted, is an example of the government's strategy to use awards to provide incentives for employers. Another example is the Improving Working Lives standard which provides a model of good human resources practice against which employers can be measured. The Workplace Wellbeing Charter (http://wellbeingcharter.org.uk/index.php [accessed 20.04.21]) sets a series of standards

for workplaces. Leadership and commitment at senior management level have been shown to be vital for effective health promotion initiatives and the creation of healthy workplaces. An organizational audit of NHS trusts in 2014 found that trusts with high levels of patient mortality had high rates of staff absence due to ill health. The health of staff is not however a priority for all NHS trusts, with 24% of trusts not monitoring the mental well-being of staff and 28% without an obesity plan for staff (Royal College of Physicians, 2015). Case Study 16.2 shows the issue of obesity and its impact on the health of employees.

Learning Activity 16.3 asks you to consider and discuss the role of employers in relation to employee health and the following Case Studies 16.2 and 16.3 outline some of the initiatives that have been undertaken.

Learning Activity 16.3 Employers and Healthy Workplaces
What might be employers' responsibilities that could encourage a healthier workplace?

CASE STUDY 16.2

Obesity in the Health Services Workplace

Obesity can impact on workplace performance of staff in a number of ways. There may be tasks which obese people find more difficult to do, or which are more dangerous due to conditions linked to obesity. For example, sleep problems may affect alertness and may pose a potential danger for employees who use machinery or technical instruments at work. Obese people often have to take more time off work than average – both short and long term – because of associated health conditions. Obesity is associated with substantially increased rates of absenteeism (i.e., more days out of work) and presenteeism (i.e., reduced productivity while at work) (Shrestha et al., 2016).

The work environment provides a range of explanations for the relatively high rates of obesity amongst some healthcare professions, such as nursing:

- Night-shift work is associated with meal irregularity; higher carbohydrate, animal fat and protein intake coupled with low dietary fibre consumption and frequent snacking (Lowden et al., 2010)
- Readily available vending machines and the common sharing of snacks may also contribute to weight gain amongst nurses (Nicholls et al., 2016)

There is limited evidence about what successfully tackles obesity within the health service (Kelly and Wills, 2018). Most interventions address individual behaviour change through improving dietary choices or increasing physical activity (Proper and van Oostrom, 2019). System-level interventions, such as releasing staff to participate in exercise sessions during the working day, are rare.

Occupational Health Staff

In many European countries occupational health is a statutory part of healthcare and is prioritized as shown in Case Study 16.3. In the UK there is no requirement for employers to provide an occupational health service, other than first aid. Occupational health nurses (OHNs), who are specialist nurses with post-qualification training, are an important element of occupational health staff. OHNs are responsible for the health and well-being of employees in the workplace.

The main functions of an occupational health service are:

- surveillance of the work environment, for example, the health effects of new technologies
- initiatives and advice on the control of hazards

CASE STUDY 16.3

European Agency for Safety and Health at Work Campaigns

The European Healthy Workplaces campaigns raise awareness of issues related to occupational safety and health including noise, dangerous substances and stress. Their website (see end of box) includes a short film about a young baker who develops asthma linked to flour dust. It promotes healthy working practices such as nose rinsing.

Recent campaigns include 'Lighten the Load' to promote an integrated approach to tackling musculoskeletal disorders (MSDs), which are the most common form of work-related illness in Europe. In the EU, 25% of workers suffer from backache and 23% from muscular pains (https://osha.europa.eu/en/campaigns/index_htm/).

- surveillance of the health of employees, for example, assessment of fitness to work, analysis of sickness absence
- organization of first aid and emergency response facilities
- adaptation of work tasks and the working environment to meet workers' needs.

The workplace has experienced considerable change and uncertainty in the last 20 years. There has been a rapid growth in the service sector, a fragmentation of large organizations, a huge increase in information technology and, during the COVID-19 pandemic, a huge shift to people working from home. Working from home will demand changes in work practices including: role clarity, workload, performance indicators, technical support, facilitation of co-worker networking and training for managers. The provision for health in companies thus needs to be seen alongside employment policies, the work environment, and overall company policies.

Health and Safety Officers and Environmental Health Officers

Health and safety officers (HSOs) and environmental health officers (EHOs) are responsible for ensuring that workplaces conform to safety legislation. HSOs and EHOs have the power to force workplaces to comply with health and safety regulations, and to impose penalties in the case of non-compliance. Responsibility for workplaces is divided between the HSE and EHOs employed by local authorities.

Worker participation is an important contributor to managing health and safety, and safety representatives prevent many injuries and work-related illnesses every year. Yet safety representatives are not universal. Only 46% of workplaces (92% of public sector and 39% of private sector) and 68% of employees (98% of public sector and 59% of private sector) have employee representation.

HEALTH PROMOTION IN THE WORKPLACE

There are two approaches to health promotion in the workplace, and examples are illustrated in Case Study 16.4. The most common approach is to target individual lifestyles and behaviour within a workplace setting. This approach sees the workplace primarily as a site through which programmes can be delivered. The more challenging, but potentially more effective, approach is to target the workplace and its organization and culture. Health promotion in the workplace falls into the following categories:

- first aid and medical treatment
- screening, for example, bone-density scanning
- protection from accidents
- control of hazards and infections
- education and advice about healthy lifestyles and practices
- policies and regulations to provide a healthier environment, for example, a no-smoking policy
- provision of services, for example, exercise facilities, screening, counselling and support for smoking cessation.

Reviews of the evidence on the effectiveness of workplace health promotion (e.g., Lutz et al., 2019; Pieper et al., 2019; Proper and van Oostrom, 2019; Schröer et al., 2014) all conclude that the heterogeneity of the interventions and the settings make conclusions about what might be the most effective interventions difficult. In common with all interventions in various settings, effectiveness depends on the nature and the delivery of the interventions.

Changing organizational culture and practice, for example, through more flexible working hours and break times, has a more significant impact than programmes that focus on individual changes such as offering relaxation classes after working hours. Research Example 16.3 considers the issue of the 12-hour shifts around which the work of nurses and midwives is organized. The whole-organization approach has been recognized

---

CASE STUDY 16.4
Examples of Healthy Workplace Initiatives

- Provision of an online personalized health advice and information service.
- Provision of an 'MoT' clinic at a railway station during rush hours, to encourage women and especially men to attend for health check-ups (Dooris and Hunter, 2007).
- Initiating physical activities in the workplace during lunch breaks, for example speed walks.
- Encouraging healthy lifestyles through, for example, the provision of cycle racks, shower rooms and stair prompts to encourage staff to walk up the stairs rather than take the lift, and providing healthy options in staff canteens and vending machines.
- Changing the physical environment of the workplace to encourage exercise, for example, situating key locations at a distance from one another to encourage brief bouts of walking to shared spaces such as mail and lunch rooms.

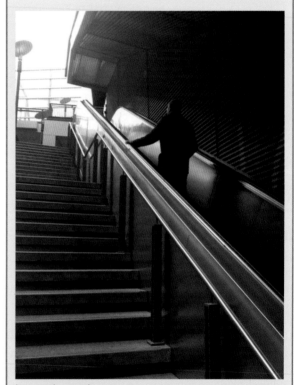

Increasing stair use

Stair use among the able-bodied can be encouraged by providing a conveniently located stair for everyday use, posting motivational signage to encourage stair use, and designing visible, appealing and comfortable stairs

RESEARCH EXAMPLE 16.3
Nursing Shifts and Health

Nurses commonly work 12-hour shifts. This schedule gives nurses a 3-day work week, potentially providing better work–life balance and flexibility. Numerous studies have explored the impact of longer shifts on stress, burnout and patient safety.

Baillie and Thomas' (2018) study compared two older people's wards, one using the common 12-hour shifts, and the other using overlapping 8-hour shifts, and found no differences in patient views or the quality of interactions. Nursing staff believed that tiredness could affect care and communication, but had varied views about which shift pattern was most tiring. Nurses believed continuity of care was important, especially for older people, but had mixed views about which shift pattern best promoted care continuity. Another study (Suter et al., 2020) found that 12-hour shifts offered fewer opportunities for social support, with reports of individuals pacing their work to preserve their emotional and physical stamina.

and endorsed at the highest level and by international bodies (e.g., the ENWHP adopted the Luxembourg Declaration on Workplace Health Promotion in 1997). This declaration states that successful initiatives should follow these guidelines:

- participation – all staff should be involved
- integration – embedding health in all organizational areas, policies and decisions
- project management – programmes to follow a problem-solving cycle of needs analysis, planning, implementation and evaluation
- comprehensiveness – embracing initiatives focused on individuals and the environment.

To maximize its impact, workplace health promotion needs to shift from an individually focused lifestyle approach to a more comprehensive approach that includes whole-organization activities.

REFLECTION ON PRACTICE

- Think of a workplace with which you are familiar. What areas would you prioritize to promote health, and why? Are there different workforces or work patterns (e.g., shift work) that you would target? Who would you involve, and how?

CONCLUSION

The workplace is recognized as a key setting in which to promote health, due to both its reach (three-quarters of the working-age population are employed) and its importance in contributing directly and indirectly to people's health. Traditionally the focus has been on individually targeted programmes centred on workplace hazards and the prevention of ill health linked to poor diets, lack of physical activity and excessive alcohol intake. The challenge today is to broaden this focus to include the whole organizational setting, and to move from the prevention of ill health to the promotion of positive health and well-being. There is a developing evidence base demonstrating that such a comprehensive and multicomponent approach is effective. The proven benefits include better employee health and increased productivity, leading to economic benefits for industry and the whole of society. Many different groups, including workers, managers, employers, occupational health staff, HSOs and EHOs, play a role in promoting health in the workplace.

SUMMARY

This chapter has looked at the potential benefits to be gained from implementing health promotion within the workplace setting. The tension between interventions that focus on individual lifestyles and those that address the whole organization has been discussed. Evaluation studies have demonstrated that the whole-organization approach is effective. The role of different partners in workplace health promotion has been identified and discussed.

FURTHER READING AND RESOURCES

European Network for Health Promotion at https://www.enwhp.org/.
This website is a useful resource for up-to-date information.
National Institute for Health and Care Excellence (NICE) at https://www.nice.org.uk/.
NICE has produced various documents synthesizing research evidence of effective health promotion practice in the workplace and what constitutes healthy workplaces:
Management practices (NG13) – recently updated to include recommendations specifically focused on older employees
Mental well-being at work (PH22)

Workplace health: long-term sickness absence and incapacity to work (PH19)

Physical activity in the workplace (PH13)

Smoking: workplace interventions (PH5)

Workplace practice at https://pathways.nice.org.uk/pathways/workplace-health-policy-and-management-practices.

Health at Work network at https://www.nhshealthatwork.co.uk/health-wellbeing.asp.

Policy on occupational health in the health service

Black, C., 2008. Working for a Healthier Tomorrow. TSO, London.

Institute of Health Equity, 2015. Promoting good quality jobs to reduce health inequalities. Available at: https://assets.publishing.service.gov.uk/government/uploads/system/uploads/attachment_data/file/460700/2a_Promoting_good_quality_jobs-Full.pdf

Department for Work and Pensions, 2013. Improving Health and Work: Changing Lives the Government's Response. Department of Work and Pensions, London.

These two reviews identify the impact of work on health, and discuss the effect of reforms on sickness, unemployment and early interventions.

▶ FEEDBACK TO LEARNING ACTIVITIES

16.1. The benefits of work include pay, the contribution of work to an individual's identity and social status and the opportunities work provides to meet people. However, work can also be detrimental to an individual's health, due to work-related hazards, job insecurity and long working hours.

16.2. Task and work reorganization is the most successful form of intervention. It describes various system solutions to improve communication, the creation of autonomous work groups and whole-organization interventions to restructure relations between management and unions. These interventions do not obviate the need for individual support, but follow an earlier stage of raising staff awareness of stress and its causes.

16.3. Employer responsibilities might be:
- making healthy choices easier for staff to adopt
- creating flexible working arrangements that are compatible with employees' home lives
- ensuring a smoke-free work environment
- ensuring that any catering offered on-site has healthy options
  - mental health awareness for managers
  - an active travel plan to encourage physical activity
  - a 24-hour canteen for shift workers.

The Wellbeing Charter standards focus on three areas: leadership, culture and communication.

REFERENCES

Baillie, L., Thomas, N., 2018. Changing from 12-hr to 8-hr day shifts: a qualitative exploration of effects on organising nursing care and staffing. J. Clin. Nurs. 28 (3), 148–158.

Black, C., 2008. Working for a Healthier Tomorrow. TSO, London. Available at: https://www.gov.uk/government/uploads/system/uploads/attachment_data/file/209782/hwwb-working-for-a-healthier-tomorrow.pdf.

Department of Health, 2004. Choosing Health: Making Healthy Choices Easier. TSO, London. Available at: http://webarchive.nationalarchives.gov.uk/+/dh.gov.uk/en/publicationsandstatistics/publications/publicationspolicyandguidance/dh_4094550.

Dooris, M., Hunter, D.J., 2007. Organisations and settings for promoting public health. In: Lloyd, C.E., Handsley, S.,

Douglas, J. (eds.), Policy and Practice in Promoting Public Health. Sage and the Open University, London.

ERS Research and Consultancy, 2016. Health at Work Economic Evidence. Available at: file:///Users/willsj/Downloads/health_at_work_economic_evidence_report_2016.pdf.

European Network for Workplace Health Promotion, 1997. The Luxembourg Declaration on Workplace Health Promotion in the European Union. European Network for Workplace Health Promotion, Luxembourg. Available at: https://www.enwhp.org/resources/toolip/doc/2018/05/04/luxembourg_declaration.pdf.

Foresight, 2008. Mental Capital and Wellbeing: Making the Most of Ourselves in the 21st Century. Government Office for Science, London. Available at: https://www.gov.uk/government/publications/mental-capital-and-wellbeing-making-the-most-of-ourselves-in-the-21st-century, Sudbury, HSE books.

Health and Safety Executive, 2012. The Causes of Stress. Available at: http://www.hse.gov.uk/stress/furtheradvice/causesofstress.htm.

Institute of Health Equity, 2015. Local Action on Health Inequalities: Promoting Good Quality Jobs to Reduce Health Inequalities. Available at: https://www.instituteofhealthequity.org/resources-reports/local-action-on-health-inequalities-promoting-good-quality-jobs-to-reduce-health-inequalities-.

Kelly, M., Wills, J., 2018. Systematic review: What works to address obesity in nurses? Occup. Med. 68 (4), 228–238.

Lowden, A., Moreno, C., Holmbäck, U., Lennernäs, M., Tucker, P., 2010. Eating and shift work — effects on habits, metabolism, and performance. Scand. J. Work, Environ. & Health 36 (2), 150–162.

Lutz, N., Taeymans, J., Ballmer, C., Verhaeghe, N., Clarys, P., et al., 2019. Cost-effectiveness and cost-benefit of worksite health promotion programs in Europe: a systematic review. Eur. J. Public. Health 29 (3), 540–546.

Marmot, M., 2010. Fair Society, Healthy Lives. Institute of Health Equity, London. Available at: https://www.instituteofhealthequity.org/resources-reports/fair-society-healthy-lives-the-marmot-review.

Marmot, M., Allen, J., Boyce, T., Goldblatt, P., Morrison, J., 2020. Health equity in England: The Marmot Review ten years on. Institute of Health Equity, London. Available at: https://www.instituteofhealthequity.org/resources-reports/marmot-review-10-years-on.

Marmot, M., Wilkinson, R., 2003. The Social Determinants of Health: The Solid Facts, second ed World Health Organisation, Geneva. Available at: http://www.euro.who.int/__data/assets/pdf_file/0005/98438/e81384.pdf.

Nicholls, R., Perry, L., Duffield, C., Gallagher, R., Pierce, H., 2016. Barriers and facilitators to healthy eating for nurses in the workplace: an integrative review. J. Adv. Nurs. 73 (5), 1051–1065.

Pieper, C., Schröer, S., Eilerts, A.L., 2019. Evidence of workplace interventions-a systematic review of systematic reviews. Int. J. Env. Res. Public. Health 16 (19), 3553.

Proper, K.I., van Oostrom, S.H., 2019. The effectiveness of workplace health promotion interventions on physical and mental health outcomes - a systematic review of reviews. Scand. J. Work. Env. Health 45 (6), 546–559.

Royal College of Physicians, 2015. Work and Wellbeing in the NHS: Why Staff Health Matters to Patient Care. Available at: https://www.rcplondon.ac.uk/guidelines-policy/work-and-wellbeing-nhs-why-staff-health-matters-patient-care.

Shrestha, N., Pedisic, Z., Neil-Sztramko, S., Kukkonen-Harjula, K.T., Hermans, V., 2016. The impact of obesity in the workplace: a review of contributing factors, consequences and potential solutions. Curr. Obes. Rep. 5 (3), 344–360. https://doi.org/10.1007/s13679-016-0227-6. PMID: 27447869.

Schröer, S., Haupt, J., Pieper, C., 2014. Evidence-based lifestyle interventions in the workplace—an overview. Occup. Med. (Lond.) 64 (1), 8–12.

Shain, M., Kramer, D.M., 2004. Health promotion in the workplace: framing the concept; reviewing the evidence. Occup. Environ. Med. 61, 643–648. Available at: http://oem.bmj.com/content/61/7/643.full.pdf+html.

Stuckler, D., Basu, S., Suhrcke, M., Coutts, A., McKee, M., 2009. The public health effect of economic crises and alternative policy responses in Europe: an empirical analysis. Lancet 374, 315–323.

Suter, J., Kowalski, T., Anaya-Montes, M., Chalkley, M., Jacobs, R., et al., 2020. The impact of moving to a 12h shift pattern on employee wellbeing: a qualitative study in an acute mental health setting. Int. J. Nurs. Stud. 112, 1–9.

Waddell, S., Burton, A.K., 2006. Is work good for your health and well being? Occup. Health Rev. 24, 30–31. Available at: https://www.gov.uk/government/uploads/system/uploads/attachment_data/file/214326/hwwb-is-work-good-for-you.pdf.

Wanless, D., 2004. Securing Good Health for the Whole Population. Stationery Office, London. Available at: https://webarchive.nationalarchives.gov.uk/+/http://www.dh.gov.uk/en/Publicationsandstatistics/Publications/PublicationsPolicyAndGuidance/DH_4074426.

Wilhelm, K., Koves, V., Rios-Seidel, C., Finch, A., 2004. Work and mental health. Soc. Psychiatr. Epidemiol. 39 (11), 866–873.

Health Promoting Neighbourhoods

LEARNING OUTCOMES

By the end of this chapter you will be able to:
- define what is meant by a neighbourhood
- discuss neighbourhoods as settings for health promotion
- distinguish between interventions in a neighbourhood and a settings approach
- understand what is meant by a place-based approach.

KEY CONCEPTS AND DEFINITIONS

Community A group of people living in the same place or sharing a common characteristic (e.g., the gay community).

Neighbourhood A geographically defined community within a larger area (e.g., city, town, suburb or rural area). There is often a high level of social interaction and networking between people in a neighbourhood.

Place A physical setting and social context.

Place-based approach An approach that brings together different stakeholders, including the local community, to address issues and needs related to a specific location.

Social capital The social networks linking people, characterized by shared values and behaviour and mutually advantageous cooperation.

IMPORTANCE OF THE TOPIC

As we have seen in other chapters in this part of the book, healthy settings are physical and social settings which serve as supportive environments for health and health promotion activities. This chapter examines the concept of neighbourhood and how different factors, for example, physical (e.g., green space), social (e.g., violence) and economic (e.g., work opportunities), contribute to the potential of neighbourhoods to be health promoting. The popularity of neighbourhoods in different policy and practice arenas has waxed and waned and the emergence of place and place-based approaches is discussed. The neighbourhood is an important setting because:

- The planning, design, construction and management of the built environment can help to provide access to healthier goods, services and lifestyles such as food or walkability.
- The neighbourhood can alleviate or prevent poor health arising from issues such as air pollution.
- The built and social environment can help create social cohesion and connectivity, or exacerbate social divisions and loneliness.

Neighbourhoods include different levels or structures, such as the neighbourhood environment, services and people, which may all be used as a springboard for health promotion. Evaluating such a multidimensional strategy poses many challenges, and issues regarding the evaluation and evidence base for neighbourhood-based health promotion are discussed.

Healthy Cities is one of the best-known and largest of the settings approaches. The programme is a long-term international development initiative that aims to place health high on the agendas of decision-makers and to promote comprehensive local strategies for health improvement and sustainable development.

The Healthy Villages programme in rural areas addresses similar issues. Health is defined by the area's residents; however, the generally accepted definition of a healthy village includes a community with low rates of infectious diseases, access to basic healthcare services and a stable, peaceful social environment (see http://www.who.int/healthy_settings/types/en/index.html).

In addition, the neighbourhood provides a link between the holistic and multifaceted linking of activities that characterize the settings approach and is used in schools, workplaces, hospitals, markets, islands and homes (discussed in other chapters in Part III). Learning Activity 17.1 asks you to clarify the concept of neighbourhood and distinguish it from the concept of community which was discussed in Chapter 11.

 Learning Activity 17.1 Neighbourhood or Community?

The terms neighbourhood and community are frequently used. Are they the same thing?

DEFINING NEIGHBOURHOODS

Neighbourhoods are defined as small localities with a distinct identity forged by a community of people who know each other, and the provision of essential services such as post offices, shops and health centres. Neighbourhoods are often bounded by geographical features such as major roads, railways or green areas, and may be urban or rural. The key factor is that neighbourhoods are defined by their residents, who feel they have an investment in its future, the services provided and its appearance. In the modern world, where transactions are more frequently fragmented and anonymous, and where the overarching symbols of community, such as religion and nationhood, are less cohesive and meaningful, the role of the neighbourhood in promoting identity and self-esteem is increasingly important. Neighbourhoods provide the immediate physical and social environment where people live, work and play, and for many more vulnerable groups, such as older people and those on low income, most of their lives are lived in one neighbourhood.

Neighbourhood identity is largely based on residents' socio-economic status, which in turn is often based on employment patterns, as well as physical characteristics

such as housing. Neighbourhoods are often internally differentiated, and the sense of community is based on everyday social interactions and networks of friends, families and neighbours. Neighbourhoods therefore combine objective and subjective components.

There are many ways to get to know neighbourhoods, ranging from the gathering of objective statistics to the collection of people's subjective thoughts, feelings and memories. Local statistics on topics such as housing and crime are collected (see www.ons.gov.uk) and can be used to compare different neighbourhoods. Community profiles or observation walks, where notes are taken of local facilities, the physical environment, transport routes and social networking opportunities, provide a more holistic picture of neighbourhoods.

WHY NEIGHBOURHOODS ARE A KEY SETTING FOR HEALTH PROMOTION

Having considered many other settings in the previous chapters, Learning Activity 17.2 asks you to think about in what ways a neighbourhood is a setting and then consider and discuss how it can be a route to reducing inequalities in health.

 Learning Activity 17.2 Can Neighbourhoods Be Used as a Setting to Address Inequalities?

The Marmot Review on inequalities (Marmot, 2010) had a policy objective to create and develop healthy and sustainable places and communities. Why might neighbourhoods be identified as a key route through which to tackle health inequalities?

Neighbourhoods are a key setting for health promotion because they provide the infrastructure for health. Neighbourhoods are where physical and social environments interact with service provision to provide an overall environment which has enormous potential to support people's health. Neighbourhoods have several aspects:

- *The physical environment*, for example, the degree of air and noise pollution, quality of housing including its energy efficiency, amount of traffic and the availability of green space.
- *The social environment* – the amount of social interaction between residents, the number of community

or voluntary groups or organizations operating in the area and the extent of mutual self-help activities. The concept of social capital, which refers to relationships of trust and regard among people, and between people and organizations, is relevant to both the social environment and services provided.

- *Services* provided in neighbourhoods include places such as shops, post offices, health services, places of worship, sports facilities and community halls. Services also cover transport systems and outreach workers from statutory agencies, for example, housing and welfare officers' weekly sessions held in a community hall.

There are many aspects of a neighbourhood or place that have an impact on well-being. Fig. 17.1 from the Health Foundation suggests a combination of our surroundings and the sense people have of friendliness,

safety and quiet impacts on health. In addition to providing the context for health, neighbourhoods are a popular setting because they are seen as a means to engage people in addressing their own health needs. A neighbourhood focus therefore fosters empowerment and independence, which are themselves health promoting.

A healthy place, according to the Ministry of Housing, Communities and Local Government in England (https://www.gov.uk/guidance/health-and-wellbeing #achieving-healthy-and-inclusive-communities), is one which:

1. Supports and promotes healthy behaviours and environments and a reduction in health inequalities for people of all ages. It will provide the community with opportunities to improve their physical and mental health, and support community engagement and well-being.

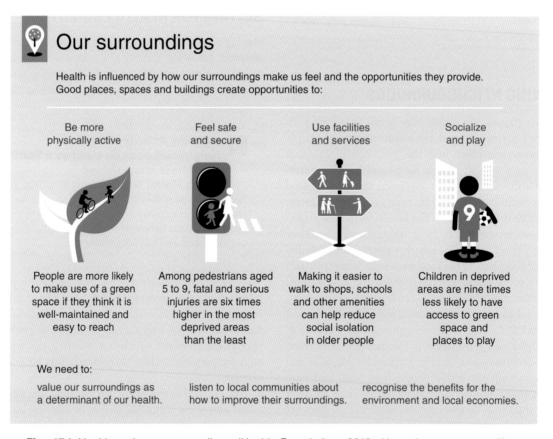

Fig. 17.1 Health and our surroundings (Health Foundation, 2019. How do our surroundings influence health. Available at: https://www.health.org.uk/infographic/how-do-our-surroundings-influence-our-health.)

2. Is inclusive and promotes social interaction in design and spaces that can be shared by all residents.
3. Meets the needs of children and young people to grow and develop, as well as being adaptable to the needs of an increasingly elderly population and those with dementia and other sensory or mobility impairments.

Our surroundings can have a negative as well as a positive impact on health. Fig. 17.2 shows some of the linkages and how, for example, blocking roads, while promoting walking, can also restrict opportunities for socializing. Similarly, Case Study 17.1 considers neighbourhood high streets and what might make them more health promoting.

The Physical Environment

Many aspects of the physical environment, such as buildings and land use, affect health, as do transport patterns and car usage. Cars contribute to climate change and have a negative impact on individuals' health. For example, in one rapidly developing area of China, those who bought a car gained on average 1.8 kg in weight

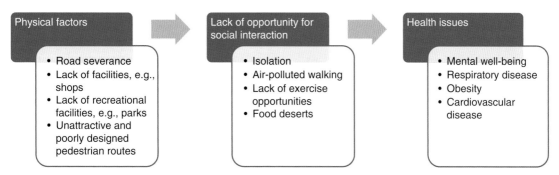

Fig. 17.2 How does the physical environment impact on health?

CASE STUDY 17.1
Healthy High Street

High streets are very important but declining features within communities. High streets are critical for economic growth, and are where some of the highest levels of social interaction and activity take place. There are multiple physical, economic and social pathways by which the high street impacts on health. Improved local economies can provide access to employment, in turn facilitating access to better housing and environmental conditions. Secure financial circumstances also reduce the likelihood of stress and enable improved material conditions, including adequate food and heating. Secure employment and income provide the resources, and sometimes the impetus, to give up health-harming behaviours such as poor diet, smoking and excessive alcohol consumption. High streets also enable and encourage people from different communities and backgrounds to meet and become more socially engaged and integrated. This leads to activating communities to create healthier environments in which to build social,

environmental and economic capital. These are the building blocks of better health outcomes. Consequently, local high streets should be considered an existing community asset, which can be used to promote and improve health, helping to make the healthy choice the easiest choice.

A healthy high street should:
- be inclusive to people from all walks of life
- be easy to navigate, including road crossings
- provide shade, shelter and places to stop and rest
- be walkable and provide options for cycling
- have low levels of noise
- have health-promoting retail offers
- have low levels of air pollution
- provide things to see and do
- ensure people feel relaxed and safe
- consider the local context of the high street, its features and current use, and how all these factors interact with one another.

From Institute of Health Equity and Jessica Allen, 2018. Healthy high street: good place making in an urban setting report. Available at: https://assets.publishing.service.gov.uk/government/uploads/system/uploads/attachment_data/file/699295/26.01.18_Healthy_High_Streets_Full_Report_Final_version_3.pdf.

(Rice and Grant, 2007). Tackling issues such as dependence on private cars can seem a daunting proposition. UK car users, although a smaller percentage of the population than in other European countries, use their cars more frequently. However, the importance of weaning ourselves away from overdependence on cars is being recognized. Goals include ensuring the provision of high-quality routes for walkers and cyclists, and making public spaces and the countryside seem more attractive. Local authorities in England are required to produce local transport plans; increasingly, these focus on sustainable transport and active travel. Case Study 17.2 considers the benefits of walking for health.

There is plenty of evidence that an environment rich in natural vegetation – trees, plants and open space – has a positive impact on our mental health and well-being, as well as being beneficial for air quality, shade and energy sustainability (Public Health England, 2020). Green and open space is necessary for physical activity as well as for socializing and play.

Poor housing can contribute to ill health in a cycle of effects, for example, damp may contribute to asthma or bronchitis, leading to time off work, leading to loss of income. Poor-quality housing is often sited in deprived neighbourhoods with few local amenities. Graffiti, litter, boarded-up premises and dog mess are all signs of a neglected environment which, in turn, affects people's perception of the safety of their neighbourhood and hence their willingness to be active participants within it. These issues often rank high on community agendas. Part of the health disadvantage in relation to housing relates to the quantity of affordable housing. As rents increase, the amount of social housing declines. Cold housing is also a health risk. Cold is the main explanation for the excess winter deaths that occur each year in England and Wales. Being able to afford a warm house is clearly a factor. Half of single pensioners and two-thirds of households with no one in work experienced fuel poverty in 2007–2008, and were spending more than 10% of their income on fuel (Marmot, 2010).

The Social Environment

The quality of life in a community is a powerful determinant of health and there follows a well-known case study (Case Study 17.3) that describes how social capital and social connectedness is beneficial for health.

📋 CASE STUDY 17.2
Walking for Health

Walking for Health (https://www.walkingforhealth.org.uk/) was launched by the British Heart Foundation and the Countryside Agency to encourage people to take part in locally designed walks. Healthcare professionals are encouraged to 'prescribe' pedometers to act as an incentive:

- Walking is the most accessible physical activity, and already the most popular. It is also accessible to people from groups who could most benefit from being more active – such as older people or those on low incomes.
- Walking is an effective form of moderate exercise.
- Walking is a cost-effective intervention delivering benefit-to-cost ratios of between 3 to 1 and 20 to 1. The costs of walking per quality year of life gained are considerably less than those thought reasonable for clinical interventions.
- As a form of active travel, walking is the most sustainable form of transport and has a key role to play in reducing congestion, pollution and climate change.
- Walking for Health provides opportunities for social contact and benefits mental health. Social contact is the top motivator for many participants.

From https://www.walkingforhealth.org.uk/sites/default/files/Walking%20works_LONG_AW_Web.pdf.

📋 CASE STUDY 17.3
Quality of Life in Communities

The small town of Roseto, Pennsylvania, USA (1600 inhabitants) is cited as an example of a community with markedly lower death rates from heart attacks than neighbouring areas. The population of Roseto is made up of Italian-Americans descended from migrants from the town of Roseto in southern Italy. It differed from other towns because it was 'remarkably close knit... with a sense of common purpose... [with] a camaraderie which precluded ostentation... [and] a concern for neighbours ensuring no one was ever abandoned... the family as the hub and bulwark of life provided a security and insurance against any catastrophe.' Roseto's considerable health advantage only seems explicable in relation to these social characteristics. As the younger people moved away, community and family ties broke down and people became more concerned with material values and conspicuous consumption (Bruhn and Wolf, 1979, cited in Wilkinson 1996, p. 116).

Social capital refers to social cohesion and the cumulative experience of relationships characterized by mutual trust, acceptance, approval and respect. People are social beings, and high-quality social interaction is vital to both personal and communal well-being. Social capital provides the foundation for collective action in the public sphere for the public good. The main indicators of social capital are:

- social relationships and social support
- formal and informal social networks
- community and civic engagement, including with voluntary associations
- trust and neighbourliness
- a sense of belonging for all communities
- appreciation and valuing of the diversity of people's backgrounds and circumstances
- similar life opportunities for those from different backgrounds
- the development of strong positive relationships between people from different backgrounds.

Community networks may be built around activities associated with school, leisure or living in a particular locality. Parents, especially mothers, have been identified as particularly active in forging neighbourhood links (Robertson et al., 2008). Buildings such as schools and leisure facilities are often used to host community events and networks. The closure of services such as schools and post offices therefore has a negative impact on neighbourliness, which might help explain the strength of feeling voiced whenever communities are threatened with the closure of such amenities.

Putnam (2000) argued that social capital mitigates the inequality among marginalized groups citing the example of Chinese garment industry in New York. However, if people are preoccupied with the basics of survival (i.e., ensuring they are fed, warm, sheltered and safe), they will be unable to focus on broader communal issues. The fact that social capital is not always benign also has to be acknowledged. Drug dealing and criminality on many housing estates relies on strong closely integrated networks. Neighbourhoods with less social capital differ from those with more social capital in many ways, for example, there is likely to be less volunteering, the neighbourhood is perceived to be less safe, and there will be less socializing and trust in others. This is discussed in Research Example 17.1.

Both crime and the fear of crime are health hazards associated with negative effects, including depression

RESEARCH EXAMPLE 17.1
Social Capital and Health

As the Marmot Review, 'Fair Society Healthy Lives' (Marmot, 2010, p. 126), points out, 'we live, grow, learn, work and age in a range of environments, and our lives are affected by residential communities, neighbourhoods and relational communities and social structures'. Section E2.3 summarizes the evidence linking social capital with health. It cites Wilkinson and Pickett (2009), stating that the most powerful sources of stress are low social status and a lack of social networks. Low levels of social integration and loneliness increase mortality rates. Social capital provides a source of resilience and social support and acts as a buffer against poor health and other difficulties. Several studies show that social networks act as a protective factor against dementia and cognitive decline. Living longer with more complex health needs means older people will be more reliant on social support systems and networks. People's participation in their communities gives added control over their lives, which contributes to their psychosocial well-being and other positive health outcomes.

and mental ill health. It has been suggested that negative effects are both direct, for example, stress and depression, and indirect, for example, mental ill health linked to social isolation and feelings of vulnerability. Excessive noise or petty disputes with neighbours, although less severe than violence or the threat of violence, can have a big impact on people's quality of life.

The National Planning Policy Framework in the UK (https://www.gov.uk/government/publications/national-planning-policy-framework--2) states that to achieve sustainable development there needs to be strong, vibrant and healthy communities. Also required are a sufficient number and range of homes to meet the needs of present and future generations, and the fostering of a well-designed and safe built environment, with accessible services and open spaces that reflects current and future needs and supports communities' health, social and cultural well-being. Case Study 17.4 shows how new place planning can prioritize a healthier built environment.

Services

An adequate service infrastructure including primary care is essential to the health and life of a neighbourhood. If essential services such as shops and post offices are not available locally, people are forced to travel outside the area, leading to a loss of social contacts as well as incurring additional time and travel costs. This has been recognized by many communities fighting to retain local schools or shops. In particular, the increase in out-of-town supermarkets has had a severe impact on both small local shopping outlets and traffic rates. One in four food eateries in England is a fast food outlet and guidance for local authorities (https://www.gov.uk/guidance/health-and-wellbeing) advises restrictions in:

- locations where children and young people congregate such as schools, community centres and playgrounds
- areas with high levels of obesity, deprivation and general poor health
- areas with an over-concentration and clustering of outlets.

Evaluating Neighbourhood Work

Numerous activities such as housing regeneration and the creation of community facilities take place *in* neighbourhoods with the aim of improving them, and Case Study 17.5 discusses the evidence of health benefits that arise from community gardens and gardening. There is great potential for integrating health into community activities such as adult education and leisure and cultural activities. Learning Activity 17.3 asks you to consider how to evaluate neighbourhood projects.

It could be argued that any neighbourhood development work has the potential to promote health by increasing social contacts and trust, or building social capital. Additional spin-offs in terms of direct support for healthy lifestyles are common, as the following example shows.

CASE STUDY 17.4
The Healthy New Towns Programme

The Healthy New Towns Programme was launched in 2015 to explore how the development of a new place can lead to a healthier built environment, with strong connected communities and integrated health and social care services. Ten demonstrator sites were chosen to receive funding and technical support: Darlington, Whyndyke Garden Village, Halton Lea, Northstowe, Bicester, Barton, Barking Riverside, Ebbsfleet Garden Village, Whitehill & Boredon, and Cranbrook. The sites have explored the 'how-to' of healthy placemaking, and worked with the National Health Service (NHS), Public Health England, the Town and Country Planning Association, The King's Fund, PA Consulting and The Young Foundation to draw out their key lessons and share these with others via

publications. The ten key principles for a healthy placemaking are discussed in a Kings Fund (2019) report:

1. Plan ahead collectively.
2. Assess local health and care needs and assets.
3. Connect, involve and empower people and communities.
4. Create compact neighbourhoods.
5. Maximize active travel.
6. Inspire and enable healthy eating.
7. Foster health in homes and buildings.
8. Enable healthy play and leisure.
9. Provide health services that help people stay well.
10. Create integrated health and well-being centres.

CASE STUDY 17.5
Community Gardens

Community gardens exist in urban and rural areas in many nations. Community gardens may fulfil a number of functions, including the provision of leisure gardens, school and children's gardens, healing and therapy gardens, demonstration gardens and gardens concerned with ecological restoration. These gardens are actively supported by specific communities, reflecting some form of mutual aid and communal reciprocity. Community gardens probably required a fair degree of altruism in getting started and are very often supported by charities or municipal grant aid. Community gardens may also be grassroots

initiatives aimed at revitalizing low- to moderate-income neighbourhoods in urban settings. Community gardens have been shown to improve health by increasing participants' access to fruit and vegetables, providing the opportunity for regular exercise and communal interaction, and enabling economic self-reliance through using the gardens for training and recreation purposes and selling surplus produce. The figure in this case study shows the impact on health of community gardens, based on evidence from a systematic review of studies and evaluations (Lovell et al., 2014).

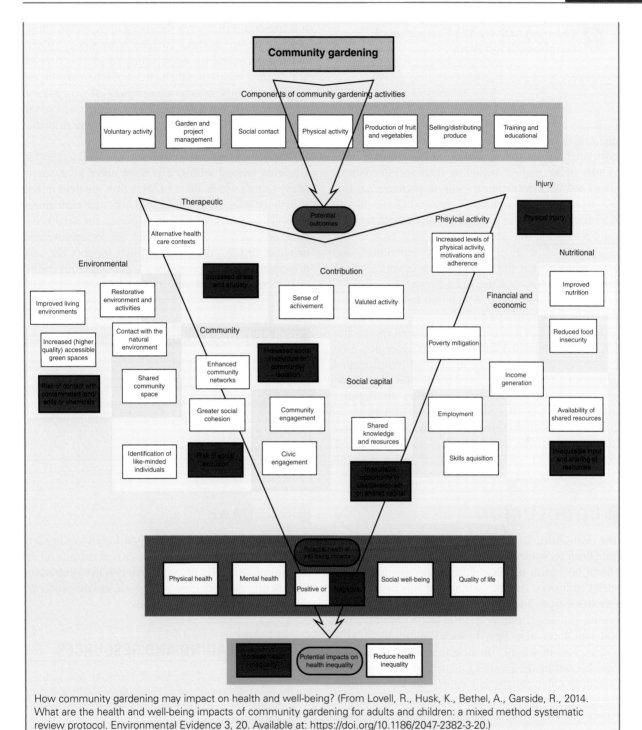

How community gardening may impact on health and well-being? (From Lovell, R., Husk, K., Bethel, A., Garside, R., 2014. What are the health and well-being impacts of community gardening for adults and children: a mixed method systematic review protocol. Environmental Evidence 3, 20. Available at: https://doi.org/10.1186/2047-2382-3-20.)

> **Learning Activity 17.3 Evaluation of Neighbourhood Work**
>
> What might be some of the challenges in the evaluation of neighbourhood development programmes?

In any consideration of the effect of neighbourhoods on health it is very difficult to separate the effects of compositional factors (those relating to the kinds of individuals being studied, including their socio-economic status and lifestyles) from the effects of contextual factors (those relating to the environment) (Kawachi and Berkman, 2003). There is a clear bias in research towards considering the impact of compositional factors. The complexity of relationships between individuals and environments, plus the long timescale in which effects become apparent, militates against research investigating whether differences in health outcomes result from the characteristics of a place.

It is unclear just how effective place-based approaches are, due to the relative lack of substantive evidence on impact, which in turn is due to a lack of well-designed evaluations. Nevertheless, most reviews do suggest the effectiveness of place-based approaches in improving outcomes (e.g., Baczyk et al., 2016; Crimeen et al., 2018; McBride, 2018; Taylor and Buckly, 2017). As Crew (2020, p. 9) states, 'the uncertainty around results is more an issue of "absence of evidence" rather than the "evidence of absence".'

It is important that when focussing on neighbourhood settings or, to use the current terminology 'place-based approaches', the opportunity to address people's self-defined needs is taken. It would be easy to use neighbourhoods merely as a means of professional outreach work, but this would be to neglect one of the great strengths of this setting – its focus on priorities defined by residents.

While there are many advantages to working within a neighbourhood setting, it is not a universal panacea. Many factors which affect people's lives are determined at national level, for example, level of benefit entitlement or availability of employment. However, the neighbourhood setting does offer opportunities for creative and imaginative ways of working which support the core principles of health promotion – participation, equity, empowerment and collaboration.

> **REFLECTIONS ON PRACTICE**
>
> - Think of your neighbourhood. What are its health promotion resources and assets?
> - Many members of the primary care team (especially health visitors and general practitioners) regard themselves as working with neighbourhood communities. How might their role change if they were to focus on place-based approaches?

CONCLUSION

The relationship between people, place and health has long been recognized, for example, in the detrimental effects on health of poor physical environments and social exclusion. The recognition that this health inequity stems from location, geography and place is more recent. The neighbourhood is not just a physical environment, but is also a psychosocial environment, as is a workplace or school. The neighbourhood provides a valuable setting for accessing many vulnerable groups, including older people and people on low incomes. Neighbourhoods are real-life settings with the potential for priorities to be defined by residents rather than professionals. Addressing health on a neighbourhood basis means addressing core determinants of health, such as the social fabric and quality of people's lives.

SUMMARY

This chapter has identified neighbourhoods as a key setting for health promotion and discussed reasons for its popularity. Examples of innovative practice centred on neighbourhood work have been given, and the problems of evaluating such work discussed.

FURTHER READING AND RESOURCES

Barton, H., Thompson, S., Burgess, S., Grant, M. (eds.), 2015. The Routledge Handbook of Planning for Health and Well-being: Shaping a Sustainable and Healthy Future. Routledge, Oxford.
An invaluable edited text with chapters on a range of issues including the obesogenic environment, active travel and safer communities.

Government departments have neighbourhood strategies: https://www.gov.uk/government/organisations/ ministry-of-housing-communities-and-local-government.

https://www.gov.uk/government/publications/health-inequalities-place-based-approaches-to-reduce-inequalities.

Public Health England, 2017. Spatial planning and health: an evidence resource for planning and designing healthier places. Available at: https://assets.publishing. service.gov.uk/government/uploads/system/uploads/. attachment_data/file/729727/spatial_planning_for_health.pdf.

Useful websites include the following:

Joseph Rowntree Foundation (https://www.jrf.org.uk/ cities-towns-neighbourhoods/neighbourhoods) which conducts research into neighbourhoods and communities.

London Healthy Urban Development Unit (www. healthyurbandevelopment.nhs.uk), which works to create healthy sustainable communities through the use of planning regulations and processes.

➤ FEEDBACK TO LEARNING ACTIVITIES

17.1. Neighbourhood and community are often used interchangeably. Neighbourhood refers to a geographical area and the people living within that area. Community refers to people who share a common characteristic, which may be the geographical area they live in but may be another shared characteristic, such as religion or ethnicity (as in the Christian or Black communities). The phrase 'place-based approaches' is also used to describe strategies that address complex determinants of health within a specific location.

17.2. The Marmot Review (2010) identified the following aspects of a neighbourhood as having a significant impact on health: pollution, green and open space, transport, food, housing and community participation. People living in the poorest neighbourhoods will, on average, die 7 years earlier than people living in the richest neighbourhoods (Marmot, 2010).

Tackling inequalities through neighbourhood interventions can be a cost-effective strategy, reaching a large number of people who might otherwise be hard to reach.

17.3. Evaluation of neighbourhood and community work is extremely difficult for several reasons. Firstly, neighbourhood work involves long-term processes to promote social cohesion and regeneration. Funding long-term evaluation projects and maintaining continuity of focus and resources are difficult. Many projects are set up under time-limited funding initiatives which then compromise their sustainability. Projects may find they are diverted from their core business into fundraising in order to keep going. Funding streams may also specify certain activities or outcomes, leading to the neglect of long-term activities to build community capacity and networks.

REFERENCES

Baczyk, M., Sckenk, K., McLaughlin, D., McGuire, A., Gadsden, S., 2016. Place-based approaches to joint planning, resourcing and delivery. An overview of current practice in Scotland. Available at: https:// www.improvementservice.org.uk/__data/assets/pdf_file/0016/10744/place-based-approaches-report.pdf.

Bruhn, J.G., Wolf, S., 1979. The Roseto Story. University of Oklahoma Press, Norman, OK.

Crew, M., 2020. The effectiveness of place-based programmes and campaigns in improving outcomes for children. A literature review. Available at: https://files.eric.ed.gov/fulltext/ED607978.pdf.

Crimeen, A., Bernstein, M., Zapart, S., Haigh, F., 2018. Place-based interventions: a realist informed literature review. Available at: https://chetre.org/wp-content/ uploads/2018/06/Place-based-Interventions-Literature-Review.pdf.

Institute of Health Equity and Jessica Allen, 2018. Healthy high streets: good place-making in an urban setting. Available at: https://assets.publishing.service.gov.uk/ government/uploads/system/uploads/attachment_data/ file/699295/26.01.18_Healthy_High_Streets_Full_Report_Final_version_3.pdf.

Kawachi, I., Berkman, L.F. (eds.), 2003. Neighbourhoods and Health. Oxford University Press, Oxford.

Kings Fund, 2019. Creating healthy places: perspectives from NHS England's Healthy New Town's Programme. Available at: https://www.kingsfund.org.uk/publications/ creating-healthy-places.

Lovell, R., Husk, K., Bethel, A., Garside, R., 2014. What are the health and well-being impacts of community gardening for adults and children: a mixed method systematic review protocol. Environ. Evid. 3, 20. https://doi.org/10.1186/2047-2382-3-20.

Marmot, M., 2010. Fair Society, Healthy Lives. London Institute of Health Equity. Available at: https://www.instituteofhealthequity.org/resources-reports/fair-society-healthy-lives-the-marmot-review.

McBride, M., 2018. Place-Based Approaches to Support Children and Young People. Children's Neighbourhoods Scotland, Glasgow. Available at: https://childrensneighbourhoods.scot/wp-content/uploads/2019/04/cnsplacebasedapproachesliteraturereview.pdf.

Public Health England, 2020. Improving access to greenspace. Available at: https://assets.publishing.service.gov.uk/government/uploads/system/uploads/attachment_data/file/904439/Improving_access_to_greenspace_2020_review.pdf.

Putnam, R.D., 2000. The Collapse and Revival of American Community. Simon and Schuster, New York, NY, USA.

Rice, C., Grant, M., 2007. The Potential of Car-free Developments: Practicalities and Health Impacts. WHO Collaborating Centre for Healthy Cities and Urban Policy, Bristol.

Robertson, D., Smyth, J., McIntosh, I., 2008. Neighbourhood Identity: People, Time and Place. Joseph Rowntree Foundation, UK. Available at: https://www.jrf.org.uk/report/neighbourhood-identity-effects-time-location-and-social-class.

Taylor, M., Buckly, E., 2017. Historical review of place-based approaches. Available at: http://lankellychase.org.uk/wp-content/uploads/2017/10/Historical-review-of-place-based-approaches.pdf.

Wilkinson, R.G., 1996. Unhealthy Societies: The Afflictions of Inequality. Routledge, London.

Wilkinson, R., Pickett, K., 2009. The Spirit Level: Why Equality Is Better for Everyone. Penguin, London.

Health Promoting Health Services

LEARNING OUTCOMES

By the end of this chapter you will be able to:
- understand the concept of a health promoting health service
- discuss the potential of health services to promote health.

KEY CONCEPTS AND DEFINITIONS

Health promoting hospital A hospital which provides high-quality medical care and seeks to develop its health promoting capacity, including its organizational structure and identity, active participation from its staff and patients, its physical environment and its role within the community.

Healthy living optical practice An optical practice that emphasizes health and well-being and where the optometrist will promote public health messages.

Healthy pharmacy A pharmacy which provides high-quality pharmaceutical services, including proactive health advice and interventions within the community it serves.

IMPORTANCE OF THE TOPIC

In this part of the book we have focused on schools, prisons, neighbourhoods and workplaces, where health and health promotion are not part of the setting's core business or primary goals. Hospitals are concerned with health, yet to change a large and complex organization such as a hospital from being focused solely on treatment to being also focused on positive health gain is a major reorientation and a challenging process (see also Chapter 9). There are many other places of treatment, such as general practices, dentists, opticians or pharmacies which, instead of being focused on curing disease and patient compliance, could be places for promoting health and empowering patients, relatives, friends and staff.

Health settings are social systems with their own procedures, culture and values. In common with other settings, there is a difference between health promoting settings and health promotion being carried out within a setting. Settings usually have physical boundaries (including geographical), a range of people with defined roles and an organizational structure. As we have seen earlier in this part of the book, a settings approach is not about doing a health promotion project such as a display for World AIDS Day, nor is it about delegating health promotion to specific departmental or staff 'champions' (Johnson and Baum, 2001), although both activities may be used as part of a wider development. The settings approach to health promotion focuses on bringing about holistic organizational and practice changes to create a more health promoting environment. The process of developing a health promoting health service will thus involve the adaptation of management structures, top-level political commitment and the facilitation of greater participation by staff and patients.

In this chapter the potential of health services to promote health is examined, and examples of good practice are given to illustrate what can be achieved.

263

DEFINING A HEALTH PROMOTING HOSPITAL

The World Health Organization (WHO) definition of a health promoting hospital (HPH) (Nutbeam and Muscat, 2021) provides a useful starting point for understanding what is required:

> The whole-of-system settings approach used by health promoting hospitals draws upon and consolidates several health reform movements: patients' or consumer rights; primary health care; quality improvement; environmentally sustainable ('green') health care and health-literate organisations. The organisational development strategy of Health Promoting Hospitals involves reorienting governance, policy, workforce capability, structures, culture and relationships towards improved health outcomes for patients, staff and population groups in communities and other settings. Strategies and standards based on quality improvement philosophy and tools are used to guide action: on priority health and equity issues; to benefit specific groups of patients.

The hospital as a setting for health was validated by the launch of the HPHs initiative in 1990 by the WHO Regional Office for Europe. This network now includes 669 institutions in 39 countries.

HPHs incorporate a variety of different projects, but with the same overall aims:

- to make the hospital a healthier working and living environment for its workforce and patients
- to expand self-management, recuperation and rehabilitation programmes for patients
- to encourage participation by staff and patients
- to provide information and advice on health issues
- to act as a community resource and an agent of social cohesion
- to act in a socially responsible manner, especially in relation to environmental impact.

WHY HOSPITALS ARE A KEY SETTING FOR HEALTH PROMOTION?

Many health practitioners assume that health promotion has always been a core task of medicine in general and hospitals in particular. Yet health promotion can be at odds with the hospital context, which is based on a medical model of care with an orientation towards cure and treatment. The following examples illustrate this divergence:

- The expectation of the patient role has generally been one of passivity.
- Staff competencies, job remits and time are mainly dedicated to clinical work and care.
- Patients' contact with hospital doctors is generally based on brief 'consultations' related to their particular diseases.
- Patients in hospital are at a late stage in their diseases, and highlighting prevention may make them feel responsible and blameworthy.
- Hospitals are not in themselves healthy environments.

Yet hospitals are also a natural focus for health promotion:

- 20% of the population will visit a local hospital as a patient within a single year, and a further percentage will visit the hospital as family and friends (NHS Confederation, 2017).
- Hospitals are often the biggest employer in their community. 8% of all jobs in Europe are in the healthcare sector (https://www.statista.com/statistics/554899/hospital-employment-in-europe/).
- Contact with patients is at a time of heightened awareness about health and illness, when patients may be motivated to make major lifestyle changes.
- Hospital staff are respected and credible.

There has been a shift in recent years away from an emphasis on the compliant patient to one which is more patient-centred and acknowledges patients' concerns and expertise. Considerable evidence exists to show that patient outcomes are much improved when patients are involved in their own care and have adequate explanations and time to discuss their concerns (Shay and Lafata, 2015; www.nationalvoices.org.uk). A major proportion of hospital admissions are for patients suffering from one or more chronic diseases. These patients require support to cope with their diseases and achieve some changes in their lifestyle, to adhere to possibly complicated drug and nutrition regimens and to manage their condition. There is evidence that patients are more receptive to information and advice in situations of acute ill health reflected in the recent moves to person-centred care (Health Foundation, 2014; Coulter and Oldham, 2016). Hospitals therefore provide a 'window of opportunity' for patients to understand the potential benefits of behaviour change. Learning Activity 18.1 asks you to consider the potential health promoting role of the urgent care or an emergency department of a hospital.

Learning Activity 18.1 Emergency Care and Health Promotion

The role of an emergency department (ED) or accident and emergency (A&E) unit is to provide prompt treatment and care for the acutely ill and injured at all times. How could an ED or A&E promote health?

An HPH will also have benefits for its staff and local community. Staff sickness/absence rates are likely to be lower, and staff retention is likely to be better, in HPHs. Local communities will benefit from having a large, responsible and responsive employer in their area. HPHs will bring income into local communities (through workforce wages), demonstrate how large organizations can be environmentally aware (through, e.g., recycling and local sourcing of food) and provide an accessible and local source of expertise regarding health matters. Chapter 9 illustrates how a hospital could be an anchor institution for a community. Learning Activity 18.2 asks you to consider and discuss what might be the metrics and indicators for an HPH.

 Learning Activity 18.2 Indicators of a Health Promoting Hospital

Existing performance management measures for hospitals relate to productivity, for example, number of emergency admissions, unnecessary procedures and inpatient bed stays. What might be indicators of an HPH?

The WHO Health Promoting Hospital Network was launched in recognition of the impact that a hospital can have, and focuses on four areas (WHO, 2007).
1. Promoting the health of patients.
2. Promoting the health of staff.
3. Promoting the health of the community in the catchment area of the hospital.
4. Changing the organization to a health promoting setting.

PROMOTING THE HEALTH OF PATIENTS

The main focus of most health promotion in hospitals is disease management and prevention for patients. But even in cases of severe diseases, patients are always partly healthy (whether emotionally, socially or spiritually) when they enter the hospital, and these aspects (e.g., self-care, psychological well-being or social contact) can be maintained.

In many healthcare settings, including hospitals, health promotion strategies are often referred to as opportunistic, for example, when a chance has arisen to offer health education or other preventive advice during a clinical visit, such as the Making Every Contact Count (MECC) initiative (https://www.makingeverycontact-count.co.uk/) which is outlined in Case Study 18.1. The skills and competences required for MECC are outlined in Chapter 10. There are other opportunities for more coordinated intervention strategies, such as risk assessment for alcohol-related problems or the offer of chlamydia screening.

 CASE STUDY 18.1
Making Every Contact Count (MECC)

MECC is a national initiative in England intended to extend radically the delivery of public health advice to the public by training all National Health Service (NHS) and local authority staff in the basic skills of giving simple and timely advice to patients and service users. A short intervention, from 30 seconds to 3 minutes, is delivered opportunistically to raise awareness of, and assess a person's willingness to discuss, lifestyle issues. It is claimed that across NHS Midlands and East, for example, there are
- 288,000 staff who collectively have millions of contacts with the public every year. If each staff member delivers MECC just 10 times each year, there will be 2.88 million new opportunities to change lifestyle behaviour every year.
- If 1 in 20 of these people goes on to make a positive change to their behaviour, a total of 144,000 people would be improving their health and well-being every year.

There is an assumption that there is a 'drip drip' cumulative impact when an individual has many conversations about their health.

Opportunistic behaviour change interventions delivered by healthcare professionals can result in patient behaviour change, for example, smoking cessation, but opportunities to address health behaviours directly during clinical interactions are often missed, for example, during cancer screening. Reasons for this may include healthcare professionals' own beliefs about patient motivation to change their behaviour, healthcare professionals' perceptions about themselves as role models or organizational barriers such as lack of time and workload.

The Royal Society of Public Health (RSPH) have developed an initiative in which they encourage allied health professionals to have healthy conversations with patients and clients (https://www.rsph.org.uk/static/uploaded/58510d9a-c653-4e7a-a90133fc4c7b192e.pdf). Research Example 18.1 outlines some of the evidence on the effectiveness and challenges for staff to have such a conversation.

Most healthcare professionals play a minor role in promoting the health of their patients, with the major contributors to patients' health being themselves, their relatives and friends. Empowering patients to get involved as partners and (co-)producers of their health in decision-making and diagnostic and therapeutic processes, through the provision of information and education, is therefore an important health promotion strategy.

Actions such as co-designing pre-admission information with patients, offering computer-based decision aids for treatment options and patient involvement in infection control illustrate how health promotion principles of being equitable, empowering and participatory can become the basis of hospital practice. Maintaining patients' positive health with greater consideration of their quality of life and psychosocial functioning includes:

- securing personal privacy (e.g., data protection, curtains around beds)
- relationship-centred caring
- providing animal therapy
- providing offers and options to encourage psychosocial activities of patients (e.g., cultural activities, religious services, patient libraries, discussions, patient internet café)
- bringing humour into the hospital, for example, by clown doctors
- using art therapy
- providing adequate visiting hours for family members, friends, peers and lay carers
- providing facilities for caring relatives or friends to stay in the hospital (especially for very vulnerable groups of patients, e.g., children and the terminally ill)
- organizing visiting and lay support services for unattended patients
- providing psychological and social assistance to cope with stress or anxieties related to the hospital stay or the patient's specific disease (e.g., cancer, terminal illness), or general life situation (e.g., loss of work due to disease), delivered by specialized personnel (e.g., clinical psychologists, social workers, pastoral carers) (www.hph-hc.cc; Hancock, 2012)
- providing good nutrition and hydration (see Case Study 18.2).

Although the NHS is the only health system in the industrialized world where wealth does not determine access to care, accessing healthcare is still a concern for patients. Before the COVID-19 pandemic, which limited access, 6% of people in the UK (compared to 33% in the USA and 5% in Holland) do not see a doctor when they are sick, or fail to get a prescription, because of the

RESEARCH EXAMPLE 18.1
Healthy Conversations

Elwell et al.'s (2014) study of Birmingham's children's hospital found that there was a general concern about engaging in conversations about health. Participants felt that it was a challenge to combine clinical care with behavioural advice. In both this and another study (Keyworth et al., 2019) some clinical staff were unwilling to discuss behaviours perceived as unrelated to the patient's visit. Discipline-specific tasks were prioritized, and delivering interventions was perceived as psychologically burdensome. Staff adopted avoidance behaviours in order to maintain a positive relationship with patients or clients. They were worried about being perceived as judgmental or alienating parents, and felt that a hospital stay was an inappropriate time to talk about lifestyle changes. Participants in the study were of the opinion that if people did not want to listen to them they were not going to change. Staff reported only offering support to those families who had taken their advice or made changes in the past, and were seen as worthwhile candidates for health advice. Participants reported preferring to engage with patients or clients with whom they had already built a relationship. Nurses in this study did not see the worth of engaging in behaviour advice with patients or families with whom they might not come into contact again. More experienced health professionals found broaching certain topics easier, which in turn reduced their concerns about negative outcomes stemming from such conversations. Participants felt challenged discussing a topic where they did not have personal experience, for example, smoking cessation if they had never smoked. Others felt that social barriers could make it difficult for staff to engage with patients, and that patients may feel more comfortable talking to someone who is 'on their level', such as a healthcare assistant or pharmacy counter assistant.

Hospital Food

One of the worst aspects of hospital care frequently cited by patients is the quality of hospital food. Intake of nutritious food is crucial for patients recovering after surgery or medical interventions. The campaign for better hospital food (http://www.sustainweb.org/hospitalfood/) claims that the NHS spends about £250 million a year on food alone, or £500 million on food and catering staff costs. The NHS serves about 300 million patient meals a year in about 1200 hospitals, as well as several million meals to staff and visitors. Poor-quality food that is overcooked or lukewarm by the time it reaches patients often ends up in the bin. Uneaten meals cost about £18 million a year. If food preparation waste and labour are included, the price of uneaten food rises to over £144 million a year. Over the past few years there has been considerable concern about patient malnutrition and dehydration, and poor-quality food and poor hygiene standards among hospital food suppliers. The Council of Europe passed Resolution ResAP (2003) on food and nutritional care in hospitals, and clinical standards are now established for food, fluid and nutritional care. However, food quality is not included. The Independent Review of NHS Hospital Food in England (NHS, 2020) made eight key recommendations, including upgrading kitchens, enshrining standards for nutrition, sustainability and quality in law (as school food standards are already) and tightening up the monitoring of NHS food by empowering the Care Quality Commission to report on compliance with standards.

cost (www.commonweathfund.org). 1.4 million people miss, turn down or do not seek hospital appointments because of transport problems. With the concentration of acute facilities into fewer and larger units, such problems are likely to increase. Others may not access care because of language barriers or fears of discrimination. A low service uptake may also be due to a service not meeting needs. The articulated needs of minority groups, including Gypsies and Travellers, people with learning disabilities and new migrants, who all experience difficulties accessing healthcare, focus on communication, information and taking account of religion, dietary preferences and obtaining consent (Bhopal, 2007).

Stating that half the population in Europe has limited health literacy, the WHO has called for action in transforming healthcare into health-literacy-friendly settings, and acknowledged that the health sector must remove barriers to information, services and care (WHO, 2013). Brach et al. (2012) identified a health-literacy friendly healthcare organization as one that:

- recognizes that anyone may have difficulty accessing health services, and so offers everyone help with tasks requiring health literacy
- uses communication strategies described in Chapter 10, such as the teach-back technique, which ensures patients' understanding by asking them to repeat back the information provided. Another tool is Ask me 3, which encourages patients to ask three key questions that enable them to understand and manage their care better: What is my problem? What do I have to do? Why is it important for me to do that?
- provides easy access to health information and services and assistance with navigation, for example, using electronic patient portals
- designs printed, audio-visual and social media content that is easy to understand and act upon
- recognizes high-risk situations for people with low literacy, for example, care transitions, invasive procedures and communications about medicines.

PROMOTING THE HEALTH OF STAFF

The hospital as a physical and social setting has an impact on the health of staff. Hospitals are potentially dangerous workplaces, encompassing physical risks (e.g., exposure to biological, chemical and nuclear agents), mental risks (e.g., stress, night shifts) and social risks (e.g., night shifts have a negative effect on social life; bullying and violence against staff). Chapter 16 considered the issue of obesity for workforces and Learning Activity 18.3 asks you to consider this as an issue for NHS staff.

 Learning Activity 18.3   Obese Staff in the NHS

The chief executive of the NHS claimed in 2014 that a third of the NHS workforce are obese. If this is true, what might be the causes, and does it matter?

Other aspects of the environment that affect the health of staff are less likely to be addressed. For example, patients, staff, visitors and the local community are affected by the physical environment of the hospital setting, including its functionality and aesthetic design. In 1859 Florence Nightingale commented:

People say the effect is on the mind. It is no such thing. The effect is on the body, too. Little as we know about the way in which we are affected by form, colour, by light, we do know this, that they have a physical effect. Variety of form and brilliancy of colour in the objects presented to patients is the actual means of recovery.

(1859)

For many of today's patients, visitors and staff, however, the hospital environment remains soulless, drab and depressing. One report (Commission on Architecture and the Built Environment, 2004) highlighted the following as key factors in hospitals' poor working environment:

- fluorescent lighting
- noise
- lack of independent control over ventilation
- no facility for exercise.

The following two research examples outline some of the evidence on the impact of the environment on the health of patients (Research Example 18.2) and staff (Research Example 18.3).

THE HOSPITAL AND THE COMMUNITY

Hospitals have an impact on the health of people living and working in the surrounding neighbourhoods. In recent years the largest capital development programme in the history of the NHS has led to large car parks, energy-intensive air conditioning, heating and

---

RESEARCH EXAMPLE 18.2
Hospitals as Health Promoting Environments

A review of numerous studies (Ulrich et al., 2004) found that the physical design of hospitals can influence a variety of patient outcomes, including cross-infection rates, sleep, length of stay, privacy, communication and social support. The studies conclude that:

- single rooms lower the rate of acquired infections, improve patient confidentiality and facilitate social support
- noise levels can be reduced by sound-absorbing ceilings, noiseless paging and single rooms
- views of natural landscapes reduce stress
- improved ventilation and lighting improve patient outcomes.

RESEARCH EXAMPLE 18.3
Creating a Health Promoting Hospital

The NHS is a round-the-clock service with caring staff who perform work which is often physically and psychologically demanding and can involve risks. A needs assessment of staff at one London hospital (Institute of Health Equity/Barts and the London Trust (2011) found:

- a low percentage use a car to get to work
- low levels of physical activity, and no access to facilities to encourage physical activity at work
- low levels of consumption of fruit and vegetables, which were thought to be overpriced in work canteens; and over 50% of staff do not take a lunch break
- 10% of staff are smokers.

The report includes the following recommendations:

- improve the psychosocial environment, with a culture of concern, reward for work and rest breaks
- better management of bullying and harassment at work
- promote a cycle-to-work scheme and cycling between sites
- reduce the availability of unhealthy food in the canteen and vending machines
- have health champions to lead on public health issues
- focus occupational health and human resources services towards the prevention of ill health.

---

lighting and huge quantities of waste. The recent focus on place-based approaches (see Chapter 17) has also impacted on the NHS. Building and development programmes create local employment and training opportunities alongside upskilling the local workforce, local procurement and working in partnership with local businesses.

ORGANIZATIONAL HEALTH PROMOTION

Healthcare settings are not just sites for health promotion activities, but are social entities that create health. They must therefore incorporate the vision, concepts, values and basic strategies of health promotion (equity, empowerment, participation and collaboration, sustainability) into their structures and culture, leading to the outcome of health (as shown in Fig. 18.1).

An ecological social systems approach to developing a healthy setting requires change from both the top, in relation to organizational development and

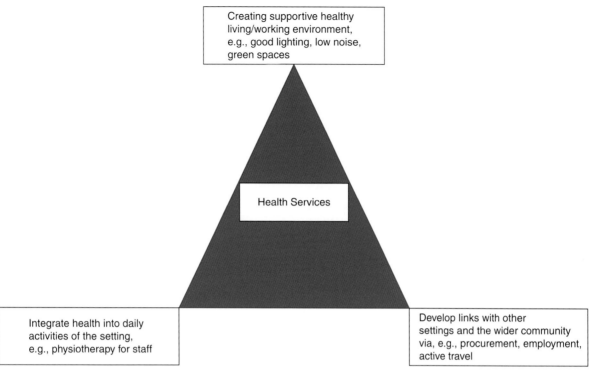

Fig. 18.1 Health promoting health services

political commitment, and the bottom, in high-visibility innovative projects, the active engagement of all users, and embedding health promotion's values into the health setting's institutional agenda and core business. This embedding into the setting's structure and philosophy can be via health promotion being linked and combined with other development strategies (e.g., health education, patients' rights, self-help movements, health at work, infection control, the ecological and sustainable development movement, strategies for personal and organizational development, and quality management) (Dooris, 2006). Learning Activity 18.4 poses a challenge, asking you to imagine yourself as a health champion or a member of a hospital board, and why and in what ways your hospital could become health promoting. Yaghoubi et al. (2019), in a review of implementation of HPHs, identified the following as important in effective development of an HPH: promotion of self-care, knowledge enhancement and patient and staff skills training, improvement of quality indicators and continuous participation of an HPH committee.

> **Learning Activity 18.4 The Arguments for Becoming a Health Promoting Hospital (HPH)**
>
> Give three reasons why a hospital should become an HPH, and three reasons why an HPH is not a good idea.

THE HPH MOVEMENT

The HPH network, launched by the WHO Regional Office in Europe in 1990, now operates in 39 countries on all continents. This initiative seeks to promote good practice by developing concepts and strategies, developing and disseminating model projects and networking via conferences and newsletters. The HPH focuses on the health of staff, patients and the local community.

Hospitals accepted into the HPH network have to meet certain conditions (WHO, 2004):
- develop a written policy for health promotion, and develop and evaluate an HPH action plan to support the introduction of health promotion into the culture

of the hospital/health service during the 4-year period of designation

- identify a hospital/health service coordinator for the coordination of HPH development and activity, and pay an annual contribution fee for the coordination of the international HPH network
- share information and experience on national and international levels, i.e., HPH development, models of good practice (projects) and the implementation of standards and indicators.

The complex organizational structures of many hospitals, and the fact that most health professionals in the hospital setting do not see health promotion as being part of their roles, makes the HPH a challenging setting. Whitehead (2004) argues that the hospital is the least visible of all the Ottawa Charter settings, and Dooris (2006, p. 57; citing McKee, 2000) states that there is 'little empirical evidence of a measurable health impact' of policies focused on creating healthy environments as part of an HPH'. A review found few studies on the benefits and effects of health promoting health services (McHugh et al., 2010), although an evaluation by Whitelaw et al. (2006) did find some positive impact from the implementation of a health promoting services framework. To realize its full potential, the HPH strategy needs to not only be implemented within limited projects but also be embedded as an integral aspect of hospital service (quality) management systems (WHO, 2004). Pelikan (2016) from the WHO Collaborating Centre for Health Promotion in Hospitals and Health Care describes this as a shift in the emphasis on quality criteria, as shown in Fig. 18.2.

HEALTH PROMOTING PHARMACIES

Pharmacies are known as places where medicines and prescriptions are collected. In the UK there is a shift for pharmacies to move from dispensing medicines to promoting health, well-being and self-care, including smoking cessation and weight management. Pharmacies will be the first port of call for minor illnesses and ailments, and will support patients with long-term conditions. Community pharmacies are well placed to do this for the following reasons:

- an estimated 1.2 million people visit a pharmacy each day
- pharmacies are located in communities
- many pharmacists have established good relationships with their regular customers, including people

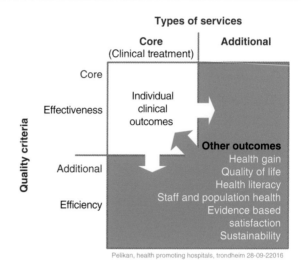

Fig. 18.2 The shift to be a health promoting hospital (From Pelikan, J., 2016. Health Promoting Hospitals: Contributions to quality of treatment and care to reorienting health services, presentation. Health Promotion Research, WHO Collaborating Centre for Health Promotion in Hospitals and Health Care, Trondheim, Norway. 28 September. Available at: https://www.ntnu.edu/documents/8445058/1271135135/Presentation+from+Jurgen+Pelikan.)

with long-term conditions and those with physical and mental disabilities

- pharmacists are acknowledged as experts in medicine by the public and health workers, putting them in an influential position to promote health and prevent ill health.

Table 18.1 suggests some of the ways for a pharmacy to promote health, but there are also obstacles to the development of health promoting pharmacies.

Obstacles to the development of health promoting pharmacies include:

- the lack of a confidential space for discussion
- the lack of training on health promotion and behaviour change for pharmacists
- the pharmacy's priority function as a commercial business.

Achieving Healthy Living Pharmacy (HLP) status is now one of the Quality Criteria for the new National Contractual Framework for pharmacies. It is now a self-accreditation process. The criteria for a HLP include staff trained as health champions; suitable facilities, for example, a private consultation area; and high-quality

TABLE 18.1   Pharmacy Services and Health Promotion

Primary Prevention	Health Education	Health Promotion
• Advice on immunizations and vaccinations • Chlamydia screening • Access to emergency contraception • Provision of statins for people who would benefit	• Maintaining medications • Advice on managing long-term conditions, e.g., asthma • Skills training, e.g., use of inhalers for asthma • Symptom management • Participation in media campaigns • Local knowledge of statutory and non-statutory services	• Tobacco cessation programmes that use nicotine replacement • Monitoring the use of antibiotic prescriptions • Pregnancy testing • Ensuring the pharmacy is user-friendly, e.g., appropriate location, opening times, welcoming staff, atmosphere

NHS services, such as emergency contraception, stopping-smoking programmes, weight management and health checks, in addition to the core services of medicine supply and self-care advice.

A systematic review was equivocal about the effectiveness of pharmacies as health promoting settings, concluding that 'Health-promotion interventions in the community pharmacy context probably improve pharmacy workers' behaviour and probably have a slight beneficial effect on health-related behaviour, intermediate clinical outcomes, and quality of life for pharmacy users' (Steed et al., 2019).

HEALTH PROMOTING DENTAL AND OPTICAL PRACTICE

Some of the same considerations about community pharmacies also apply to dental and optical practices which are also close to their communities. There is plenty of evidence for the effectiveness of health promotion

in dental healthcare settings in relation to smoking cessation, the identification of human immunodeficiency virus (HIV) and acquired immunodeficiency syndrome (AIDS) and diabetes, as well as periodontal diseases (e.g., Scottish Needs Assessment Programme, 2016). There are some highly developed local oral health promotion strategies (e.g., https://democracy.bristol.gov.uk/documents/s6367/Oral_Health_Promotion_Strategy_Appendix%20B%20KC%201st%20Aug%202016.pdf) and an oral health improvement strategy in Scotland (https://www.gov.scot/publications/oral-health-improvement-plan/pages/11/) as well as NICE guidelines on oral health promotion (https://www.nice.org.uk/guidance/ng30/resources/oral-health-promotion-general-dental-practice-pdf-1837385644741). Similarly, optical practices exist in most high streets and communities and so are easily accessible. With 13 million sight tests carried out in 2020, they offer a great opportunity to initiate conversations with individuals about health and well-being. Learning Activity 18.5 asks you to consider what might be involved in a health promoting dental or optical practice.

The Healthy Living Optical Practice (HLOP) programme started in Dudley in the Midlands following the success of the HLP project.

 Learning Activity 18.5   Look Back at Fig. 18.1 – What Would a Health Promoting Optical Practice Look Like?

What would a health promoting optical practice look like?

CONCLUSION

Although core activities of health services remain focused on medical diagnosis and treatment, the healthy settings concept has taken root and there are many examples of hospitals, and more recently pharmacies and general and optical practices, embracing health promotion principles. Health promoting initiatives occur at all levels, from individual practitioners using checklists to systematically include health promotion in client contacts, to hospital-wide initiatives to increase service user participation and reduce environmental impact. In-between lie a range of activities at ward or departmental level, including the use of arts therapies and the provision of healthy locally sourced food. All initiatives are guided by core health promotion principles: a holistic concept of health, empowerment, participation, intersectoral collaboration, equity and sustainability.

Health promoting health services need to be supported by an organizational structure: support from management, a budget, specific aims and targets and action plans for implementing health promotion as part of everyday business. All staff need to make health promotion their business. This can be a challenge, particularly for staff in acute settings, who are trained in other priorities (e.g., diagnosis and treatment). Treating health promotion as a specific quality aspect which needs to be monitored can aid its incorporation into core processes. Integrating health impact assessments into all decision-making within the hospital will also help to advance the HPH.

REFLECTIONS ON PRACTICE

- Think of a health facility you use or work in. Can you identify activities that promote equity, collaboration, participation, engagement and empowerment?
- What factors might impede the development of the service becoming health promoting? How could these factors be addressed?

▌ SUMMARY

This chapter has looked at the reasons for prioritizing health services for health promotion. Recent national and international policy developments which affect the delivery of health promotion in health service settings, and the range of professionals involved, have been identified. Ways in which the following health promotion principles may be applied in health service settings have been discussed:

- person-centred care
- using every healthcare contact as a health improvement opportunity

- staff health and well-being
- an environment where the healthier choice is the easy choice.

FURTHER READING AND RESOURCES

Various documents from the healthy hospital movement include:

Gröene, O., Garcia-Barbero, M. (eds.), 2005. Evidence and Quality Management. WHO, Copenhagen. Available at: http://www.euro.who.int/__data/assets/pdf_file/0008/99827/E86220.pdf.
Summarizes evidence on HPHs and knowledge on implementation of the concept implementation.

Hancock, T., 2012. The healthy hospital: a contradiction in terms? In: Scriven, A., Hodgins, M. (eds.), Health Promotion Settings: Principles and Practice. Sage, London, pp. 126–140.
An interesting discussion of the potential of the hospital as a health promotion setting.

McHugh, C., Robinson, A., Chesters, J., 2010. Health promoting health services: a review. Health Promotion International 25, 230–237.
A useful summary of the evidence on the benefits of health promoting services.

World Health Organization, 2004. Standards for Health Promotion in Hospitals. WHO Office for Europe, Copenhagen. Available at: http://www.euro.who.int/__data/assets/pdf_file/0006/99762/e82490.pdf.

World Health Organization, 2006. Putting HPH Policy into Action: Working Paper. WHO Collaborating Centre on Health Promotion in Hospitals and Health Care, Vienna. Available at: http://www.hph-hc.cc/fileadmin/user_upload/HPH_BasicDocuments/Working-Paper-HPH-Strategies.pdf.
Theory-driven background paper on 18 HPH core strategies, including examples and selected evidence.

World Health Organization, 2007. Integrating Health Promotion into Hospitals and Health Services Concept, Framework and Organization. WHO Office for Europe, Copenhagen. Available at: http://www.euro.who.int/__data/assets/pdf_file/0009/99801/E90777.pdf.

FEEDBACK TO LEARNING ACTIVITIES

18.1. The ED can be a suitable setting for health promotion because it is an established entry point to the health system and it tends to have good links with the community. Bensburg and Kennedy (2002) offer numerous examples of health promotion strategies, from risk assessment (young people and alcohol) to health information (triage nurses providing information to carers who are high users of emergency paediatric services, including a follow-up appointment after discharge) and health education (asthma management training and follow-up telephone calls, and using the waiting room to promote reading and literacy to children). A more recent study (Robson et al., 2020) identified constraints of time and staff capability.

18.2. An HPH would adhere to the following core principles, outlined in the Vienna Recommendations (WHO, 1997):
- acknowledges differences in the needs, values and cultures of different population groups
- promotes dignity and empowerment
- forms as close links as possible with other levels of the healthcare system and the community.

18.3. The NHS workforce is similar to the rest of the population, which also has a high level of obesity. It is estimated that 28% of the adult population are obese (https://digital.nhs.uk/data-and-information/publications/statistical/statistics-on-obesity-physical-activity-and-diet/england-2020/part-3-adult-obesity-copy). If the NHS chief executive's claims are true, NHS staff have an above-average rate of obesity. This could be due to some aspects of the NHS work environment, for example, shift work and lack of access to healthy food in work canteens. Being obese compromises health and impacts on certain aspects of care, for example, manual handling and a lack of willingness to deliver health promotion messages about diet and healthy eating. High levels of obesity among NHS staff are therefore a matter of concern for several reasons.

18.4. Reasons why there may be objections to an HPH include:
- it takes up valuable staff time
- there are no specific and skilled personnel to implement an HPH
- the purpose of a hospital is to treat patients
- any actions will be small scale, and health promotion is best taken place in the community.

18.5. Dental practices are known as places where oral ill health and disease are treated. However, they could provide many more services, including smoking cessation services and nutritional advice. There is an emerging body of evidence that periodontal disease, which is associated with chronic inflammation, may also contribute to more severe outcomes in those with COVID-19 (Marouf et al., 2021). There is an ongoing discussion about the use of behaviour change techniques to promote oral health – discussing with patients their perceived susceptibility to periodontal disease and its severity, and coaching patients to tooth brushing and flossing, using a nuanced and tailored style of communication.

Optical practices offer a sight test through which an optometrist can pick up many conditions of the eyes that are related to the patient's general health. Diabetes, hypertension and hyperlipidaemia can all be identified during a sight test. There are also lifestyle factors, such as smoking and poor diet, which have an impact on eye health as well as general health.

REFERENCES

Bensberg, M., Kennedy, M., 2002. A framework for health promoting emergency departments. Health Promot. Int. 17, 179–188. Available at: http://heapro.oxfordjournals.org/content/17/2/179.full.pdf+html.

Bhopal, R., 2007. Ethnicity, Race and Health in Multicultural Societies. Oxford University Press, Oxford.

Brach, C., Dreyer, B., Schyve, P., Herrnandez, L.M., Baur, C., et al., 2012. Attributes of a Health Literate Organization. Institute of Medicine. Available at: https://nam.edu/wp-content/uploads/2015/06/BPH_Ten_HLit_Attributes.pdf.

Commission on Architecture and the Built Environment, 2004. The Role of Hospital Design in the Recruitment, Retention and Performance of NHS Nurses in England. Queen Margaret University College, Edinburgh.

Coulter, A., Oldham, J., 2016. Person-centred care: what is it and how do we get there? Future Hosp. J. 3 (2), 114–116.

Dooris, M., 2006. Healthy settings: challenges to generating evidence of effectiveness. Health Promot. Int. 21, 55–65.

Elwell, L., Powell, J., Wordsworth, S., Cummins, C., 2014. Challenges of implementing routine health behaviour change support in a children's hospital setting. Patient Educ. Couns. 96, 113–119.

Hancock, T., 2012. The healthy hospital: a contradiction in terms? In: Scriven, A., Hodgins, M. (eds.), Health Promotion Settings: Principles and Practice. Sage, London, pp. 126–140.

Health Foundation, 2014. Person centered care made simple. Available at: https://www.health.org.uk/publications/person-centred-care-made-simple.

Institute of Health Equity/Barts and the London, 2011. Strategy for health promoting hospitals. Available at: https://www.instituteofhealthequity.org/resources-reports/barts-and-the-london-nhs-trust-health-promoting-hospitals-strategy/barts-and-the-london-nhs-trust-health-promoting-hospitals-strategy.pdf.

Johnson, A., Baum, F., 2001. Health promoting hospitals: a typology of different organizational approaches to health promotion. Health Promot. Int. 16, 281–287.

Keyworth, C., Epton, T., Goldthorpe, J., Calam, R., Armitage, C.J., 2019. It's difficult, I think it's complicated: health care professionals' barriers and enablers to providing opportunistic behaviour change interventions during routine medical consultations. Br. J. Health Psychol. 24 (3), 571–592. Available at: https://bpspsychub.onlinelibrary.wiley.com/doi/10.1111/bjhp.12368.

Marouf, N., Cai, W., Said, K.N., Daas, H., Diab, H., et al., 2021. Association between periodontitis and severity of COVID-19 infection: a case control study. J. Clin. Periodontol. 48, 483–491.

McHugh, C., Robinson, A., Chesters, J., 2010. Health promoting health services: a review of the evidence. Health Promot. Int. Available at: http://heapro.oxfordjournals.org/content/early/2010/02/23/heapro.daq010.full.pdf+html.

McKee, M., 2000. Settings 3 – health promotion in the health care sector International Union for Health Promotion and Education. The Evidence of Health Promotion Effectiveness. Shaping Public Health in a New Europe. Part Two: Evidence Book. ECSC-EC-EAEC, Brussels.

NHS Confederation, 2017. Key Statistics on the NHS. Available at: https://www.nhsconfed.org/publications/key-statistics-nhs.

NHS, 2020. Independent Review of Hospital Food. Available at: https://assets.publishing.service.gov.uk/government/uploads/system/uploads/attachment_data/file/929234/independent-review-of-nhs-hospital-food-report.pdf.

Nightingale, F., 1859. Notes on Nursing What It Is and What It Is Not 84. Lippincott, Williams and Wilkins, Philadelphia.

Nutbeam, D., Muscat, D.M., 2021. Health promotion glossary. Health Promot. Int. Available at. https://doi.org/10.1093/heapro/daab067. daaa157.

Robson, S., Stephenson, A., McCarthy, C., Lowe, D., Conlen, B., et al., 2020. Identifying opportunities for health promotion and intervention in the ED. Emerg. Med. J. https://doi.org/10.1136/emermed-2019-209101.

Scottish Needs Assessment Programme, 2016. Oral health promotion. Available at: https://www.scotphn.net/wp-content/uploads/2015/11/Oral_Health_Promotion.pdf.

Shay, L.A., Lafata, J.E., 2015. Where is the evidence? A systematic review of shared decision making and patient outcomes. Med. Decis. Making 35 (1), 114–131.

Steed, L., Sohanpal, R., Todd, A., Madurasinghe, V.W., Rivas, C., et al., 2019. Community pharmacy interventions for health promotion: effects on professional practice and health outcomes. Cochrane Database Syst. Rev. 2019 (12), CD011207.

Ulrich, R., Simring, C., Joseph, A., Choudhary, R., 2004. The Role of the Physical Environment in the Hospital of the 21st Century: A Once in a Lifetime Opportunity. Available at: https://www.healthdesign.org/chd/research/role-physical-environment-hospital-21st-century.

Whitehead, D., 2004. The European health promoting hospitals (HPH) project: how far on? Health Promot. Int. 19, 259–267.

Whitelaw, S., Martin, C., Kerr, A., Wimbush, E., 2006. An evaluation of the Health Promoting Health Service Framework: the implementation of a settings based approach within the NHS in Scotland. Health Promot. Int. 21 (2), 136–144.

World Health Organization, 1997. Vienna Recommendations on Health Promoting Hospitals. WHO, Vienna.

World Health Organization, 2004. Standards for Health Promotion in Hospitals. WHO, Copenhagen.

World Health Organization, 2007. Integrating Health Promotion into Hospitals and Health Services: Concept, Framework and Organization. WHO, Copenhagen. Available at: http://www.euro.who.int/_data/assets/pdf_file/0009/99801/E90777.pdf.

World Health Organization, 2013. Health Literacy: The Solid Facts. WHO, Copenhagen. Available at: http://www.euro.who.int/__data/assets/pdf_file/0009/99801/E90777.pdf.

Yaghoubi, M., Karamali, M., Bahadori, M., 2019. Effective factors in implementation and development of health promoting hospitals: a systematic review. Health Promot. Int. 34 (4), 811–823.

Health Promoting Prisons

IMPORTANCE OF THE TOPIC

Prisons have been identified as a health promotion setting in a variety of policy documents over the last 30 years. Over 30 European countries are now members of the World Health Organization (WHO) Health in Prisons Project (HIPP) network. Prisons have been identified as a key setting for health promotion for several reasons. Prisoners are one of the most socially excluded groups in society, so addressing their health is a means of addressing health inequalities. However, there are also challenges to promoting health within prisons, and there are many features of prison life that would seem to militate against a healthy lifestyle. There is a range of possible interventions, and a growing body of evidence for their effectiveness. As with all settings, the evidence suggests an integrated whole-systems approach works best within the prison setting to promote the health of prisoners, staff and the wider community.

WHY PRISONS ARE A KEY SETTING FOR HEALTH PROMOTION

While it may seem that health promotion runs counter to the setting of a prison, which curtails freedom and choice, there are several reasons why prisons have been identified as a suitable setting for health promotion:
- prisoners are a socially excluded group suffering from demonstrable health inequalities
- the prison population is a 'captive audience'
- prisoners typically comprise the 'harder-to-reach' segments of the population and some evidence of this is provided in Case Study 19.1
- prisoners often service multiple and short-term sentences, so improving their health will also impact on their families and communities.

The rate of ill health in the prison population is higher than in the wider community. Mental health problems and drug and alcohol issues are commonplace among prisoners. Imprisonment tends to exacerbate social exclusion and mental ill health, and increase the occurrence of risky behaviours such as the shared use of needles for drug injections. Overcrowding is an ongoing problem within prisons. The Howard League estimate that in the UK 12, 000 prisoners (out of a total prisoner population of around 75, 000) are being held two to a cell in cells designed for one (https://howardleague.org/news/revealed-the-scale-of-prison-overcrowding-in-england-and-wales/).   Overcrowding leads to unsafe and degrading conditions, increases the risk

275

CASE STUDY 19.1
Prisoners as a Socially Excluded Group

The following statistics clearly demonstrate that many prisoners have experienced a lifetime of social exclusion:

- prisoners are 13 times more likely than the general population to have been in care as a child and to be unemployed
- 20%–30% of all offenders have learning disabilities or difficulties that interfere with their ability to cope with everyday life
- one-third of prisoners were not in permanent accommodation prior to their imprisonment
- 49% of female and 23% of male prisoners suffer from anxiety and depression
- half of women prisoners have suffered domestic violence and one-third have suffered sexual abuse
- half of male prisoners have no qualifications
- nearly half of all prisoners' reading age is at, or below, the level expected of an 11-year-old
- prisoners are more likely than the general public to engage in high-risk behaviours such as smoking, hazardous drinking and unprotected sex.

From The Prison Reform Trust, 2019. Prison the Facts. Bromley Briefings. Available at: http://www.prisonreformtrust.org.uk/Portals/0/Documents/Bromley%20Briefings/Prison%20the%20facts%20Summer%202019.pdf.

of transmission of infectious diseases, and impedes prisoners' access to purposeful training opportunities, exercise and fresh air. From a health inequalities perspective, prisoners are thus a key target group. Although this chapter has highlighted the evidence for challenges to prisoners' health, Learning Activity 19.1 asks you to debate a more philosophical question about whether prisons can or should be health promoting.

Learning Activity 19.1 Health Promoting Prisons: An Oxymoron?

Is there a contradiction between using prisons as a penal system to remove people's liberty and using prisons as a health promoting setting?

BARRIERS TO PRISONS AS HEALTH PROMOTING SETTINGS

Prisons are by their nature closed communities. For some this may mean the use of prisons as a health promoting setting is a contradiction in terms, as key principles of

health promotion such as free choice and empowerment are severely restricted (De Viggiani, 2006a). The prison regime allows prisoners little opportunity to make decisions, exert their autonomy or become empowered. The monotony and boredom of prison life may predispose some prisoners towards risk-taking behaviour (such as smoking or drug use). The evidence on smoking in prisons and how it can be reduced are outlined in Research Example 19.1. Prison culture is known for its bullying, victimization and violence – all factors that contradict health promotion principles. As Woodall et al. (2014, p. 480) put it, 'The paradox is that prisons are by their nature disempowering yet are tasked with creating more

RESEARCH EXAMPLE 19.1
Smoking in Prisons

Smoking has been banned in most enclosed public spaces since 2006. However, people in custody were still allowed to smoke in their cells. Smoking prevalence among those in custody in Scotland, 72% in 2015, was three to four times higher than in the general population. There are correspondingly high co-morbidities, for example, in Australia mortality rates from smoking-related cancers for people who had been imprisoned are double that of the general population (de Andrade and Kinner, 2017).

Prisons remain one of the few UK workplaces where staff continued to be exposed to second-hand smoke (SHS) after it was banned in 2006. Several countries (e.g., Canada, New Zealand, England and Wales) have introduced smoke-free policies to reduce the burden of tobacco on people in custody and staff. Scotland's prisons became smoke-free in 2018, in part in response to evidence on SHS levels (Semple et al., 2020)

There is little consensus on the effectiveness of smoking bans and the availability of cessation programmes on smoking behaviour, either in prison or post release, and also limited evidence regarding the impact of the ban on other prisoner behaviours such as aggression (de Andrade and Kinner, 2017).

E-cigarettes (disposable and rechargeable with prefilled e-liquids) became available in all prisons in the UK in an attempt to support individuals to stop smoking or cope without tobacco, and to support prison services through challenging organizational change (e.g., to reduce aggression and violence) (Brown et al., 2021). Possible risks of allowing e-cigarettes in prison include their potential to be repurposed to charge illicit mobile phones or facilitate illicit drug taking.

empowered individuals capable of taking control of their lives on release.'

Other commentators, however, see the nature of the prison setting as offering potential to promote health, as it guarantees access to prisoners and a long-term stable environment where any changes will impact directly on inmates (Ramaswamy and Freudenberg, 2007). Targeting prisoners also potentially enables health promotion programmes to reach out beyond the prison to prisoners' families and deprived communities. The imprisonment of a family member often leads to emotional, psychological and financial stress for the rest of the family. The availability of support in prison may prompt offenders to seek help when they are released.

Finally, targeting the prison as a setting enables interventions to reach prison staff as well as prisoners. Prison staff are an important, if neglected, target group in their own right. The positive health and well-being of staff can also be expected to impact favourably on the prisoners in their charge.

HEALTH PROMOTING PRISONS

A focus on the health of prisoners and the prison setting is a relatively new phenomenon. The first-ever seminar on prison health, organized by the Council of Europe and the Ministry of Justice in Finland, was held in 1991. A European initiative, HIPP, was launched by the WHO in 1995. This programme identified three key priority areas: communicable diseases, mental health and drugs. HIPP's underlying principles included 'All prisoners have the right to health care, including preventive measures, without discrimination and equivalent to what is available in the community' (World Health Organizaton/UNAIDS, 1998).

Prison health was identified in the UK as a key public health target in the 2004 public health white paper (Department of Health, 2004) but there has been little progress (Woodall, 2016). While the settings approach is recognized as crucial to achieving positive health outcomes in other settings discussed in this part of the book, the 'whole-prison approach' to health promotion is not well understood (Health and Social Care Committee House of Commons Education and Skills, 2018).

The whole-prison approach sees the environment, structural issues, physical conditions and policy as interlinked, as shown in Fig. 19.1.

The wider determinants of health – for example, educational attainment, literacy and work experience – need to be tackled by a whole-prison approach. Yet it has been

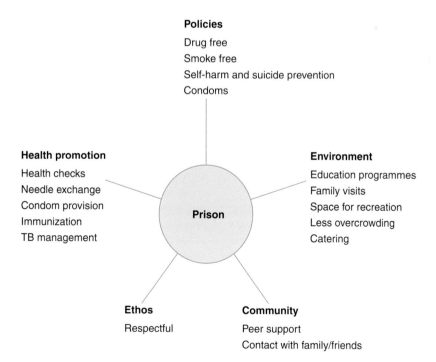

Fig. 19.1 A health promoting prison

argued that a relatively narrow medical perspective still prevails in prisons, with an emphasis on disease control, screening and testing (Woodall and South, 2012). In an analysis of prison inspection reports, Woodall and Freeman (2019) argue there is a dominant focus on lifestyle issues and projects at the cost of a social determinants approach. Yet it is clear that prisoners' health is influenced by a complexity of 'deprivation' and 'importation' factors – relating both to imprisonment itself and to circumstances pre-dating imprisonment (De Viggiani, 2006b). Furthermore, there is a contradiction between the dominant aims and culture of prisons as a place of deterrence, punishment and reform, and values central to health promotion – such as enablement and empowerment (Woodall et al., 2014). Learning Activity 19.2 asks you to consider a core health promotion value – decency – and the extent to which it is evident in the prison setting.

❓ Learning Activity 19.2   Decency and Health Promotion

The concept of decency has been identified as an important foundation for promoting health. What do you understand by this concept?

The settings approach is based on an ecological model that sees health as created in the interaction of personal, organizational and environmental factors (Dooris, 2009). A health promoting prison, just like a health promoting school, will therefore focus on all aspects of life, from individual health needs to the social community it represents for prisoners, and as a workplace for staff, as shown in Fig. 19.1.

EXAMPLES OF EFFECTIVE INTERVENTIONS

The novelty of the prison as a health promoting setting means that the evidence base for effective interventions is scarce. However, theory suggests that a whole-systems approach, involving the prison's social and physical environment as well as individual behaviours, is likely to prove most effective. Developing a whole-prison approach involves three components:
- policies that promote health, for example, no smoking, prevention of communicable diseases

- an environment that is supportive of health, for example, the opportunity to undertake meaningful work
- prevention and health education programmes, for example, avoiding sexually transmitted infections, anger management and immunization against TB and hepatitis B.

What evidence there is suggests prisons can be an effective setting for health promotion. For example, a review of needle-exchange programmes in prisons concluded that they were effective in reducing reported needle sharing and did not undermine institutional safety or security (Lines et al., 2005). These programmes remain recent and controversial, with the first trial of such a scheme in Australia in 2012. There is also evidence that substitution therapy is beneficial, and that together these measures can reduce the spread of HIV and help support the health of drug-addicted prisoners (Gatherer et al., 2005). Other projects provide a variety of opportunities for offenders to participate in gardening and cooking activities that increase physical activity and improve mental well-being (Baybutt et al., 2019).

A coordinated approach is necessary to address the multiple determinants – individual, social and environmental – that affect prisoners' health. This in turn requires an infrastructure, including supportive policies, senior support and leadership, coordination of efforts and engagement with both staff and prisoners.

▌CONCLUSION

The philosophical underpinnings of health promotion working towards empowerment, autonomy, participation, partnerships and informed choice seem at odds with prison regimes that are hierarchical, disempowering and security-focused. This is why the prison setting is the most challenging of all the WHO settings for promoting health. Yet it also presents an opportunity to tackle health inequalities and address a socially marginalized and excluded group in conditions of relative security and predictability.

Over the last 30 years the prison has been identified as a health promoting setting by the WHO, the European Community and the UK government in a number of policy and strategic documents. Various projects tackling health behaviours have been launched, but evaluation suggests the most effective programmes are those that address the whole prison system. Applying the whole-organization focus makes clear that a health promoting prison must be safe, secure and address the prison culture and its physical and social environment. A systems perspective means, according to Baybutt and Chemlal (2016), ensuring that all the parts of the prison system (not solely the healthcare service) address the range of health and social issues across the pathways of the wider criminal justice system before, during and after prison. Funding prison health promotion programmes is likely to be a sound economic investment, as it may help prevent reoffending as well as improving health.

SUMMARY

This chapter has examined the reasons why prison has been identified as a health promoting setting, and outlined some of the most important policies and strategies. The barriers to promoting health in prisons have been identified and discussed. Some examples of successful projects have been given to illustrate the potential for the prison as a healthy setting.

REFLECTIONS ON PRACTICE

'Health promotion in prisons is a contradiction in terms'. Construct an argument either for or against this proposition.

FURTHER READING AND RESOURCES

De Viggiani, N., 2006. A new approach to prison public health? Challenging and advancing the agenda for prison health. Crit. Public Health 16 (4), 307–316.
A persuasive proposal to advance prison health through moving 'upstream' to address the determinants of health.
Woodall, J., Dixey, R., South, J., 2014. Control and choice in English prisons: developing health promoting prisons. Health Promot. Int. 29 (3), 474–482. Available at: http://heapro.oxfordjournals.org/content/29/3/474.full.pdf+html.
Discusses how key elements of health promotion discourse – choice, control and implicitly, empowerment – can apply in the context of imprisonment.
World Health Organization, 2014. Prisons and Health Copenhagen. WHO. Available at: http://www.euro.who.int/-data/assets/pdf_file/0005/249188/Prisons-and-Health.pdf?ua=1.

FEEDBACK TO LEARNING ACTIVITIES

19.1. The key elements of a health promoting setting are choice and empowerment. Many would argue that health promotion is impossible in a setting which curtails freedom and choice (e.g., De Viggiani, 2006a). Woodall (2016) argues that prisoners should be conceptualized as 'citizens in prison' and equipped with the necessary skills to successfully reintegrate back into society.

19.2. It has been argued that decency underpins all aspects of prison life (Wheatley, 2001). Decency includes clean facilities, attending promptly to prisoners' concerns, protecting prisoners from harm, and fair and consistent treatment of prisoners by staff.

REFERENCES

Baybutt, M., Chemlal, K., 2016. Health-promoting prisons: theory to practice. Glob. Health Promot. 23 (1 suppl.), 66–74. https://doi.org/10.1177/1757975915614182.
Baybutt, M., Dooris, M., Farrier, A., 2019. Growing health in UK prison settings. Health Promot. Int. 34 (4), 792–802. https://doi.org/10.1093/heapro/day037.
Brown, A., O'Donnell, R., Eadie, D., Purves, R., Sweeting, H., et al., 2021. Initial views and experiences of vaping in prisons: a qualitative study with people in custody preparing for the imminent implementation of Scotland's prison smokefree policy. Nicotine Tob. Res. 23 (3), 543–549. https://doi.org/10.1093/ntr/ntaa088.
De Andrade, D., Kinner, S.A., 2017. Systematic review of health and behavioural outcomes of smoking cessation interventions in prisons. Tob. Control. 26, 495–501.
De Viggiani, N., 2006a. Surviving prison: exploring prison social life as a determinant of health. Int. J. Prisoner Health 2 (2), 71–89.
De Viggiani, N., 2006b. A new approach to prison public health? Challenging and advancing the agenda for prison health. Crit. Public Health 16 (4), 307–316.

Department of Health, 2004. Choosing health. Making healthy choice easier. Available at: https://www.yearofcare.co.uk/sites/default/files/images/DOH2.pdf.

Dooris, M., 2009. Holistic and sustainable health improvement: the contribution of the settings approach to health promotion. Perspect. Public Health 129, 29–36.

Gatherer, A., Moller, L., Hayton, P., 2005. The World Health Organization European Health in Prisons Project after 10 years: persistent barriers and achievements. Am. J. Public Health 95 (10), 1696–1700.

Health and Social Care Committee House of Commons Education and Skills, 2018. Prison health. Twelfth report of session 2017–19. London. Available at: https://publications.parliament.uk/pa/cm201719/cmselect/cmhealth/963/963.pdf.

Lines, R., Jurgens, R., Betteridge, G., Stover, H., 2005. Taking action to reduce injecting drug-related harms in prisons: the evidence of effectiveness of prison needle exchange in six countries. Int. J. Prisoner Health 1 (1), 49–64.

Ramaswamy, M., Freudenberg, N., 2007. Health promotion in jails and prisons: an alternative paradigm for correctional health services. In: Greifinger, R.B., Bick, J., Goldenson, J. (eds.), Public Health Behind Bars. From Prisons to Communities. Springer, New York, pp. 229–248.

Semple, S., Dobson, R., Sweeting, H., Brown, A., Hunt, K., on behalf of the Tobacco in Prisons (TIPs) Research Team, 2020. The impact of implementation of a national smoke-free prisons policy on indoor air quality: results from the Tobacco in Prisons study. Tob. Control. 29, 234–236. Available at: https://tobaccocontrol.bmj.com/content/tobaccocontrol/29/2/234.full.pdf.

The Prison Reform Trust, 2019. Prison the facts. Bromley Briefings. Available at: http://www.prisonreformtrust.org.uk/Portals/0/Documents/Bromley%20Briefings/Prison%20the%20facts%20Summer%202019.pdf.

Wheatley, P., 2001. Prison Service Conference Speech. HM Prison Service Internal Communications Unit.

Woodall, J., 2016. A critical examination of the health promoting prison two decades on. Crit. Public Health 26 (5), 615–621. Available at: https://www.tandfonline.com/doi/pdf/10.1080/09581596.2016.1156649?needAccess=true.

Woodall, J., Freeman, C., 2019. Promoting health and wellbeing in prisons: an analysis of one year's prison inspection reports. Crit. Public Health 30 (5), 555–566. Available at: https://www.tandfonline.com/doi/epub/10.1080/09581596.2019.1612516?needAccess=true.

Woodall, J., South, J., 2012. Health promoting prisons: dilemmas and challenges. In: Scriven, A., Hodgins, M. (eds.), Health Promotion Settings: Principles and Practice. Sage, London.

Woodall, J., Dixey, R., South, J., 2014. Control and choice in English prisons: developing health promoting prisons. Health Promot. Int. 29 (3), 474–482. Available at: http://heapro.oxfordjournals.org/content/29/3/474.full.pdf+html.

World Health Organization/UNAIDS (Joint United Nations Programme on HIV and AIDS), 1998. HIV/AIDS, Sexually Transmitted Diseases and Tuberculosis in Prisons; Joint Consensus Statement. WHO, Geneva.

Implementing Health Promotion

The final part of this book is concerned with the practical task of how to implement health promotion. Good practice depends on the coexistence of many factors: adherence to core health promoting principles, personal skills and training and the use of suitable models and frameworks to guide action. Health promotion programmes and activities should be guided by the following principles:

- Empowering, to enable individuals and communities to take control over the factors affecting their health;
- Participatory, involving all concerned in all stages of the process of development and evaluation;
- Equitable, and guided by a concern for social justice;
- Intersectoral, involving the collaboration of many sectors and agencies;
- Sustainable, such that any change can be continued once initial funding has ended;
- Multi-strategy, combining policy development, legislation and regulation, organizational change, community development, advocacy, communication and education (Rootman et al., 2001).

Good practice also depends on a systematic and structured approach to interventions, which is the focus of this part of the book. There are several stages in programme planning.

1. **Defining the problem to be addressed**. What is the problem? What are its causes and the contributory factors? What are people's needs and what is the nature of the context and communities in which people live?
2. **Solution generation**. How might the problem be solved or addressed? What is known about what works? What do practitioners believe might work? What resources are available?
3. **Intervention testing**. Did the intervention work? How do we know?
4. **Intervention dissemination**. Can the intervention or programme be repeated or should it be refined? Is it feasible to implement given the resources available? Can it be sustained?

Nutbeam (1998) shows the stages of planning in six steps with associated questions in Fig. PIV.1.

As seen in the figure, there are four major stages in carrying out interventions: needs assessment, solution generation based on evidence and theory, planning and evaluation. In Part IV we consider each of these stages in turn, devoting a chapter to each.

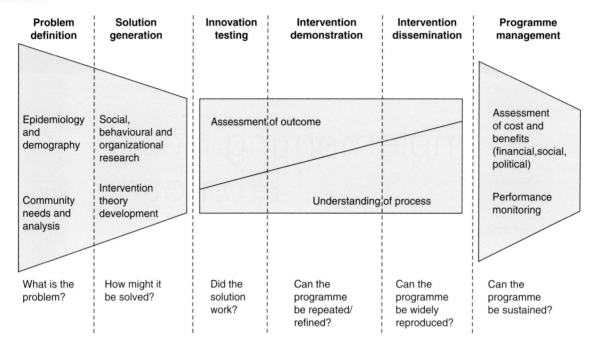

Problem definition	Solution generation	Innovation testing	Intervention demonstration	Intervention dissemination	Programme management
Epidemiology and demography	Social, behavioural and organizational research	Assessment of outcome			Assessment of cost and benefits (financial,social, political)
	Intervention theory development				
Community needs and analysis		Understanding of process			Performance monitoring
What is the problem?	How might it be solved?	Did the solution work?	Can the programme be repeated/ refined?	Can the programme be widely reproduced?	Can the programme be sustained?

Fig. PIV.1 The stages of programme planning and evaluation (From Nutbeam, D., 1998. Evaluating health promotion progress, problems and solutions. Health Promotion International 13 (1), 27–44.)

Chapter 20 explores how needs – whether identified by communities, practitioners or researchers – underpin the actions we take. The process of assessing needs includes soliciting subjective perceptions from clients as well as accessing objective factual indicators such as mortality, morbidity or service-use statistics. Needs assessment methods should be health promoting in themselves, including a variety of participatory methods to support empowerment and capacity building, and a focus on equity of inputs and outputs. Asset based approaches recognize and build on the human, social and physical resources that exist within local communities and can help ensure that public services are provided where and how they are needed. Resource and organizational constraints tend to prioritize disease-reduction targets but understanding the determinants of health will help orient health promotion activities towards 'upstream' interventions.

Evidence-based practice is a key part of the health promotion planning cycle and is explained in Chapter 21. In addition to identifying needs, we need to understand what types of interventions work and under what conditions. Looking at existing evidence helps to make decisions about what to implement to address a problem and how the intervention should be designed, based on whether a successful intervention can be transferable to your context.

A systematic approach to planning will help the health promoter to analyse clearly the problem or area of need, set appropriate aims and objectives, and identify an appropriate plan of action. Chapter 22 discusses the factors that need to be taken into account when planning a health promotion intervention at any level (individual intervention, project or strategy). Planning is an important tool for the practitioner, enabling a structured and rational approach to one's workload. It enables transparency and accountability, allowing all stakeholders to assess the proposed plan and monitor its progress. Planning also contributes towards reflective practice, enabling practitioners to develop their expertise and build their capacity to promote health.

Evaluation has long been recognized as fundamental to good practice but is often neglected. From the point of view of practitioners, reviewing progress and making changes to ensure a project or intervention proceeds as envisaged is all part of sound planning and professional practice. For other stakeholders, evaluation is a means to have their voices heard and their values and priorities recognized. Evaluation helps to build an evidence base, identifying interventions that are not only effective and cost-effective but also acceptable and sustainable. Such evidence should inform decision-making but is often missing in the field of health promotion. Evaluation is therefore a vital stage in developing professional health promotion practice. Chapter 23 discusses the importance of identifying appropriate outcomes and indicators of success, and how practitioners may evaluate their health promotion activities.

Together these four chapters provide a reflective and critical account of the practice of health promotion, combining 'how-to' information with a critique of underlying assumptions and values. The intention is to help practitioners develop effective and reflective practice that operationalizes core health promotion principles, produces the desired results and helps build a solid evidence base for health promotion.

REFERENCES

Nutbeam, D., 1998. Evaluating health promotion progress, problems and solutions. Health Promot. Int. 13 (1), 27–44.

Rootman, I., Goodstadt, M., Hyndman, B., McQueen, D.V., Potvin, L., et al., 2001. Evaluation in Health Promotion. Principles and Perspectives. WHO Europe, Copenhagen. Available at: https://www.euro.who.int/__data/assets/pdf_file/0007/108934/E73455.pdf.

20

Assessing Health Needs and Assets

LEARNING OUTCOMES

By the end of this chapter you will be able to:
- understand the concept of need
- evaluate critically different approaches to identifying needs
- discuss the ways in which policy and practice respond to, and develop, programmes that reflect needs.

KEY CONCEPTS AND DEFINITIONS

Asset The collective resources that individuals and communities have, which protect against negative health outcomes and promote health status.

Community profile A representation (written or graphical) of information regarding the characteristics of a place or community.

Need Something which is required or essential rather than merely desired or wanted.

Needs assessment A systematic process to identify needs or the gap between existing and desired conditions.

Quality-adjusted life year (QALY) The quality-adjusted life year combines both the quality and the quantity of life lived and is used as a measure of the impact of disease and in assessing the value of medical interventions.

Stakeholder An individual, group or community that has an interest in a project, intervention or assessment

Supply Provide or make available something which is wanted or essential.

Want A lack or deficiency of something.

IMPORTANCE OF THE TOPIC

The first phase in health promotion planning is an assessment of what a client, community or population group needs to enable them to become healthier. Within a neighbourhood there will be people in settings such as schools and workplaces, and population groups with specific health needs. Practitioners need to know how to assess individuals, how to manage their care and how to encourage healthier lifestyles. They also require an understanding of people's ways of life and the health problems and opportunities they experience, and they need to know how to use this understanding to systematically assess the needs of people in groups.

The term 'needs assessment' describes the process of gathering information and it is a systematic method

of reviewing the health needs and issues facing a given population leading to agreed priorities and resource allocation. The purpose of health needs assessment at national, regional or local level is to identify:
- What are the highest priority needs?
- Which actions to improve health should have greatest priority?
- Which particular groups or communities should have priority, and so help in targeting interventions and commissioning services?

Asset assessments can be separate from, or combined with, a focus on needs. A focus on assets would document existing resources, strengths and skills in a community.

National Health Service (NHS) and local government reforms have emphasized the participation of local people in setting priorities, signalling a philosophical shift from a paternalistic medical model to a participatory consumer-led model. Recognition of the right to participate in defining health needs and healthcare was also acknowledged in the 1978 World Health Organization Alma Ata Declaration, and one of the underlying principles of Health For All is community participation (World Health Organization, 1985).

This chapter considers the ways in which local health needs are assessed and applied in planning for health promotion. It should be read in conjunction with Chapter 3, which outlines the principal sources of information about health status.

DEFINING HEALTH NEEDS

The concept of need is widely used but often not well understood; Learning Activity 20.1 probes you to define 'need'. People may believe they 'need' a new coat because someone observed that their old one is worn out, or because it looks old compared to other people's coats, or simply because they would like one. A need may thus be something people want or something that is lacking in comparison to others.

 Learning Activity 20.1   Defining Health Needs

How would you define need?

Economists tend to avoid the use of the term 'needs' altogether, arguing that it is overlaid with emotion, and what is really meant by a health need is actually a matter of people's wants and demands, and these are limitless (Cohen and Flood, 2021). Identifying health needs therefore becomes a question of identifying priorities.

An alternative view is that there are universal needs and Learning Activity 20.2 asks you to consider and discuss what these might be. Maslow's (1954) hierarchy of needs suggests that all human needs, whether they are related to safety or self-esteem, are in fact health needs (Fig. 20.1).

 Learning Activity 20.2   Human Needs

- Make a list of 10 important human needs.
- Are some more fundamental than others?
- Are these needs relative to a particular country, or are they universal?

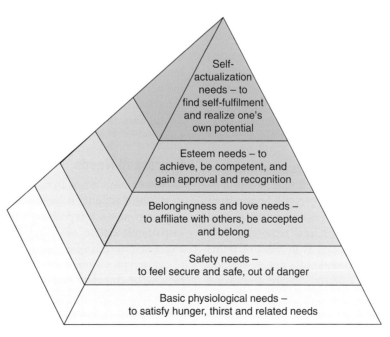

Fig. 20.1 Maslow's hierarchy of needs

For a person to be self-actualizing, physical, social and emotional needs must be met. Doyal and Gough (1992) similarly argued that the ultimate goal of human beings is to participate fully in society, and to do this the basic needs for physical health and autonomy must be met. These needs are not relative to a particular country or period of time, but are fundamental rights and include the prerequisites for health – peace, shelter, education, food, income, a stable ecosystem, sustainable resources, social justice and equity (World Health Organization, 1986) – and social security, social relations, the employment of women, respect for human rights and the alleviation of poverty (World Health Organization 1997). The United Nations Declaration of the Rights of the Child (1959, Article 6) declares that 'the child, for the full and harmonious development of his personality, needs love and understanding'. But these needs are not undisputed. How healthy do people have to be before we can say that their needs have been met?

Bradshaw (1972), in a widely used taxonomy, distinguished four types of health and social need.

1. Normative needs, as defined by experts or professional groups, for example, a patient needs an operation.
2. Felt needs, as defined by clients, patients, relatives or service users, for example, a person feels he or she needs pain relief.
3. Expressed needs, when felt needs become a demand, for example, a person who expects and seeks a service.
4. Comparative needs, identified when people, groups or areas fall short of an established standard, for example, a service should be provided as it is available elsewhere.

Normative Needs

Normative needs are objective needs as defined by professionals, who also identify the ways in which these needs can be met. A normative need reflects a professional judgement that a person or persons deviate from a required standard. This may be against some external criteria such as occupational or legal requirements – thus the manager of a restaurant is in need of training because they have not completed a course in food hygiene. Or it may be that a person deviates from what is defined by medical staff as the range of 'clinically normal' physiological indicators.

Normative needs are not absolute or objective 'facts' – they reflect the judgement of professionals, which may

CASE STUDY 20.1
Normative Needs and Child Development

Growth charts are based on data collected in different populations and time periods. The WHO growth charts (www.rcpch.ac.uk/research/uk-WHO-Growth-Charts) are meant to act as a normative standard, as they are based on children who fulfil specific criteria – being breastfed, born with a specific weight for gestational age, living in adequate socio-economic conditions and born to non-smoking mothers. The data on growth were gathered from infants in the USA, Norway, Oman, Brazil, India and Ghana, and there was a similar linear growth pattern for all the infants. However, a professional may plot a child's growth differently, for example, by not taking account of gestational prematurity or not assessing neonatal weight loss.

be different from that of their clients. Case Study 20.1 illustrates this point by reference to child development. Healthcare workers will judge a need relative to what they are able to provide. The ability to judge normative needs also contributes to the notion of professionalism and the authority and status of professionals.

Felt Needs

Felt needs are what people really *want*. They are needs identified by clients themselves and may relate to services, information or support, which can be termed service needs. Moves towards bottom-up approaches in health and social care have meant a greater acceptance of service users' views. Needs may be limited by the perceptions of an individual. Individuals may not believe themselves to be in need simply because they do not know what is available in terms of treatment or services.

Expressed Needs

Expressed need arises from felt needs but is expressed in words or action – it has become a *demand*. Thus clients or groups are expressing a need when they ask for help or information, or when they make use of a service. Expressed need is often used to measure the adequacy of service provision, even though it is not a comprehensive or complete measure. There are also objective needs which exist but are not expressed. Only a proportion of patients make contact with health services and they are merely the tip of an iceberg of potential need, as illustrated in Fig. 20.2.

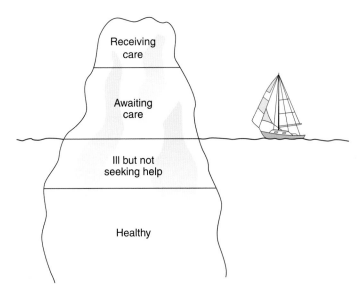

Fig. 20.2 Iceberg of healthcare needs

Sometimes people will use a service because it is all that is available, even if it does not adequately meet needs. The best example of expressed need (and unmet demand) is the waiting list. Some needs are not expressed, perhaps because of an inability or unwillingness to articulate the need. This could be due to language difficulties or a lack of knowledge. Expressed needs should not be taken as an indicator of demand because they also exclude needs which are felt but not expressed. Tudor Hart's (1971) inverse-care law has been of vital importance in showing that just because a service or treatment is used less does not mean that it is needed less. Those who could most benefit from a service are often those least likely to use it. People may express different needs, and there is a tendency to listen to those with loud and powerful voices, such as views which come from an established group or which appear to express a popular need. Responding to expressed needs may also therefore have the effect of increasing inequalities in service provision.

Comparative Needs

Individuals or groups are said to be in need if their situation, when compared with that of a similar group or individual, is found wanting or lacking with regard to services or resources. For example, if a person with dementia in area A is living in sheltered accommodation and receiving day care, but in area B this was not available, we would say that people with dementia in area B were in need. In the NHS, although people may be assessed to be in absolute need (normatively), in practice comparative needs assessment will often dictate whether their needs will be met. Areas may be compared on the basis of provision of services or length of waiting lists to see if the health needs of their populations are being met. In a sense, then, comparative need is about equity, or equal provision for equal need. As stated by Nutbeam (1998, p. 7): 'Equity is about fairness. Equity in health means that people's needs guide the distribution of opportunities for wellbeing.' This kind of analysis of need does, of course, also assume that those in receipt of a service are receiving adequate provision and that their needs are being met. Yet health services are provided in a market environment and are more likely to be led by demand rather than need.

The NHS uses the term 'health gain' in association with health needs to signal that the meeting of needs is related to a person's ability to benefit. Health gain is defined as:
- adding years to life by reducing premature mortality
- adding life to years by enhancing the quality of life and improving well-being.

The concept of health gain is rooted in a medical model, which defines health quite narrowly as the absence of disease. Consequently, health needs tend to be defined as problems which may be successfully met by services or

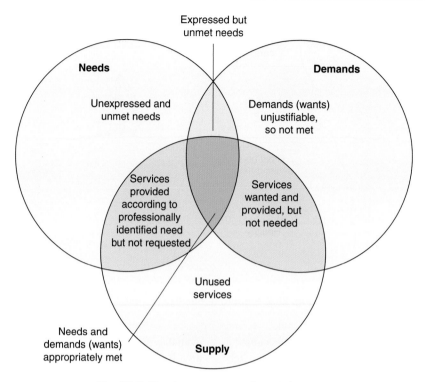

Fig. 20.3 Needs, wants, supply and demand

treatment, and the gain is measured by concepts such as quality-adjusted life years (QALYs) or disability-adjusted life years (DALYs) (these are discussed in Chapter 3). Because need is seen as infinite and resources as limited, health authorities confine themselves to what is known to be effective care. Yet community surveys often show that the public define ill health far more broadly than simply problems requiring treatment by health services. Many priorities for health go beyond the narrow outcomes encompassed by adding 'years to life' and require health authorities to take account of the structural influences on health, such as housing, community safety and transport links. The meeting of needs is also related to what can be offered (what the state can supply). Health economists thus distinguish need from supply. As we have seen, need is influenced by contemporary culture; demand is influenced by the abilities of a person or group to express needs and by the media; supply may be influenced by political pressure. These differing interpretations are illustrated in Fig. 20.3. When demand outstrips supply, people will not be able to access the services they want or even that healthcare professionals believe that they need.

Different groups in society, whether the public, professionals or commissioning or providing organizations, all hold different definitions of need. We can see that needs are not objective and observable entities to which we must just match our interventions. This point is the focus of Learning Activity 20.3 in which you are asked to consider and discuss need in relation to innovation and service development. The concept of need is a relative one, and is influenced both by values and attitudes and by other agendas including political ones.

 Learning Activity 20.3   Needs and Health Service Interventions
Consider these interventions available to women in childbirth. Has medicine created these needs or are they needed improvements in technology?
• Prostaglandin to induce labour.
• Epidural to reduce pain.
• Electronic foetal monitoring.
• Belt monitoring of contractions.
• Elective caesarean section.

What is clear from this discussion is that definitions of need vary depending on whose interpretation and values are used. People's health needs are not the same as those of 20 years ago – the nature and prevalence of diseases may change, as do the expectations of the population and the capacity of health services to meet them.

THE PURPOSE OF ASSESSING HEALTH NEEDS

The process of assessing needs is integral to a basic process approach to planning. Needs assessment, including the collection of data is the first step, from which subsequent aims will be derived. Assessing the health and social needs of local populations is a means of obtaining accurate and appropriate information on which to base priorities, and ensures that decisions are based on solid information and evidence. This overall purpose can be broken down into different elements:
- to direct interventions appropriately
- to identify population needs and reduce inequalities
- to identify and respond to the specific needs of minority and socially excluded or disadvantaged groups
- to allocate resources.

To Direct Interventions Appropriately

Within clinical practice assessing needs is routine and accepted. Assessment takes place to determine what care is required through the gathering of data about:
- the individual, for example, age
- health history, for example, medical, surgical, activities of daily living
- current health, for example, self-reported symptoms
- current health measurement, for example, blood pressure, pain assessment, oxygen saturation.

An integrated care pathway gives a single record of assessment for all the many professionals and agencies who may be involved with a patient, and also provides a map of care for all patients with a similar set of symptoms or diagnosis. It is intended to reduce variations in interpretations of need and treatment offered. The 'common assessment framework' is an assessment tool shared across all children's services and areas in England. Its aim is to identify a child's additional needs which may not be met by the services they are receiving.

For those practitioners who work with individual clients, there is increasing recognition of the importance of client participation in the assessment of needs. Nursing practice, for example, has frequently been criticized for being too inflexible and routine – doing things *to* people rather than *with* them. Prescription has now given way to negotiation, alongside the move from sick nursing to health nursing. Understanding the thoughts, feelings and experiences of individuals has become an important part of the therapeutic and nursing process and some of the associated challenges are considered in Learning Activity 20.4.

 Learning Activity 20.4   Expressed Needs

For what reasons might clients find it difficult to express their needs in a clinical situation?

The needs of patients may not accord with the needs identified by professionals, who may be confined by what they feel they can provide. There are many examples where needs are expressed very differently. For example, the main goal of sanitation programmes in low-income countries is to improve health and reduce diarrhoeal diseases, but according to the summary of the evidence by Mara et al. (2010), householders rarely adopt and use toilets for health-related reasons. Instead, needs in relation to sanitation include the desire for privacy and convenience, to avoid embarrassment, wanting to be modern, to avoid the discomforts or dangers of the bush (e.g. snakes, pests, rain and risk of rape or attack for women) and wanting social acceptance or status. The meeting of a patient's needs is the focus of Learning Activity 20.5.

 Learning Activity 20.5   Meeting Patient Needs

A male patient who is young and fit has a heart attack. The nurse on the ward offers the patient advice on cardiac rehabilitation and information on healthy eating, exercise and safe drinking.
- Is the nurse meeting the patient's needs?
- Is health education information an appropriate intervention?

To Identify Population Needs and Reduce Inequalities

To meet community health needs it is essential to have a clear understanding of what the needs are, what capacity communities have for addressing these needs and

CASE STUDY 20.2

Health Profiles

Local Health (www.localhealth.org.uk) is produced by Public Health England. It provides health information at small-area and local authority levels. It includes:

- the total resident population and the numbers of people in different age groups
- the percentage of the population who cannot speak English well or at all
- the percentage of the population living in income-deprived households
- the crude rate of births per 1000 females of childbearing age
- the percentage of children aged 0 to 15 living in income-deprived households.

Fingertips (https://fingertips.phe.org.uk/) is a rich source of data. You can choose to view by life-course stage (e.g., child health profiles) or view by theme (e.g., perinatal mental health). You can also compare local areas to a range of comparators within the profiles.

Consultation with the community can provide qualitative insights into the health needs of the population that cannot be elicited from data alone. Community consultation is essential in order to obtain information about the perceived needs of local communities and individuals, insight into the experiences of patients, consumers and carers, and their perspectives on barriers to positive health and wellbeing, as well as to ascertain how satisfied the local community is with existing health service provision and identify which health service provision could be improved to better meet their needs.

CASE STUDY 20.3

Health Equity Audit of Diabetic Eye Screening

A review by Public Health England (https://www.gov.uk/government/publications/nhs-population-screening-a-health-equity-audit-guide/diabetic-eye-screening-hea-example) looked at whether demographic factors (e.g., age, sex, ethnicity, language and literacy, deprivation); patient condition (e.g., ambulatory status, diabetes type); service provider (e.g., clinical commissioning group (CCG), registered GP and provider of screening) resulted in inequity. There was significant variation in uptake by the GP practice, CCG and screening location and significant inequity in screening attendance associated with deprivation.

To Identify and Respond to the Specific Needs of Minority and Socially Excluded or Disadvantaged Groups

There are recognizable social, demographic or identity-based groups who have traditionally avoided, or been excluded from, service needs assessments. Such groups may think that services do not care about them, do not listen or are irrelevant. They are sometimes referred to as 'underserved'.

Needs assessments may help to identify populations who are underserved, and also groups at particular risk. The concept of risk groups has emerged as a means of directing health promotion activities to people who are most in need. A risk group may be defined as a population group vulnerable to certain diseases or conditions. A risk group's vulnerability may be due to genetic, lifestyle, economic, social or environmental characteristics. Normative needs derived from epidemiological research, which identifies groups with poorer than average health, are often used to establish target groups. For example, lower socio-economic groups at most risk from ill health and premature death are a commonly identified risk group. Comparative need is used to identify at-risk groups who have low take-up rates of services.

However, a focus on high-risk groups can lead to 'victim blaming'. Health problems are seen as specific to particular groups, who may also be seen as responsible through their behaviour for their own ill health. For example, young people are the subject of numerous targeted health promotion campaigns; yet it is not being young that is a risk, but certain activities. Gay men were

whether particular groups face specific challenges in meeting their needs. Case Study 20.2 outlines some of the information that is routinely collected and available to identify health needs.

A health equity audit (HEA) is a requirement of planning in which local strategic partnerships and other organizations systematically review the role of inequities in the causes of ill health and the access to services for defined population groups (NICE, 2003). The HEA is a process used to examine whether resources are distributed fairly, relative to the health needs of different groups. The overall aim is not to distribute resources equally but rather, relative to health need. It is used to identify and address inequalities, by enabling a systematic review of inequities in ill health or in access to effective services. An example of an HEA is outlined in Case Study 20.3 of diabetic eye screening.

barred from blood donation in many countries until recently, but similarly, it is not being gay that is a risk but certain activities. Many health promoters also reject the notion of targeting because they prefer to work in partnership with groups and communities on the issues *they* define as important.

To Allocate Resources

The NHS was predicated on the notion that there was an untreated pool of sickness which, once treated by a national health service, would diminish. Experience shows that there can be unlimited demand for healthcare. As healthcare is provided, so expectations rise; as technology improves, people with disabilities and chronic conditions live longer and demand more healthcare. General improvements in health and living conditions have led to people living longer and an increase in the percentage of older people in the population. It will not be possible to meet all these needs, as resources are limited.

Most healthcare workers accept that some kind of priority setting or rationing of healthcare is inevitable. There have always been waiting lists, but rationing is a more far-reaching concept. It entails decisions about how much money should be put into different forms of care or treatment. Not only does this raise issues about justice and equity, it also poses the huge dilemma about who decides the priorities for investment. Public views may be very different from those of doctors. For example, infertility treatment may have a high value to individuals but not to society as a whole. Osteoporosis screening (bone-density measurement) may be rated highly by the public but not by doctors, who have access to more information and are therefore able to question its effectiveness.

While the 'postcode lottery' of accessing drugs such as herceptin on the NHS is frequently highlighted, there are also considerable variations in local spending. This is only partly explained by the age and needs of the population and the local cost of services. In Oregon, USA, a health commission of healthcare workers and the public devised a complex formula in the 1990s to prioritize health services, and decided there were certain services that they would not provide. Despite a free and available service in the UK, health authorities are beginning to consider particular services which will not be provided as part of the NHS. Cosmetic surgery, for example, is not provided free for cosmetic reasons alone, but may be allowed for the correction of congenital abnormalities,

injuries and other special criteria determined locally. Learning Activity 20.6 asks you to consider a hypothetical scenario of decision-making about resources.

> **Learning Activity 20.6   Deciding Priorities**
>
> Consider the following typical costs (not actual amounts) of interventions. What factors would you take into account in deciding priorities?
>
> | | |
> |---|---|
> | Home visit by community psychiatric nurse | £50 |
> | Tonsillectomy | £250 |
> | Hip replacement | £1000 |
> | Place in group home for someone with learning difficulties | £30,000 per year |
> | Pregnancy termination | £200 |
> | Brief intervention of psychotherapy (10 weeks) | £1500 |
> | Day care for an older person with mental ill health | £200 per week |

HEALTH NEEDS ASSESSMENT

Needs assessment can be carried out from the perspectives of professionals, the lay public or key informants (members of the community with a particular viewpoint, such as teachers or police officers). It can be carried out at different levels, from that of the individual to specific groups (e.g., population groups, such as older people or people with specific health problems), local geographic communities or national populations. It can inform general practice profiles, community profiles, intervention planning or service design.

Wright (1998) describes three approaches to health needs assessment.

1. Epidemiological (the focus is on the size and nature of the problem).
2. Corporate (the focus is on the views of stakeholders).
3. Community (uses a variety of methods to enable communities to identify, prioritize and decide what actions to take to meet health needs).

In all cases, health needs assessment is a systematic and explicit process identifying issues affecting a population that can be addressed. Health needs assessment is:
- about health not just disease
- about needs not just demands
- an assessment not just a response.

Health needs assessment should be guided by these common questions:
- What information is needed?
- How can I find out this information?
- What am I going to do with the information when I obtain it?
- What scope is there to act on the information?

What Information Is Needed?

Chapter 3 discussed the different sources of information used to measure and assess health and wellbeing: epidemiological data on the rates of mortality and morbidity from a particular problem and its distribution; health related behaviours; socio-economic data.

The first step in a needs assessment is to define the relevant population group or community, including its demographic and social characteristics; behaviours, values and lifestyles; cultural environment; and historical circumstances. Community nurses are often involved in compiling community profiles to identify the health of a community and what resources are needed to enable it to achieve health and stay healthy. A community profile has been described as:

> A comprehensive description of the needs of a population that is defined, or defines itself, as a community, and the resources that exist within a community, carried out with the active involvement of the community itself, for the purpose of developing an action plan or other means of improving the quality of life in the community.
>
> **Hawtin and Percy Smith (2007, p. 5)**

Community profiles do not follow a standard format. Fig. 20.4 shows a schematic representation of the main elements:
- the composition of the community, for example, its age profile, social networks, the way the community is organized and its capacity in relation to skills and organizations
- socio-ecological environment, for example, extent of economic activity and unemployment, private car ownership, housing, transport links, green areas, air pollution
- availability, effectiveness and impact of health and social service provision
- local strategies for health, for example, health improvement programmes, planning projects.

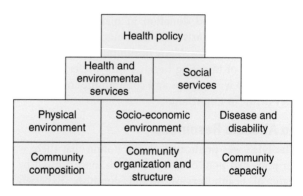

Fig. 20.4 Community information profile (From Annett, H., Rifkin, S., 1990. Improving Urban Health. World Health Organization, Geneva.)

Gathering Information and Public Participation

Routine information that is already available (e.g., census, NHS and local authority data) will give a picture of the potential needs of a community and what is available to meet those needs. It may give an idea of areas of unmet need and identify groups experiencing inequities of healthcare provision. The community's perceptions of its own health needs and expectations of services or interventions are a vital part of planning, as are the views of professionals about the nature of health needs, best practices and existing service delivery.

Since the NHS reforms of the 1990s, engaging with service users and local people is central to the provision of public health services. Planning guidance emphasizes that there will be different needs and priorities within each community. It also highlights that listening to views is as important as using epidemiological or survey data. There are many reasons for this shift to patient and public involvement:
- ethical – people have the right to a voice
- pragmatic – where people have identified the solution it is more likely to be appropriate and used
- political – experts and professionals may have vested interests in a particular provision and limited understanding of people's needs.

The aim of gathering information from communities is to understand issues from their perspective. As we saw in Chapter 11, interventions based on such information are more likely to be effective than if they are suggested by outside experts or professionals, whose interpretations of need may be based on general interpretations and impressions of the community.

The gathering of community knowledge can take place in different ways. Chapter 11 discussed this in more detail. There may be a formal exercise of consultation conducted in a top-down way. Frequently the consultation is confined to issues relating to patient satisfaction with services, and particularly the hotel aspects of care. Ong and Humphris regard this as inadequate:

It is not sufficient to see users as consumers who are satisfied or dissatisfied with services. The place of users is in the joint definition of need, priority setting and evaluation. This approach means a paradigm shift whereby the community perspective will be used as the guiding principle for setting priorities in health care.
(1994, p. 89)

The term 'co-production' is used to describe a way of working whereby citizens and policy makers, or people who use services, carers and service providers, work together to create a decision or service which works for them all. Co-production is built on the principle that those who use a service are best placed to help design it. It does not view people as the passive providers of information, but as active participants in the process. Public participation in needs assessment can range from tokenistic consultation where the results may seemingly be ignored, and the timing, location and publicity for public meetings may lead to a poor turnout, to community control – as we saw in the ladder of participation in Chapter 11. Public participation needs to be carefully planned and its initiators need to be motivated to listen and include, and to act on people's views.

Many health and local authorities are using a range of methods to achieve a wider picture of community needs. These approaches represent a move away from traditional epidemiological data gathering towards techniques which reflect the importance of social and environmental factors and the involvement of the community in data collection. These include:
- public meetings and forums
- interviews with users and key informants
- focus groups
- using local media such as radio phone-ins
- community health panels and citizens' juries
- research techniques such as rapid appraisal, ethnographic studies and observation
- participatory appraisal.

Rapid appraisal is a research technique applied to both urban and rural settings and is the focus of Learning Activity 20.7. It is geared to identifying the health needs and priorities of a target population quickly and without great expense. It uses secondary data already available, and then researchers interview people with knowledge of the area to identify problems and solutions. Key informants are:
- people who work in the community and have a professional understanding of local issues (e.g., teachers, health visitors, police)
- people who are recognized community leaders and represent a section of the community (e.g., religious leaders, councillors, leaders of self-help groups)
- people who are important in informal networks and play a role in local communication (e.g., shopkeepers, bookmakers, lollipop men and women).

 Learning Activity 20.7   Rapid Appraisal

List some of the advantages and disadvantages of rapid appraisal as a method of community needs assessment.

Participatory appraisal (e.g., as shown in Fig. 20.5) uses members of the community as data gatherers, valuing their knowledge and experience. A range of methods may be used to capture the ways in which people describe local issues, for example, mapping, community walks, timelines, photography and life histories. These techniques focus on mapping community assets and resources.

The advantages of participatory appraisal are:
- its underlying ethos of shared ownership of research
- it can build capacity in people undertaking the training to carry it out
- it may describe issues differently from the usual professional viewpoint
- it can focus on assets as well as deficits in the community.

The disadvantages of participatory appraisal are:
- the views of local people may not be as valued as epidemiological data
- it is time-consuming
- it may raise false expectations among the community that identified issues will be acted upon.

Collecting data where there are low levels of literacy demands different techniques. Participatory appraisal

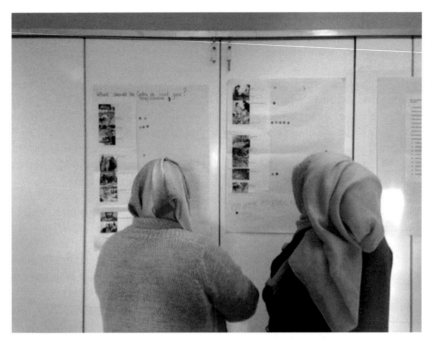

Fig. 20.5 Participatory appraisal ranking exercise used in a community event to assess health needs

methods are highly visual and use a range of activities to elicit and triangulate the same information. Tools used in participatory interviews or group meetings include brainstorming, mapping, ranking, sequencing and diagramming. Mapping exercises, for example, can locate specific community assets or identify areas for community change. Methods of ranking or matrix scoring can indicate priorities for the development of health needs.

Whose Needs Count?

Moves to participation in either community affairs or healthcare cannot involve everyone, and it is important that participation does not favour those with the most influence and loudest voices.

The involvement of service users and carers in decision-making is now a statutory requirement, including those who previously might have been excluded, such as children, people with mental ill health issues and people with learning difficulties. There are many guides as to how to involve service users and children effectively (e.g., https://www.nwleics.gov.uk/files/documents/guide_to_involving_children_and_young_people/Guide%20to%20Involving%20Children%20and%20Young%20People.pdf).

Patient and public involvement and engagement (PPIE) is now an accepted principle in research and service assessments and Research Example 20.1 illustrates

> **RESEARCH EXAMPLE 20.1   The Needs of Pregnant Women Who Have Been Sexually Abused**
>
> Pregnancy, birth, and parenthood can present particular challenges for those who have experienced childhood sexual abuse. Re-traumatization during the perinatal period is common and can occur in ways that may not be anticipated by those involved.
>
> A participatory needs assessment and coproduction of a resource for women whose voices may not be heard was undertaken. To encourage participation from this hidden population, data were collected by a variety of means including focus groups, telephone interviews and an on-line survey. The final resource is hosted on The Survivors Trust Website (https://www.thesurvivorstrust.org/pbpaftercsa). The process of developing the resource used trauma-informed principles and it speaks with women's words in a peer-to-peer voice.

From Montgomery, E., Seng, J.S., Chang, Y.S., 2021. Co-production of an e-resource to help women who have experienced childhood sexual abuse prepare for pregnancy, birth, and parenthood. BMC Pregnancy Childbirth 21, 30.

this in relation to pregnant women and sexual violence. The term 'stakeholder' is often used to refer to those individuals, groups or communities who have an interest in, and are likely to be affected by, the findings of a project, intervention or assessment. Important stakeholders can include service users, carers, wider family members, healthcare professionals, service managers and commissioners as well as policy makers. There are groups in society who are minorities or socially excluded. Such groups were often referred to as 'hard(er) to reach' but more accurately such groups may be described as 'seldom heard' and underserved in relation to services and resources.

 Learning Activity 20.8   Harder to Reach or Seldom Heard

- What reasons can you think of to explain why certain groups are harder to reach or seldom heard?
- Can you think of any such groups?
- Why might they prefer not to be described as 'harder to reach'?

SETTING PRIORITIES

The traditional public health approach for setting priority areas includes the following criteria:

1. *Impact* – The issue should be a major cause of premature death or avoidable ill health in the population as a whole or among specific groups of people.
2. *Inequalities* – There are marked inequalities in those who suffer ill health or premature death.
3. *Changeability* – What can most easily be changed?
4. *Acceptability* – What are the most acceptable changes needed to achieve the maximum impact? What do people want or need?
5. *Resource feasibility* – What is most able to be achieved with least resource?

The public health priorities identified in the NHS Long Term Plan launched in 2019 (https://www.longtermplan.nhs.uk/) include:

- *smoking*: embedding cessation into patient pathways
- *obesity*: enabling access to weight management for people with diabetes, BMI >30, hypertension
- *diet*: flour fortification with folic acid, salt tax
- *alcohol*: teams in inpatient facilities
- *mental health and learning disability*: health checks for people with severe mental illness and people with autism
- *gambling support.*

The priorities relate to target groups (people with mental illness or learning disability, people with obesity;

problem gamblers); specific lifestyle/behaviours (alcohol, smoking, diet). Other strategies have included the targeting of stages of the life course (e.g., older people) or specific diseases and conditions (e.g., diabetes).

The medical origins of public health are apparent in the focus on communicable diseases and chronic conditions and non-communicable diseases that impact on quality of life and longevity. This is reflected in various service frameworks that may have been developed in partnership with a range of service providers and service users. Public health refers to the health of the whole population, but within that category, certain groups of people may be prioritized. The rationale for focusing on specific groups is usually that their health potential is not being met. This often emerges from research or needs assessments that demonstrate that a specific population group has a high level of health needs that are often unmet due to problems with service access and availability (e.g., asylum seekers, migrants and Gypsy and Travellers). Targeting can, however, stigmatize groups. HIV, for example, is concentrated in social groups that are already marginalized, such as commercial sex workers, injecting drug users and men who have sex with men. It can also lead to oversimplification in categorizing the target group. Black, Asian and minority ethnic (BAME) groups, for example, are frequently treated as a homogeneous category for interventions. Priorities may also seek to address risk conditions – those social determinants – that are associated with worse health such as housing or polluted environments but far more commonly it is certain health behaviours that have come to be seen associated with negative health outcomes such as physical inactivity or excessive drinking that become priorities. Targeting lifestyles which are deemed amenable to change is therefore viewed as both an effective and an efficient strategy to promote health even though the public themselves may not prioritize personal change in the face of more pressing concerns.

We have seen in this chapter that people's identified needs may be taken as the first step in the planning process. However, this subjective interpretation may be tempered by economic and political priorities. People may express a need for interventions or treatment whose effectiveness is in doubt (e.g., antibiotics for simple colds or ear infections). For health promoters, therefore, a simple needs assessment may not be an adequate basis for setting priorities. A range of other influences may determine what is included in a local health promotion plan as discussed in Chapter 22:

- national targets of reducing disease
- a national theme, for example, World AIDS Day
- a major determinant of health in the area, for example, air pollution or poverty
- pragmatism on the basis of available skills and interests
- cost and staffing
- longer-term strategy
- existing activity
- cost-effectiveness and what is amenable to change and evaluation
- client choice
- professionals' views.

CASE STUDY 20.4

Questions to Ask When Planning a Needs Assessment

- What defines the scope of the health need to be addressed? Are you interested in the whole population or a particular subsection, such as older people or women?
- What is the size of the problem? How many people share the health need?
- What are the views of patients, carers and the local community? What is known from previous work? Who do you need to talk to locally?
- How do your figures compare with local and national averages? How important is the problem compared with other issues?
- What interventions are already taking place? Do you have a response to the problem? What are other agencies doing?
- What has worked elsewhere? Is there any relevant literature available or projects which can be visited? Are there examples of best practice in the area in which you are interested?
- What could and should you be doing in future? Consider all options, prioritize and develop an action plan, as described in Chapter 22.

CONCLUSION

This book has shown that there are several tensions or 'pulls' in health promotion described in Chapter 5. One of these 'pulls' can be illustrated in relation to the type of information used to plan interventions:

- identifying needs through participatory, bottom-up and negotiated approaches versus professionally led top-down approaches
- using types of data that are subjective, individual or community-held views versus objective, primarily epidemiological, data.

The selection of an approach and of methods to measure needs will depend on the purpose and context. The process of encouraging participation in public services by identifying and understanding individual and community needs has led to attempts to make such services more flexible. So, for example, we find, as part of the nursing process, clients being encouraged to identify aspects of their situation that they deem harmful to their health. We find health organizations using a variety of methods to ascertain the views, beliefs and health behaviours of their population, in addition to the objective measures yielded by epidemiology. We find voluntary and community groups being required as part of their funding to monitor not only their clients' use of the service but also their health needs.

The public sector, including the NHS, is seeking to integrate public views into the planning process. However, most of the information used to assess needs is gathered from a professional perspective which assumes a direct relationship between certain indicators and needs, and which is embedded in a medical model of health. For example, if health statistics show an above-average incidence of coronary heart disease, local health planners may well assume a need for greater provision of cardiac treatment and rehabilitation services, and a health promotion programme to address risk factors for coronary heart disease. Health promoters have an important role to play in ensuring that needs assessment which feeds health needs into planning takes account of public views and self-defined needs, and uses indicators to measure a social model of positive health. For those with client caseloads, it is a vital task to know the health status of patients/clients and how this may differ from the broader community in order to plan appropriate interventions.

Assessing health needs is important both in terms of promoting health and in determining priorities. For health promoters, the process of identifying needs is not, however, the only basis for setting priorities. Resource constraints will limit what is available and what is deemed amenable to change. Professional views, practice wisdom and existing activity will provide boundaries to what is considered possible.

- Think about a current priority in your work: Who decided this should be a priority? (e.g., Your clients/ service users? National guidance? Public views? Epidemiological trends?)
- What evidence is there that there is a need for intervention?
- What was the response to the identified need?

■ SUMMARY

This chapter has discussed the ways in which need is defined. We have seen that perceptions of need vary according to whether these are client or professional views, and how the assessment is made – clients' expressed views, levels of service use or epidemiological and social data. The chapter concludes that need is relative, and influenced by values and attitudes as well as the historical context. It also considers the role of health promotion in identifying and meeting certain needs.

FURTHER READING AND RESOURCES

Green, J., Cross, R., Woodall, J., Tones, K., 2019. Health Promotion: Planning and Strategies, fourth edn. Sage, London. *A useful text illustrating approaches to promoting health. Chapter 5 discusses needs assessment.*

Cavanagh, S., Chadwick, K., 2005. Health Needs Assessment: A Practical Guide. Health Development Agency, London. Available at: https://ihub.scot/media/1841/health_needs_assessment_a_practical_guide.pdf. *A step by step guide that is easy to follow. Guidance exists for specific practitioners, for example, recent guidance for health visitors and school nurses at* https://www.gov.uk/government/publications/commissioning-of-public-health-services-for-children/population-health-needs-assessment-a-guide-for-0-to-19-health-visiting-and-school-nursing-services.

⚡ FEEDBACK ON LEARNING ACTIVITIES

20.1. Need relates to the experience of a problem which requires a response. There are two different understandings of what constitutes a health need. It can be seen as:
  - a subjective, relative concept which is judged by an expert or professional and is influenced by whether the need can be met
  - an objective and universal concept which is a fundamental right.

20.2. Important human needs include those shared with all living bodies (e.g., food, water and shelter), and those which are unique to humans (e.g., the need for a social network, social recognition, liberty and freedom of expression). Maslow (1943) proposed a hierarchy of needs, with the most fundamental need being physiological, followed by safety, love and belonging, esteem and self-actualization. Human needs are shared by all people, regardless of their country.

20.3. At first sight these developments may be seen as the consequence of medical advances. However, medical interventions in childbirth can also be seen historically as an attempt to establish doctors' control over that of midwives. The range of interventions may, on the one hand, alienate women and make childbirth an uncomfortable and distressing experience; on the other hand, the very availability of these services may create a need for them.

A very different list of needs may be compiled by pregnant women (see for example, Downe et al., 2018), including:
  - the same known midwife to be present throughout labour and birth (continuity of care)
  - water births
  - partner to be present during birth
  - home births.

  These felt or expressed needs may or may not be acknowledged and met by service providers.

20.4. Increasingly, healthcare workers seek to identify clients' views and perceptions about their health as part of their assessment. What they often find is that their perception differs from that of the client. Clients' need for information is often underestimated, and in healthcare settings this may mean that information is confined to ward or clinic routines. Despite the greater emphasis on being client-centred, practitioners tend to assess needs in relation to the service they provide. Practitioners may interpret client needs as information needs because it is possible to provide this, whereas the satisfaction of physical needs (as in Maslow's hierarchy) may seem beyond their scope.

20.5. The medical and individualistic approach is adopted because it is a well-understood part of the nurse's professional role. The nurse understands coronary heart disease prevention as focusing on risk factors, even though they may not be relevant to this situation. The patient may have other health needs, such as a concern about getting back to work or when he might be sexually active again. Assessing individual health needs means starting with the patient's own concerns.

20.6. Some of the factors you might take into account are as follows.

- Costs – the relative costs of different services, and the opportunity costs (e.g., if the money is spent on this, what is it not being spent on?).
- Numbers – how many people will benefit from the service, and will it provide the greatest good for the greatest number?
- Effectiveness – what are the likely outcomes of providing care or treatment? Will it promote health, prevent ill health or improve or cure ill health?
- Quality – what areas of health-related quality of life (physical, mental, social, well-being, perception of pain, self-care) will be most affected by the service?

20.7. Rapid appraisal is useful if virtually nothing is known about the needs and priorities of the target population. It can give a deep understanding of the problems and issues in a community and provide a sense of local ownership. But it does not provide the quantitative analysis of the size of the problem which many public health departments require. It may also be difficult to get beyond personal agendas to find out the community's views.

20.8. It is very difficult to get a cross-section of a community, and there are some groups of people who are harder to reach. These may include homeless people, unemployed people, refugees, migrants and some groups, such as people from Black and minority ethnic groups, may be seldom heard. Some groups comprise individuals who may have a similar experience of health services because of a defining characteristic, for example, being unemployed or homeless, but who do not have a collective voice or means of expressing their views. Other groups may be informal, with no recognized meeting place. Many groups may be wary of formal and statutory bodies.

REFERENCES

Annett, H., Rifkin, S., 1990. Improving Urban Health. WHO, Geneva. Available at http://apps.who.int/iris/bitstream/10665/62112/1/WHO_SHS_NHP_88.4.pdf.

Bradshaw, J.R., 1972. The taxonomy of social need. In: McLachlan, G. (ed.), Problems and Progress in Medical Care. Oxford University Press, Oxford. Available in a collection at: http://www.york.ac.uk/inst/spru/pubs/pdf/JRB.pdf.

Cohen, D., Flood, C., 2021. Health economics. In: Naidoo, J., Wills, J. (eds.), Health Studies: An Introduction, fourth edn. Palgrave/Macmillan, Basingstoke.

Downe, S., Finlayson, K., Oladapo, O.T., Bonet, M., Gülmezoglu, A.M., 2018. What matters to women during childbirth: a systematic qualitative review. PLoS One 13 (4), e0194906. https://doi.org/10.1371/journal.pone.0194906.

Doyal, L., Gough, I., 1992. A Theory of Human Need. Macmillan, London.

Hart, T., 1971. The inverse care law. Lancet 1, 405.

Hawtin, M., Percy-Smith, J., 2007. Community Profiling: A Practical Guide. Auditing Social Needs, second edn. Open University Press, Buckingham.

Mara, D., Lane, J., Scott, B., Trouba, D., 2010. Sanitation and health. PLoS Med. 7 (11), e1000363.

Maslow, A., 1943. A theory of human motivation. Psychol. Rev. 50, 370–396.

Maslow, A.H., 1954. Motivation and Personality. Harper & Row, New York.

NICE, 2003. Health Equity Audit. A Guide for the NHS. Available at: http://webarchive.nationalarchives.gov.uk/20130107105354/http://www.dh.gov.uk/prod_consum_dh/groups/dh_digitalassets/@dh/@en/documents/digitalasset/dh_4084139.pdf (accessed 09.03.21).

Nutbeam, D., 1998. Evaluating health promotion progress, problems and solutions. Health Promot. Int. 13 (1), 27–44.

Ong, B.N., Humphris, G., Annett, H., Rifkin, S., 1991. Rapid appraisal in an urban setting: an example from the developed world. Soc Sci Med. 32 (8), 909–915.

Wright, J. (ed.), 1998. Health Needs Assessment in Practice. BMJ Publishing, London.

World Health Organization, 1985. Targets for Health for All. WHO Regional Office for Europe, Copenhagen.

World Health Organization, 1986. Ottawa Charter. WHO, Geneva. Available at: http://www.who.int/healthpromotion/conferences/previous/ottawa/en/.

World Health Organization, 1997. The Jakarta Declaration. Leading Health Promotion into the 21st Century. Available at: http://www.who.int/healthpromotion/conferences/previous/jakarta/declaration/en/.

21

Finding and Using Evidence for Health Promotion

LEARNING OUTCOMES

By the end of this chapter you will be able to:
- define evidence-based practice in public health and health promotion
- understand what constitutes evidence for health promotion practice
- understand the skills required for evidence-based practice: finding, appraising and synthesizing evidence.

KEY CONCEPTS AND DEFINITIONS

Evidence Facts used to support a conclusion.
Evidence based Decision-making based on evidence. The term evidence-informed is often preferred, suggesting that decision-making is enhanced by, but not limited to, research.

IMPORTANCE OF THE TOPIC

Evidence-based practice (EBP) is a key constituent of the health promotion planning cycle. In addition to identifying needs (see Chapter 20) we need to understand what types of interventions work and under what conditions. An important aspect of building evidence for health promotion practice is the evaluation of interventions; evaluation methodologies are explored in Chapter 23. Looking at existing evidence helps to make decisions about what to implement to address a problem, and how the intervention should be designed, based on whether a successful intervention is transferable to your context. There are a number of considerations that underpin practice, including effectiveness, cost effectiveness and the acceptability of an intervention to the public or a patient. EBP claims to provide an objective and rational basis for practice by scrutinizing available evidence about what works, in order to determine current and future practice. As such, EBP should be differentiated from other influences on practice as shown in Fig. 21.1 and those identified in Learning Activity 21.1:

- tradition ('this is what and how we have always done it')
- experience ('in my experience and judgement this is how it should be done, and this is what has worked')
- values ('this is what we ought to do, and this is the right thing to do')
- economic considerations ('this is what we can afford to do within the budget').

Learning Activity 21.1 Influences on Decision-Making

Think of an example of your practice where you have changed what you do. Has this change been brought about by:
- policy and/or management imperatives
- colleagues' advice
- technological advances
- cost
- evidence-based practice recommendations
- your own assessment and reflection
- users' requests and feedback.

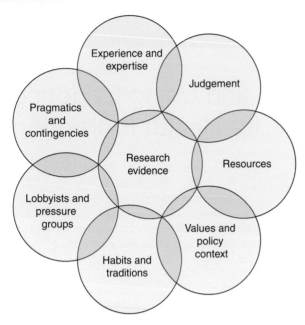

Fig. 21.1 Factors influencing decision-making

There are countless examples of therapies that have proved effective in clinical practice, such as low-dose aspirin for acute myocardial infarction, yet their uptake into routine practice has sometimes been slow. Similarly, there are assumptions about what works to promote health, such as shock-horror campaigns to dissuade people from smoking, which have been continued until rigorous evaluations revealed that the results were not as intended.

The nature of what defines 'evidence', or how it should be used to drive changes in practice and policy, is hotly contested. This chapter outlines current thinking about evidence, the reasons for pursuing evidence-based practice and policy, and the skills needed in order to become evidence-based practitioners. Evidence-based policy and practice take place in a complex context where other factors, such as custom, acceptability or ideology, may be more important than evidence in determining what is done. It is for this reason, and because there are numerous challenges faced in accessing and translating research into practice, that the term evidence-informed is often used to describe decision-making that is enhanced by research evidence, but not limited to it. This chapter focuses on evidence that informs practice, and the challenges this poses for practitioners.

INTRODUCTION

Good practice requires the use of explicit research evidence and non-research knowledge (tacit knowledge or accumulated wisdom). The process is uncertain and frequently no 'correct' decision exists, especially in the complex field of health promotion where there may be few direct outcomes. However the evidence we use to support decision-making needs to be:

- convincing and rigorously collected
- of high quality so we can have confidence in it, applicable and transferable beyond its original context and setting.

EBP was first applied to medicine, when it was defined as: 'The conscientious, explicit and judicious use of current best evidence in making decisions about individual patients based on skills which allow the doctor to evaluate both personal experience and external evidence in a systematic and objective manner' (Sackett et al., 1996, p. 71). In the 1970s, Archie Cochrane, a physician, became aware that there were substantial variations in medical practice on a range of issues, and many practices were unsubstantiated by evidence of their effectiveness. Cochrane instituted the drive to use research evidence to inform practice, and the first repository for evidence in 1993 was named after him: the Cochrane collaboration, which has now reached issue 7 (Cochrane Database of Systematic Reviews, 2019).

EBP offers the promise of maximizing expenditure by directing it to the most effective strategies and interventions. The exponential rise of information technology, and almost instant access to a multitude of sources of information, makes EBP a more realistic possibility. However it is unrealistic to expect practitioners to track down and critically appraise research for *all* relevant topics. It can be difficult for individual practitioners to know what is happening in the research world, and pre-searched pre-appraised resources, such as the systematic reviews of the Cochrane Collaboration (https://www.cochrane.org/), can offer an already synthesized and aggregated overview of the most up-to-date research findings for the busy practitioner.

Being an Evidence-Based Practitioner

There is an expectation for healthcare professionals to be evidence based and to always practise in line with the best available evidence. Being evidence based means having both the knowledge and the confidence to tackle issues effectively. To become an evidence-based practitioner means adopting a critical view with regards to research and evidence, and being willing to change your practice if the evidence suggests this is worthwhile. The practitioner who seeks to become evidence based needs to acquire the knowledge and skills to find out and access, critically appraise, synthesize and apply relevant evidence. Evidence includes research as well as more anecdotal and developmental accounts linking inputs to outputs.

Being evidence based requires an open and critical mind to reflect on your own knowledge about an issue, and assess competing claims of knowledge. Many interventions are implemented despite a lack of certainty about the evidence for their effectiveness, because practitioners act on intuition or respond to pressure to do something. Cummins and Macintyre (2002) refer to 'factoids' – assumptions that get reported and repeated so often that they become accepted. They describe the way in which food deserts (areas of deprivation where families have difficulty accessing affordable, healthy food) have become an accepted part of policy because they fit with the prevailing ideological approach, although there is little evidence to support their existence. Equally, some interventions are not implemented despite evidence of their effectiveness, because they are not politically or socially acceptable.

It is this uncertainty that has led to the production of evidence-based briefings that appraise current evidence of effective interventions in a digestible form for practitioners and policy makers. Evidence-based briefings select recent good quality systematic reviews and meta-analyses, and synthesize the results. Clinical guidelines are an example of this, in which evidence is translated into recommendations for clinical practice and appropriate healthcare that can be implemented in a variety of settings. Clinical guidelines are a top-down strategy to produce practice in line with available evidence of what works, and to ensure comparable standards nationwide and reduce variations in practice. Recommendations are graded according to the strength of the evidence and their feasibility. So recommendations supported by consistent findings from randomized controlled trials (RCTs) that use available techniques and expertise would be graded more highly than recommendations supported by an expert panel consensus that rely on scarce expertise and resources. The National Institute for Health and Care Excellence (NICE) publishes guidance on public health interventions (https://www.nice.org.uk/guidance/published?type=ph). Such guidance makes recommendations for populations and individuals on activities, policies and strategies that can help prevent disease or improve health. The guidance may focus on a particular topic (e.g., smoking), a particular population (e.g., schoolchildren) or a particular setting (e.g., the workplace). Recent guidance (with their reference numbers) includes digital and mobile health interventions [NG183], indoor air quality in the home [NG 149] and alcohol interventions in secondary and further education [NG 135]. Learning Activity 21.2 asks you to consider and discuss the usefulness of guidelines for health promotion.

> ### ❓ Learning Activity 21.2   Guidelines for Health Promotion Practice
>
> If guidelines are 'systematically developed statements to assist decision making about appropriate interventions for specific circumstances', is it feasible to produce them for public health and health promotion?

Adopting an evidence-based approach follows five key stages, shown in Fig. 21.2:
- turning a knowledge gap into an answerable question
- searching for relevant evidence
- extracting data/information for analysis
- appraising the quality of the information/data
- synthesizing appraised information/data.

ASKING THE RIGHT QUESTION

Being clear about what you need to know is a vital first step. It is this process that starts the search for relevant evidence and the process of appraisal. Asking the right question means finding a balance between being too specific (asking a question that is unlikely ever to have been researched), and being too vague (asking a question that will produce a mass of research studies, many of which will be inapplicable to the context and circumstances you are interested in). Questions can address specific interventions (do they work?) or ask about any intervention that works to address the problem in question. Learning Activity 21.3 considers two different scenarios of a practitioner wanting to find evidence before planning an intervention.

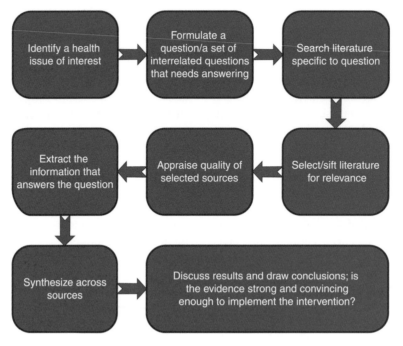

Fig. 21.2 Steps in evidence-informed practice

Learning Activity 21.3   Designing an Intervention

1. A midwife wants to find out if bottle-fed babies are more likely to be obese in adulthood.
2. A smoking cessation coordinator is concerned at the rising rates of smoking among young women. The coordinator wants to extend the cessation service to young people in secondary school who wish to quit.

   Consider these scenarios and describe for each:

   • What is the target group or population?
   • What is the intervention?
   • What is the change or outcome that is sought?

WHAT COUNTS AS EVIDENCE

Evidence may be of many different types, ranging from systematic reviews and meta-analyses to collective consensual views to individual experiences and reflections. All types of evidence have their uses as is illustrated in Research Example 21.1. EBP traditionally reifies science relying on:

• written accounts of primary research in refereed academic and professional journals

• academic and professional texts (which have been reviewed)
• independently published reports
• unpublished reports and conference papers and presentations (grey literature).

However, the use of evidence to inform practice is broader than this and encompasses:

• information about an intervention's effectiveness in meeting its goals
• information about how transferable (to other settings and populations) this intervention is thought to be
• information about the intervention's positive and negative effects
• information about the intervention's economic impact
• information about barriers to implementing the intervention (Supplement to American Journal of Preventive Medicine, 2000, p. 36, cited in McQueen, 2001).

The scientific medical model has gained dominance in the debate about defining evidence. This model states that evidence is best determined through the use of scientific methodologies which prioritize quantitative objective fact finding. The use of scientific models of evidence leads to a search for specific inputs causing specific outputs, regardless of intervening or contextual factors

> ### RESEARCH EXAMPLE 21.1
> **Types of Evidence**
>
> 'Scared Straight' is a programme in the USA that brings at-risk or already delinquent children, mainly boys, into prison to meet 'lifers'. The young people are told stories about prison life and the choices of the inmates that led to imprisonment. Inmates, the lifers themselves, the juvenile participants, their parents, prison governors, teachers and the general public were very positive about the programme in all studies, concluding that it should be continued. However in a systematic review, seven good-quality randomized control trials showed that the programme increased delinquency rates among the treatment group (Petrosino et al., 2000). This evidence suggests that the intervention is ineffective as a deterrent to juvenile offending.
>
> Participants may not tell the same story as the outcome evaluation for many reasons, but their views on the process are valid and constitute important data in their own right. Participants' views on the appropriateness and accessibility of the programme are essential in deciding whether or not to adopt programmes.

See https://whatworks.college.police.uk/toolkit/Pages/Intervention.aspx?InterventionID=2#:~:text=Scared%20Straight%20involves%20organised%20visits,prison%20life%20with%20the%20juveniles.

such as socio-economic status, beliefs or a supportive environment. Such intervening factors, which mediate and moderate the effect of inputs, are viewed as 'confounding variables' and study designs try to eliminate their effect. The RCT, using the experimental method, is viewed as the most robust and useful method for achieving results which qualify as evidence, and is viewed as the 'gold standard'. The criteria relevant for RCTs are outlined in Chapter 23.

There is now a well-established 'hierarchy of evidence', shown in Fig. 21.3, which grades research findings according to how valid and reliable the research methodology is deemed to be. Valid means that appropriate methods to answer the question are selected and correctly performed, and therefore the results are generalizable to other populations. Reliable means that the research methodology is transparent and unbiased and could be replicated, with the same results, by other researchers.

The hierarchy of evidence has evolved in the context of individual care and treatment carried out within one disciplinary paradigm – scientific medicine. Public health and health promotion, which focus on communities and populations, provide a very different subject for research. They are multidisciplinary bodies of knowledge, and the evidence they draw upon is correspondingly varied. The use of evidence within health promotion has been likened to the judicial notion of evidence, which is typically a mixture of witness accounts, expert testimony and forensic science (McQueen, 2001). Using this concept of evidence, individual stories which relate processes, interpretations and outcomes, such as those described in Research Example 21.1, are as valid as scientific trials which seek to determine the effect of single causal factors.

This more inclusive notion of evidence, with its combination of accounts that vary in terms of what they construct as the truth, seems more appropriate to public health and health promotion. The scientific model of evidence could be viewed as disabling multidisciplinary practice through its prioritization of scientific evidence and its discounting of other forms of evidence. However using a more inclusive notion of evidence does not mean abandoning the concept of methodological rigour and quality.

Different research paradigms will focus on different research questions, even about the same issue, such as ageing. Positivist research views ageing as a real phenomenon, measurable through objective scientific tools, for example, measurement of bone loss associated with the ageing process. Positivist research into caring for the elderly might produce projected population profiles and extrapolate the possible extent of certain age-related diseases, for example, dementia or arthritis. Positivist research might also attempt to measure the projected costs of caring for an ageing population in the future. Research findings are viewed as objective and generalizable. Interpretivist research, by contrast, seeks to explore the meanings and context of ageing among older and younger populations. The connotations of ageing would be identified and explored. The factors that help or hinder older people's coping mechanisms would be researched, for example, social networks and religious beliefs. Research would study the perceived benefits of an ageing population (e.g., grandparents providing childcare for working parents) as well as its disadvantages. Research findings are specific to the population being studied (e.g., its gender, social class, ethnicity), although findings might be transferable to other similar populations. Learning Activity 21.4 asks you to consider and discuss what might be some key research questions warranting investigation in relation to immunization.

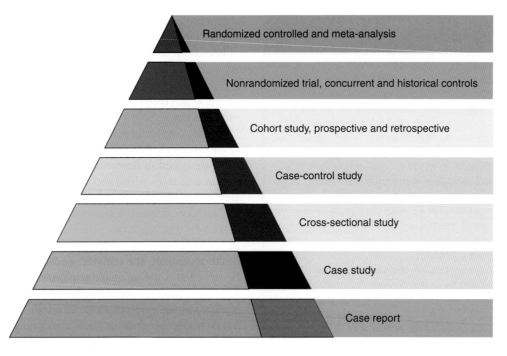

Randomized controlled and meta-analysis

Nonrandomized trial, concurrent and historical controls

Cohort study, prospective and retrospective

Case-control study

Cross-sectional study

Case study

Case report

Randomized controlled trial:
This method compares a group experiencing an intervention with a similar control group which does not.

Nonrandomized controlled trial:
This method compares between a group receiving intervention and one which does not. Participants are allocated by researcher.

Cohort study:
These studies observe a group over time to see if there is any association between particular behaviours or characteristics and patterns of disease. For example, the Framingham Heart Study in Massachusetts began in 1948 and is now studying the third generation of participants to identify risk factors for heart disease.

Case-control study:
These studies investigate the causes of a condition by comparing a group with the condition with a control group.

Cross-sectional studies:
These studies determine the prevalence or patterns of conditions or behaviours in populations or groups at one point in time. For example, the Health Survey for England was started in 1991 to investigate changes in the health and lifestyles of adults and children. Around 8000 adults and 2000 children take part in the survey each year. Information is collected through an interview and, if participants agree, a visit from a specially trained nurse.

Case study:
This is a research approach used to generate an in depth, multifaceted understanding of a complex issue in its real-life context.

Case report:
This is an exploration of a phenomenon or patient or service-user sharing their characteristics and often focusing on the efficacy of an intervention.

Fig. 21.3 Hierarchy of evidence

Learning Activity 21.4   Research Questions

Consider the example of immunization. What might be some of the questions that warrant exploration? Locate the questions generated in either positivist or interpretivist perspectives (or perhaps both).

FINDING THE EVIDENCE

The key to EBP is that evidence is collected systematically. This means that a full search of all available sources of information is undertaken, and full details are given of how the search has been conducted. This includes citing:

- keywords
- databases that have been accessed
- criteria used to include or exclude research studies.

Systematic reviews, for example, typically exclude large numbers of studies that fail to meet their criteria for rigour. Such criteria include full details of non-respondents, before and after measurements, and the use of a control group. Searches for evidence are also usually only undertaken for English language materials and are often confined to research carried out in developed Western countries. It has been claimed that this omission leads to systematic bias and a lack of relevance for developing countries (McQueen, 2001).

The internet has greatly expanded the amount of information that can be accessed, and it is easy to waste time collecting information that is not relevant. In order to avoid this, systematic searches should be:

- explicit – use key terms, record your search and ensure it is transparent so others can assess its value and it can be repeated
- appropriate – look where the evidence is likely to be
- sensitive – collecting all the information which is relevant to your question
- specific – collecting only information that is relevant to your question
- comprehensive – include all available information.

Internet search engines such as Google are useful in the early stages of finding literature about a chosen question because they use software to interpret natural language, and so will find information based on your thinking, but they can also find a lot of irrelevant material. It is likely however that the major source of evidence will be in online databases. These act as indexes to published literature and include thousands of journals.

Such databases tend to be organized around the literature of a particular subject, for example:

Medline covers medicine, dentistry and veterinary science. It can be searched for via *PubMed* which is freely available.

CINAHL (Cumulative Index to Nursing and Allied Health Literature) covers nursing and allied health professions.

PsychInfo covers psychology.

Public health and health promotion literature could be in any or all of these databases. Some databases will include access to the full text of journal articles, while others will only include a list of titles and abstracts. Searching a database means using keywords and their synonyms. Keywords are the words most associated with the question or issue that you are investigating. Synonyms are alternative words that mean the same thing. Most journal articles include a list of keywords after the title, so you are able to see which are the words most commonly used in relation to your topic of interest. Most databases provide tools to make this easier, such as truncation symbols – where a word is shortened to its stem, enabling a search for all variants with a minimum of typing. It is usually possible to search for a phrase by enclosing it in speech marks (e.g., "National Health Service"). The database can be searched using free text or subject headings. Using free text means that the database searches for the words that are typed in and gathers up all the articles that mention the typed words. The other way of searching is using the database's own subject headings, which is like a dictionary that collects together all the articles that are about a specific topic.

In addition to the online databases there are many other means of searching sources of evidence. These include:

- searching online repositories of reviews (e.g., cochranelibrary.com) or the evidence policy and practice institute (https://eppi.ioe.ac.uk/cms/)
- searching online databases of unappraised primary research
- online searching of relevant websites for unpublished articles and information
- library searches of indexed and non-indexed sources
- manual searching of academic and professional journals
- manual searching of theses and independently published reports
- contacting dedicated information clearing houses and acknowledged experts.

Grey literature is the term used to describe any literature that is hard to find. It includes conference proceedings, unpublished dissertations, policy documents, internal reports and blog entries. The internet has made the task of searching for grey literature much easier, as well as increasing its quantity. Many organizations publish research findings on their websites or support their own online journals.

Case Study 21.1 is an example of a search for evidence of effectiveness of a particular intervention. Because evidence is regularly published, it will only be correct and exhaustive at a specific point of time. Learning Activity 21.5 asks you to conduct a similar search on cyclists and alcohol consumption.

> **? Learning Activity 21.5 Searching for Evidence**
>
> If you wanted to find evidence on the behaviour of cyclists towards alcohol consumption:
> - what keywords would you use?
> - what databases and other sources would you search?
> - how would you decide which papers (articles) to exclude?

APPRAISING THE EVIDENCE

The evidence that has been found now needs to be assessed or appraised. Judging the usefulness of information is a task undertaken every day – does this information help to answer my questions? Is it detailed enough? Can it be trusted? Does it apply to my situation? Not all evidence is useful for planning public health and health promotion activities. Some interventions have not been rigorously evaluated so it is difficult to know if they are worth repeating elsewhere. Assessing the value of evidence is a skilled task, which is called critical appraisal. Traditionally critical appraisal in EBP determines the quality of the research study and whether it is believable and dependable:

- Believable: how transparent were the means by which conclusions were made? This relates to the design, methods and procedure, how the conclusions were reached and whether there is an audit trail of actions and decision-making.
- Valid: does the information collected measure what it purports to measure? Self-reporting may be biased and not give valid responses.
- Reliable: if the study was repeated using the same research instruments would it give the same results?

📋 CASE STUDY 21.1
Searching for Evidence

Obesity in children is a recognized and increasing problem. While there is considerable research into predisposing factors, most interventions that aim to control and reduce weight gain are poorly evaluated. In the USA, residential weight-loss 'fat' camps have been running for three decades. In order to ascertain whether to introduce 'fat' camps to the UK evidence is needed on:
- their effectiveness in reducing weight in children
- their efficiency in relation to other family-centred methods
- their acceptability to children and parents
- the factors that influence their success.

One of the main problems when searching for evidence is being too broad in the search of online databases. A search using the keywords "child" and "obesity" would be likely to yield an excessive amount of 'hits'. Successful searching systematically limits and combines key terms, and may use exclusion criteria such as English language and a year period. A search using keywords of fat OR obese OR 'weight loss' AND children AND camp AND residential found 98 published papersRestricting the search.

to the past 5 years found 22 results, but this removed some of the most relevant results. Although having a limited time frame will reduce the number of results, there must be a clear justification for only searching over a shorter time, for example, a change of policy. Examples of studies found in the search include Fonseca et al. (2014), Gately et al. (2005), Gately (2014), McGregor et al. (2016) and Wong et al. (2013). The Cochrane library may yield a systematic review that has synthesized the available evidence, and in this case there is a recent review on interventions for preventing obesity in children (Brown et al., 2019) but it only included the Gately et al. (2005) study. A hand search of journals might include the *International Journal of Human Nutrition and Dietetics* or *International Journal of Obesity*. A web search using a search engine such as 'Google' for key experts found a chapter by Gately (2014).

Appraising the evidence can seem a daunting prospect when there are so many sources of evidence available in various formats. It is important to obtain the relevant information from research reports:

- identification (title, date, authors, publishers, funding)
- the population, settings and activities (what, how, where, when and with whom was the intervention carried out?)
- the outcomes
- data collection and analysis techniques.

Critical appraisal for public health and health promotion may be defined as the systematic and structured evaluation of the relevance of a study. Its purpose is to find in the evidence anything of value that will help you make a better decision. Five key questions are:

1. What did the research set out to find? (Are there specified aims or questions?)
2. With whom was the study conducted? (Is there a clear rationale for the sample?)
3. What methods were used? (Were the methods appropriate for the question? Were the methods carried out correctly?)
4. What were the findings? (What methods were used to analyse the data and is this adequately described? Are the findings reported in full?)
5. What does it mean? (Are the findings relevant to your problem? Are they applicable to your setting?)

There is a large body of literature on critical appraisal skills as well as several useful guides (e.g., CASP, https://casp-uk.net/). Critical appraisal guides provide questions that enable the appraiser to assess the methodological rigour of different types of research study. Questions are grouped under three main headings:

- Are the results of the study valid?
- What are the main results?
- Will the results be of help locally?

Critical appraisal aims to identify useful, rigorous, high-quality research and exclude irrelevant or flawed research. This is a question of degree, for it is usually possible to identify flaws in published research studies, and ways in which the context of the research and one's own practice differ. Critical appraisal is a pragmatic process whereby research is screened so that only studies that reach a certain standard of rigour and relevance are taken into account.

WIDENING THE EVIDENCE BASE

Reviews of evidence privilege certain forms of knowledge and information over others. However, to achieve practical results, practitioners and users need to be persuaded that the outcomes they value will be affected by an intervention. This means incorporating their views in the evidence base and Learning Activity 21.6 asks you to consider and discuss how this might be achieved.

 Learning Activity 21.6   Different Views and Evidence-Informed Decision-Making

How can expert, practitioner and user views be incorporated into evidence-informed decision-making?

Because quantitative methods involve counting real phenomena – a process that can be verified – they are often assumed to be more objective, reliable and therefore 'better' or more 'desirable' than qualitative methods. A more realistic view is that all research involves both the 'facts' and the theoretical frameworks that determine which facts count and how they are interpreted. This stance may be termed the inclusive approach to research and evidence. Although evidence may never be completely objective or neutral, it is still important to assess its validity, reliability and robustness according to appropriate criteria. There may be subjectivity or bias involved in a researcher's decisions about which studies to include and exclude in a systematic review which can, for example, be limited by using more than one researcher and a common data extraction form. Research Example 21.2 highlights how choosing certain methodologies can introduce bias in findings.

SYNTHESIZING THE EVIDENCE

Systematic reviews and meta-analyses are both forms of secondary research that take primary research studies as their object of study. A systematic review identifies all the relevant information available on a specific topic, critically appraises its quality and summarizes its results using an appropriate scientific methodology. The 'systematic' aspect of the review means that it is undertaken in a structured, objective and thorough manner, and that it is written up in a transparent manner that enables someone else to reproduce the study and reach the same findings. Systematic reviews synthesize research findings in a form which is easily accessible to those who have to make decisions regarding policy or practice. In this way, systematic reviews reduce bias.

Despite the widespread and recognized value of qualitative studies, the criteria for inclusion within systematic reviews of health promotion have tended to be similar to those used by evidence-based medicine, with a dominance of experimental studies. Inclusion tends to be based on the quality of the study rather than the quality of the intervention. Their usefulness for public health and health promotion practitioners and policy makers is limited, due to insufficient information about the process of implementing an intervention, and a focus on a narrow range of outcomes.

Contextual factors such as the enthusiasm or commitment of organizations and practitioners; population characteristics (e.g., social stability and cohesion); and geographical factors (e.g., declining or renewing areas), will all have a significant impact on outcomes. This means that key aspects of the intervention may vary widely from study to study. For example, research into the effectiveness of brief interventions to promote physical activity in primary care have used very different definitions of 'brief' from 5 to 40 minutes (Lamming et al., 2017). It could be argued that there is a significant difference between 5 and 40 minutes of one-to-one consultation and advice. This example demonstrates the importance of investigating processes as well as outcomes in order to identify factors leading to success. This in turn makes the case for including qualitative as well as quantitative evidence. A useful framework is the realistic evaluation framework proposed by Pawson and Tilley (1997) described in Chapter 23. Realistic evaluation recognizes that key features of an intervention relate to the specific context, which therefore needs to be taken into account.

In pulling the evidence together, the practitioner will need to:
- weigh the strength and direction of the evidence in relation to a question
- identify areas of uncertainty
- identify what is likely to be effective in particular populations and institutional contexts
- identify how the intervention works, why, and for whom.

This value of systematic reviews is illustrated in Research Example 21.3, which makes conclusions about the strength of evidence about a particular intervention and makes recommendations about implementation.

RESEARCH EXAMPLE 21.2
Smoking in Pregnancy

A systematic review reported increases in birthweight and a reduction in stillbirths following smoking cessation in pregnancy programmes. A letter to the author of the review commented on: 'the need for trials to address broader outcome measures such as the impact on other family members, the benefits to women's health, whether non-smoking is sustained, the impact of failing to stop smoking, stress levels, the emotional impact of having a low birthweight baby after taking part in a strategy to stop smoking and self-esteem'. Oliver reports that the resulting revised review incorporated observational and qualitative research as well as small-scale consultations with health promotion practitioners and health service users. These methods broadened the content of the work and influenced the criteria used to judge the effectiveness of the programmes. For research to be instrumental in changing practice, evidence on programmes' effects and outcomes needs to be acceptable and relevant to those delivering and receiving such programmes.

From Oliver, S., 2001. Making research more useful: integrating different perspectives and different methods. In: Oliver, S., Peersman, G. (eds.), Using Research for Effective Health Promotion. Open University Press, Buckingham.

USING EVIDENCE-BASED PRACTICE TO DETERMINE COST-EFFECTIVENESS

In any discussion about effectiveness the issue of resources is likely to occur. Real-life decisions take place within an economic context and are made with reference to costs and competing claims. It is not enough to argue that an intervention is effective; it also has to be cost-effective (producing desired outcomes at least cost). The expanding field of health economics addresses these issues and seeks to evaluate interventions by comparing costs with benefits.

Economic evaluation examines whether limited resources are used in the best possible way. The most rigorous economic evaluations examine both costs and consequences for two or more alternatives (one of which may be the existing status quo). There are five main types of economic evaluation:

1. Cost-minimization analysis – used when there is strong evidence that two or more interventions are equally effective. This technique compares the costs to determine the least costly alternative.
2. Cost-effectiveness analysis – investigates the best way of achieving a single objective (e.g. life years

RESEARCH EXAMPLE 21.3
Childhood Vaccination Uptake

A systematic review about whether face-to-face interventions to inform or educate parents about routine childhood vaccination in low- and middle-income countries (LMIC) would improve uptake, undertaken as part of the commvac project (http://www.commvac.com/), concluded that:

The limited evidence available is low quality and suggests that face to face interventions to inform or educate parents about childhood vaccination have little to no impact on immunisation status, or knowledge or understanding of vaccination. There is insufficient evidence to comment on the cost of implementing the intervention, parent intention to vaccinate, parent experience of the intervention, or adverse effects. Given the apparently limited effect of such interventions, it may be feasible and appropriate to incorporate communication about vaccination into a healthcare encounter, rather than conduct it as a separate activity.

Kaufman et al. (2018)

gained; improved social capital) by measuring costs and benefits of different interventions to arrive at a cost per unit of benefit. The least costly intervention is then determined and prioritized.

3. Cost-consequences analysis – similar to cost-effectiveness analysis but used to evaluate interventions with more than one outcome, and can include a range of benefits including social outcomes.
4. Cost-utility analysis – measures the effects of an intervention in terms of utilities (e.g., the quality-adjusted life year or QALY, described in Chapter 3) and focuses on minimizing costs or maximizing benefits.
5. Cost–benefit analysis – examines the costs and benefits, expressed in monetary terms, of an intervention in order to determine its desirability. A desirable intervention is one where benefits exceed costs.

Research Example 21.4 is of the cost-effectiveness of an intervention in which debt advice is offered in a GP practice.

PUTTING EVIDENCE INTO PRACTICE

Although evidence-based public health and health promotion are often portrayed as the key to effective professional practice, there remain significant questions and dilemmas for practitioners seeking to incorporate evidence into their everyday practice. Common dilemmas for practitioners include:

- How much evidence is required before introducing an intervention?
- Does the research describe situations that are comparable to their own (including comparable caseloads or communities, organizations, staff and resources)?
- Does the evidence include the views of all relevant stakeholders?
- What to do when the evidence goes counter to personal intuition, judgement or values?
- Whether evidence can ever claim to be objective or neutral?

Finding and appraising evidence is a skilled task, and the findings may go counter to one's judgement, intuition or customary behaviour. For example, midwives used to advise parents to put babies to sleep in the prone (tummy down) position because this was similar to the recovery position, and this practice continued until the mid-1990s. Research proving that this sleeping position is associated with an increased risk of sudden infant death syndrome was available but it was not widely disseminated. Indeed a systematic review in 2005 concluded:

Advice to put infants to sleep on the front for nearly half a century was contrary to evidence available from 1970 that this was likely to be harmful. Systematic review of preventable risk factors for SIDS from 1970 would have led to earlier recognition of the risks of sleeping on the front and might have prevented over 10,000 infant deaths in the UK and at least 50,000 in Europe, the UK and Australasia.

Gilbert et al. (2005, p. 874)

It was a major public media campaign called 'back to sleep' that helped to change practice.

The government advice to use the triple vaccine for measles, mumps and rubella (MMR) is founded on strong research evidence, yet many parents reject this vaccine and opt for single vaccines, even if they have to pay. Giving a child a vaccination that might have harmful effects may be viewed as more unacceptable than taking no action and the child contracting the disease. The difference would seem to lie in the action/omission

RESEARCH EXAMPLE 21.4

Providing Debt Advice to Protect Mental Health

Evidence cited in a report by Public Health England (2017) on commissioning cost-effective services for the promotion of mental health and wellbeing, and the prevention of mental ill health, used the example of advice about debt.

Using various data the report estimated that 16.1% of UK adults (8.25 million people) were over-indebted, conservatively defined as regularly missing monthly payments in at least 3 of the last 6 months, or finding meeting financial commitments a heavy burden. Unmanageable financial debt has been associated with an increased risk of poor mental health and suicide. The impact of debt related stress and depression also impacts on health and legal systems (including creditors), and leads to lost productivity due to absenteeism and reduced employment.

The model explores the cost-effectiveness of an intervention in which volunteers deliver debt advice in a GP surgery, targeted at working age adults without mental health problems but at risk of unmanageable debt. Over 5 years, from a societal perspective there is a Return on Investment (ROI) of at least £2.60 for every £1 invested in face-to-face debt advice services.

Return on investment for face-to-face debt advice services delivered in a GP surgery.

Based on Public Health England, 2017. Commissioning Cost-Effective Services for Promotion of Mental Health and Wellbeing and Prevention of Mental Ill-Health. Available at: https://assets.publishing.service.gov.uk/government/uploads/system/uploads/attachment_data/file/640714/Commissioning_effective_mental_health_prevention_report.pdf.

dichotomy, whereby an action is seen as more blameworthy than an omission. A parent's decision on what is best for their child takes into account factors that are invisible in large trials of treatments. So an individual child's risk of an adverse reaction to MMR vaccination might be assessed using their previous history of allergic reactions and any unusual syndromes or the reactions and behaviour of siblings. The undoubted benefits to the population of adequate levels of MMR vaccination do not apply to individuals. In addition, the severe effects of contracting measles, mumps or rubella are often downplayed because they are so rarely seen nowadays. Parents who reject the triple vaccine would undoubtedly argue that they are making the best judgement for their child, based on their knowledge of individual circumstances, rather than accepting the blanket advice of health professionals to be vaccinated.

CONCLUSION

Health promotion and public health are multidisciplinary and recognize the validity of differing types of evidence, including context-specific and subjective views. Their multidisciplinary nature leads to complexity and ambiguity in the search for evidence, as different disciplines have their own rules of evidence. Attempting to consolidate these differences into an over-arching holistic body of evidence is a challenging task.

One means of consolidating available evidence would be to use the hierarchy of evidence that privileges the RCT as providing the best evidence. However there is on-going debate about whether or not RCTs should remain the 'gold standard' for public health and health promotion interventions. Proponents of the RCT argue that they are feasible in the area of health promotion and do provide the best available evidence on which to base practice (Oakley, 1998). Critics respond by arguing that RCTs are inappropriate for population-based, multicomponent interventions where there may be a considerable time lag between the interventions and the outcomes (Nutbeam, 1998). There is also a strong argument that, in line with underlying health promotion and public health values of equity, participation and autonomy, the views of practitioners and users deserve to be valued as a source of evidence in their own right.

The most useful stance for practitioners to take appears to be adopting the inclusive concept of evidence that acknowledges and values a range of different kinds of evidence including RCTs, qualitative process research, and users' views and accounts. Adopting the inclusive concept of evidence facilitates the involvement of different partners, including the public, and seeks to persuade people to implement interventions because they lead to valued outcomes. The evidence-based practitioner has an important role liaising between clients and the research community. Practitioners can disseminate to clients and communities knowledge and skills about the evidence gathering process as well as the evidence itself, and feed back their concerns to researchers, organizations and colleagues. In order to undertake this role, practitioners need to be confident about their critical appraisal skills. The term evidence-informed is beginning to be used, in recognition that decision-making in health promotion is informed by evidence, not directed by it. The move to evidence-based, or evidence-informed, practice is established, and offers practitioners the prospect of greater confidence and effectiveness. For clients, it offers the prospect of interventions based on the best available knowledge and evidence, rather than the preoccupations or biases of individual practitioners. However, evidence will only ever be one of several drivers of practice. The role of ethics, ideology, theory and resources as independent drivers of practice remains, alongside evidence.

Different concepts of evidence need to be recognized and valued, as shown in the guidelines for making decisions and using evidence in health promotion outlined by Raphael (2000):

1. Be as explicit as possible regarding the principles and values that you bring to your health promotion activities.
2. Recognize the tensions and interactions between structural and individual determinants of health, and between values and facts.
3. Whenever possible, use multiple sources of evidence.
4. Use truth criteria associated with each form of knowledge.
5. Show awareness of the decisions you make concerning evidence by being a reflexive practitioner.

> ### REFLECTIONS ON PRACTICE
>
> - What reasons do practitioners in your work setting give for the way things are done?
> - What evidence, and to what extent, is used routinely in decision-making?
> - Are there opportunities for the sharing of research evidence?

SUMMARY

This chapter focuses on the role of evidence in determining what interventions are likely to be effective to meet needs and improve health. Evidence-based or evidence-informed practice is a key part of the competences for health promotion practice. Key skills are the ability to use online technology to search for evidence and having the research skills to appraise that evidence. Interventions in health promotion are both complex and context dependent and so it is also important to be able to interpret the evidence to understand the conditions under which an intervention may work and for whom.

FURTHER READING AND RESOURCES

Aveyard, H., 2018. Doing a Literature Review in Health and Social Care: A Practical Guide, fourth edn. Open University Press, London.
  A key text for all students who are required to undertake a literature review, covering developing a question, finding relevant literature, searching, appraising and analysing the findings and making recommendations.
Campbell Collaboration at http://www.campbellcollaboration. org.
  An international collaboration which produces systematic reviews of studies researching the effectiveness of social and behavioural interventions.
Cochrane Collaboration at http://www.cochrane.org/.
  An international collaboration which produces systematic reviews of the effects of health care interventions covering a wide range of health care topics.
Craig, J.,V., Smyth, R.L. (eds.), 2014. The Evidence-Based Practice Manual for Nurses, third edn. Churchill Livingstone, Edinburgh.
  An accessible and easy to follow guide to becoming an evidence-based practitioner.
Critical Appraisal Skills Programme at https://casp-uk.net.
  The website for the Critical Appraisal Skills Programme provides checklists on how to evaluate different kinds of research studies.
Evidence for Policy and Practice Information Centre at https://eppi.ioe.ac.uk/cms.
  A UK centre using innovative methods for systematic reviews, mostly related to health promotion interventions for young people.
NICE, 2020. Developing NICE Guidelines: The Manual. Available at: https://www.nice.org.uk/process/pmg20/ chapter/the-scope
  A clear outline of how NICE guidelines are developed.

FEEDBACK TO LEARNING ACTIVITIES

21.1. Any decision about changes that are made or what to do is made up of:
- a balanced consideration of what we know
- what we think might plausibly work
- what we think we ought to do
- what we think we can do.

In other words, when we make a decision we use information in the form of data about the issue, theories about why things are the way they are, values and opinions about what we should do, and we also take into account a context of limited resources and practical constraints around what people want.

21.2. Promoting health is complex and it is sometimes difficult to provide evidence of effectiveness for single interventions. Addressing many of the issues that affect public health, such as obesity, demand a combination of interventions and thus are often termed complex. Complex interventions may include a range of different actions including advocacy, education and communication campaigns, regulation and legislation.

21.3. It is often advised that questions for literature searches are categorized as PICO – population, intervention, comparator (if relevant), and outcome. Learning Activity 21.3 asks you to identify two different scenarios, the target group, the intervention and the outcome or change sought. The PICO framework for each scenario is shown in the table.

Popula-tion	Interven-tion	Compara-tor	Out-come
Babies	Bottle-feeding	Breast feeding	Adult obesity
Young female smokers in school	Cessation group	Health education	Quit attempts and successful quits

21.4. It might be important to understand how communicable diseases spread in communities, and how effective immunization programmes are. It might also be important to understand levels of the uptake of immunization. Qualitative research would be invaluable in providing answers to the 'how' and 'why' questions (e.g., knowledge about unimmunized groups in society, whether this is a deliberate choice and, if so, the reasons for it). Vaccine hesitancy is a complex phenomenon and qualitative research is important in helping to understand it.

21.5. Possible keywords include:

Population AND	Exposure AND	Outcome
Cycling OR Cyclist OR	'Alcohol' OR 'Alcohol consumption' OR	'Attitude'
Bicycle OR Bicyclist OR	'Alcohol influenced' OR 'Under the influence' OR	'Behavi#r'
'Pedal cycle'	*'Drink' OR 'Drunk'	'Risk Behavi#r'

In many search engines there are shortcuts which are explained in section 'Finding the Evidence' in this chapter: speech marks are used for phrases such as "under the influence", an asterisk indicates that there may be associated words such as 'drinker', a hashtag (#) may be substituted where there are different spellings, such as behaviour/behavior.

This topic includes a crossover of disciplines including medicine, psychology, social policy but should be captured in Medline, CINAHL and PsychInfo.

21.6. There are a number of ways in which practitioners' and users' views can feed into this process, including evaluations of users' views, inputs into research design, and representation on committees and bodies that construct and use evidence. For example, INVOLVE (www. involve.org.uk) examines the ways in which research is prioritized, commissioned, undertaken and disseminated.

REFERENCES

Brown, T., Moore, T.H.M., Hooper, L., Gao, Y., Zayegh, A., et al., 2019. Interventions for preventing obesity in children. Cochrane Database Syst. Rev. 7, CD001871.

Cummins, S., Macintyre, S., 2002. 'Food deserts' – evidence and assumption in policy making. Br. Med. J. 325, 436–438.

Fonseca, H., Palmeira, A.L., Martins, S., Ferreira, P.D., 2014. Short- and medium-term impact of a residential weight-loss camp for overweight adolescents. Int. J. Adolesc. Med. Health 26 (1), 33–38.

Gately, P.J., Cooke, C.B., Barth, J.H., Bewick, B.M., Radley, D., et al., 2005 Children's residential weight-loss programs can work: a prospective cohort study of short-term outcomes for overweight and obese children. Pediatrics. 116 (1), 73–77.

Gately, P.J., 2014. Residential weight loss camps for children and young people. In: Haslam, D.W., Sharma, A.M., le Roux, C.W. (eds.), Controversies in Obesity. Springer, London, pp. 221–227.

Gilbert, R., Salanti, G., Harden, M., See, S., 2005. Infant sleeping position and sudden infant death syndrome: systematic review of observational studies and historical review of recommendations from 1940-2002. Int. J. Epidemiol. 34 (4), 874–887. 2005.

Kaufman, J., Ryan, R., Walsh, L., Horey, D., Leask, J., et al., 2018. Face-to-face interventions for informing or educating parents about early childhood vaccination. Cochrane Database Syst. Rev. 5, CD010038. Available at https://www.cochranelibrary.com/cdsr/doi/10.1002/14651858.CD010038.pub3/full.

Lamming, L., Pears, S., Mason, D., Morton, K., Bijker, M., et al., 2017. What do we know about brief interventions for physical activity that could be delivered in primary care consultations? A systematic review of reviews. Prev. Med. 99, 152–163.

McGregor, S., McKenna, J., Gately, P., Hill, A.J., 2016. Self-esteem outcomes over a summer camp for obese youth. Pediatr. Obes. 11 (6), 500–505.

McQueen, D., 2001. Strengthening the evidence base for health promotion. Health Promot. Int. 16 (3), 261–268.

Nutbeam, D., 1998. Evaluating health promotion: progress, problems and solutions. Health Promot. Int. 23, 27–44.

Oakley, A., 1998. Experimentation and social interventions: a forgotten but important history. Br. Med. J. 317, 1239–1242.

Oliver, S., 2001. Making research more useful: integrating different perspectives and different methods. In: Oliver, S., Peersman, G. (eds.), Using Research for Effective Health Promotion. Open University Press, Buckingham, pp. 167–180.

Pawson, R., Tilley, N., 1997. Realistic Evaluation. Sage, London.

Petrosino, A., Turpin-Petrosino, C., Finckenauer, J.O., 2000. Programs can have harmful effects! Lessons from experiments of programs such as Scared Straight. Crime Delinquency 46 (1), 354–379.

Public Health England, 2017. Commissioning Cost-Effective Services for Promotion of Mental Health and Wellbeing and Prevention of Mental Ill-Health. Available at: https://assets.publishing.service.gov.uk/government/uploads/system/uploads/attachment_data/file/640714/Commissioning_effective_mental_health_prevention_report.pdf (accessed 09-05-21).

Raphael, D., 2000. The question of evidence in Health promotion. Health Promot. Int. 14 (4), 355–367.

Sackett, D.L., Rosenberg, W.M., Gray, J.A., et al., 1996. Evidence-based medicine: what it is and what it isn't. Br. Med. J. 150, 1249–1255.

Supplement to American Journal of Preventive Medicine, 2000. Introducing the guide to community preventive services: methods, first recommendations and expert commentary. Am. J. Prev. Med. 18, 35–43.

Wong, W.W., Barlow, S.E., Mikhail, C., Wilson, T.A., Hernandez, P.M., et al., 2013 Jann. A residential summer camp can reduce body fat and improve health-related quality of life in obese children. J. Pediatr. Gastroenterol. Nutr. 56 (1), 83–85.

Planning and Implementing Health Promotion Interventions

By the end of this chapter you will be able to:
- understand the value of careful planning and preparation
- understand what is required to translate a needs assessment into effective action
- distinguish project activities from outcomes
- identify realistic aims and objectives for health promotion interventions.

Aims Broad goals or statement of what is to be achieved.

Contingency plan A plan for an organization to respond coherently to an unusual event.

Milestones Key events with dates that mark progress.

Objectives Specific activities that need to be done in order for a project to achieve its aims.

Outcomes Changes, effects or results.

Outputs What is done or produced.

Plan How to get from your starting point to your end point, and what you want to achieve.

Policy Guidelines for practice which set broad goals and the framework for action.

Programme An umbrella term for all activities.

Stakeholders Those directly affected by an intervention or whose support is necessary.

Strategy A broad framework for action which indicates goals, methods and underlying principles. It derives from evidence, identified needs and experience. It may be used at all levels, as in a programme strategy or an implementation strategy.

IMPORTANCE OF THE TOPIC

We saw in Chapter 20 how needs assessment and targeting may be carried out, and the importance of undertaking this process and being clear about the context in which it is done. This chapter builds on the discussion of the first stage of planning – needs assessment – in Chapter 20. It is important to be clear why you are carrying out an intervention or project, and what changes or improvements are expected. Funders, managers, commissioners and other stakeholders will want to know this as well as the activities that may take place. In determining the best approach, you may need to work with others, use the available resources to best effect, and set out a clear action plan of who does what and when. Planning at different levels, from broad strategic planning through project planning to small-scale health education planning, is considered in this chapter. Quality and audit issues, and how these relate to planning, are then considered.

REASONS FOR PLANNING

Health promoters usually have no problem in finding things to do which seem reasonable. Work areas are inherited from others, delegated from more senior members in the workplace, or demanded by clients. It is possible to be kept very busy reacting to all these pressures, and planning health promotion interventions may seem a luxury or a waste of time. However, there are sound reasons for planning health promotion or being proactive in your work practice. Planning is important because it helps direct resources to where they will have most impact. Planning ensures that health promotion is not overlooked, but is prioritized as a work activity.

Planning takes different forms and is used at different levels. It may be used to provide the best services or care for an individual client, as in the nursing process, or it may be used for group activities, such as antenatal classes. Planning may also refer to large-scale health promotion interventions targeted at whole populations.

The degree of formality of the planning process also varies. When planning a one-to-one intervention, the process is informal and may involve no one else. Planning for a group intervention may involve liaising with other professionals as well as the target group, to find out what their aims and objectives are and what sorts of methods and resources are available and acceptable. A written plan may be produced to act as a guide and a statement of agreed outcomes and methods. Planning a large-scale intervention will usually involve more long-term collaborative activity. Often a working group (or task force or local forum) will be established early on to identify interested groups or stakeholders and gain their support and expertise. The plan will outline not only objectives and methods but also a timescale of what is to be achieved and when, funding details and a budget, who is responsible for which tasks, and how the intervention will be evaluated, any targets monitored and the findings reported back.

There has been much greater emphasis on systematic planning in recent years due to a need for greater economic accountability, more focus on targets and their achievement, and the need to include evidence as part of project development. It is particularly important for practitioners to be clear about the rationale for interventions, the goals and the approach that is adopted.

HEALTH PROMOTION PLANNING CYCLE

Planning involves several key stages or logical stepping stones which enable the health promoter to achieve a desired result. The benefit is being clear about what it is you want to achieve, i.e., the purpose of any intervention. Planning entails the following seven steps:
1. An assessment of need.
2. Setting aims – what it is you intend to achieve.
3. Setting objectives – precise and measurable outcomes.

4. Deciding which methods, interventions or strategies will achieve your objectives.
5. Identifying the resources needed.
6. Evaluating outcomes in order to assess the effectiveness of methods and make improvements in the future.
7. Setting up an action plan including the assessment of milestones.

Some planning models are presented as a linear process. Others show a circular process to indicate that any evaluation feeds back into the process, as illustrated in Fig. 22.1.

Fig. 22.1 outlines a seemingly rational and simple approach which describes how decisions should be made. It does not take into account that there may not be agreement on objectives or the best way to proceed, and that in real-life planning is often piecemeal or incremental. There is no grand design, but circumstances dictate many small reactive decisions. Learning Activity 22.1 asks you to consider this planning cycle and where might be the best starting point for a project or intervention.

 Learning Activity 22.1   The Planning Cycle

What do you think would be the best starting point for planning an intervention or programme? Why?

Think of any planned activities you have been involved with. What was the starting point? Why?

LOGIC MODELS

The following famous quote is attributed to the American Yogi Berra:

If you don't know where you're going, how are you gonna know when you get there?

This neatly sums up the challenges of planning and the importance of knowing what we hope to achieve. All sorts of assumptions underlie what we do, for example, what we think is the problem or situation to be addressed; who are the participants and how they learn or what might motivate them; what resources are needed; and yet these are rarely made explicit. In particular, assumptions are made that if there is a specific end goal, certain activities are going to make that happen, and that doing x will lead to certain outcomes.

A logic model is a depiction or map of a project or programme showing the relationship between its resources, activities and intended results. It tests the logic of the programme through a series of 'if–then'

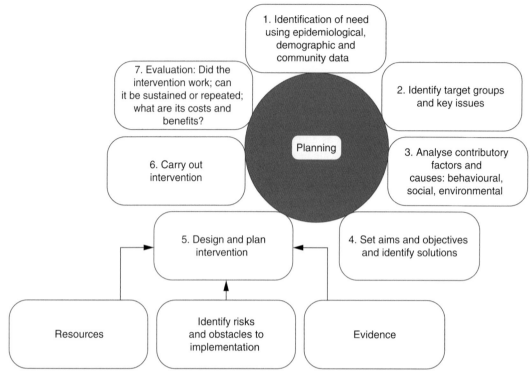

Fig. 22.1 Health promotion planning cycle

relationships that lead to the desired outcomes. These if–then relationships express the programme's theory of change, and how and why a set of activities is expected to lead to early, intermediate and long-term outcomes over a specified period. Thus if we do these activities, then this output will be achieved; if we deliver these outputs, then this purpose will be achieved; if the purpose is achieved, then this will contribute to the goal, as shown in this example:

IF we want to achieve a reduction in obesity

THEN we should reduce the consumption of high fat, sugar and salt (HFSS) foods

IF we want to reduce consumption of HFSS foods

THEN we need to encourage/persuade the public not to eat them

IF we want to encourage a change in consumption

THEN we need to restrict advertising.

Fig. 22.2 illustrates this logical chain of connections showing what the programme sets out to accomplish.

Logic models, increasingly used in programme planning, start with the end in mind. Everything else flows from the outcomes so it is important to work with

stakeholders to generate a shared understanding of the end goal and what success will look like. This helps to avoid any flaws in the logic chain, such as anticipated outcomes being too distant from the planned activities. Outcomes are usually framed as 'immediate or short term' and 'medium to longer term' outcomes. Not all logic models include outputs but if they do, they are the quantifiable end product of the activities and can be likened to the 'milestone deliverables'. The activities element is a very important part of the model i.e. IF you do these things then you will get that result. Inputs are the resources required to put into practice planned activities.

STRATEGIC PLANNING

Strategy tends to be used as an umbrella term to cover a broad programme. It may therefore have several different objectives and projects. Practitioners often do not start with a blank sheet but have to work in a wider policy context where issues are determined nationally. Strategies may be local as well as national, and involve many

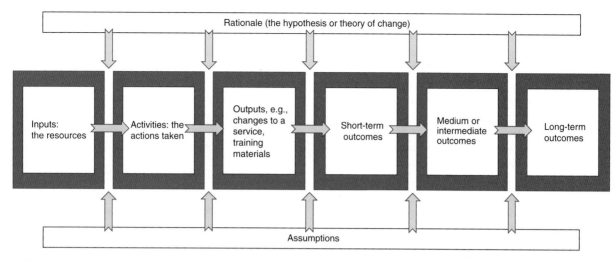

Fig. 22.2 The logic chain

stakeholders. A stakeholder analysis helps to identify relevant partners and their interests regarding the issue. For example, all local authorities are required to have a strategy to tackle obesity that includes the following:

- a detailed specification of services, projects and activities;
- identification of costs, inputs and quality standards;
- expected outcomes. These are expressed as present-day goals rather than targets which specify how and when an objective will be measured. For example, a target for health services to reduce childhood obesity may be to increase the percentage of 5–16-year-olds participating in at least 2 hours of intensity sport per week to over 90% by a specified date.

Bearing this in mind consider Learning Activity 22.2 which asks you to begin the planning for a local strategy on alcohol use.

> **Learning Activity 22.2   Planning a Strategy**
>
> You are involved in a working group drawing up a local strategy to reduce alcohol use.
> 1. Who would you involve in the project planning?
> 2. What would influence the choice of goals that you adopt?
> 3. If you decided to control availability, what might be achievable outcomes?
> 4. What might be an appropriate activity or intervention?
> 5. What factors may affect what you want to achieve?

PROJECT PLANNING

Project planning is a smaller-scale activity, and refers to planning a specific project which is time limited and aims to bring about a defined change. Examples of small-scale health promotion projects include a project to raise awareness among university students about meningitis; a project to train school nurses in presentation skills; and a project to map safe routes to school for young children.

> **Learning Activity 22.3   Carrying Out a Project**
>
> The strategy outlined in Learning Activity 22.2 might include a project centred on training GPs and practice nurses to identify the problematic use of alcohol at an early stage. This project, which is part of the overall alcohol reduction strategy, would require careful and detailed planning, including the following:
> - Setting appropriate objectives. For example, would it be appropriate to set an objective of reducing problem drinking in the practice population? Why?
> - How might objectives best be achieved? For example, should training be unidisciplinary or multidisciplinary? Should the training be accredited? Who would be the best person to run the sessions? What venue, day and time would be most acceptable? How would the sessions be funded? How long will the project last?
> - How would you evaluate the project? What criteria would you use to demonstrate success?

The kind of planning most health practitioners will be involved in will be on a small scale. For example, you may want to plan a health education session with an individual client, or a series of sessions with a small group around a specific issue. Using the example above, you might want to plan a single session in detail. This would require you to:

- set detailed objectives for participants to achieve by the end of the session, for example, being aware of symptoms and behaviours (e.g., poor attendance and time-keeping at work, especially in the mornings) which might be due to problematic alcohol use
- investigate the range of resources available and select resources to use in the session
- plan the session showing different activities and time allocated for each activity
- plan a means of evaluating the session.

Planning Models

Planning, whatever the scale of the activity, requires systematically working through a number of stages that relate to the following questions.

- What is the nature of the problem?
- Who is affected?
- What are the causes and contributory factors?
- What needs to be done to tackle the problem?
- How should any intervention be carried out?
- How will we know if it is successful?

One of the most well-known models for planning is the PRECEDE-PROCEED model (Green and Kreuter, 2005), which is shown in Fig. 22.3.

PRECEDE stands for predisposing, reinforcing and enabling causes in educational diagnosis. This model recognizes the multiple determinants of health and starts with an assessment of the quality of life, which is the ultimate goal. Health contributes to quality of life. The model then works 'backwards' in a sequence of diagnostic phases to identify the environmental and organizational factors that influence health behaviour, including health service utilization. It considers the *predisposing factors*, personal factors such as individual motivation, knowledge, attitudes and beliefs; *reinforcing factors*, the attitudes and behaviours of role models, peers and employers; and *enabling factors*, resources and skills that either support or hinder change in behaviour or environment. As well as diagnosing what needs to be addressed, the capacity for implementation of a proposed programme is also considered.

The model may be broken down into phases. Priority targets for intervention are established through each phase of the assessment process (phases 1–4) on the basis of their causal importance in the chain of health determinants, their prevalence and their changeability. The results of this assessment process guide the development of the intervention (phase 5). The evaluation (phase 6) then tracks the impact of the intervention on factors identified as important targets in the assessment process.

Phases of the PRECEDE-PROCEED Model

Phase 1. Identify desirable outcomes regarding health status and quality of life – the identification of a population's felt concerns and problems relating to their quality of life, for example, unemployment, crime.

Phase 2. Identify desirable outcomes regarding lifestyle and environment – the identification of a population's health practices, for example, service utilization, self-care and management, lifestyles and environmental factors.

Phase 3. Identify required education, skills and ecology, for example, beliefs, values and attitudes that affect motivation to change; skills and resources; and social factors, for example, income, social norms and social support.

Phase 4. Identify the administrative and financial policies that are needed. How well does the implementation of the programme meet these needs?

Phase 5. Implementation of the intervention follows logically from the previous phases. The management and administration of the intervention are also considered at this stage. Administrative diagnosis includes assessment of resources and organizational relationships, and the production of a timetable.

Phase 6. The impact and outcomes of the programme are used in the evaluation of the intervention, although Green and Kreuter (2005) stress that this should be an integrated activity addressed throughout the planning process.

The intention is that using the PRECEDE-PROCEED model will guide the health educator to the most effective type of intervention. Using knowledge drawn from epidemiology, social psychology, education and management studies, the health educator can arrive at an optimum intervention. The model is said to be based on a complementary mix of expertise drawn from these different disciplines. In practice, the model is often modified and is rarely used as illustrated (see Green's own website for an account of the application of the model,

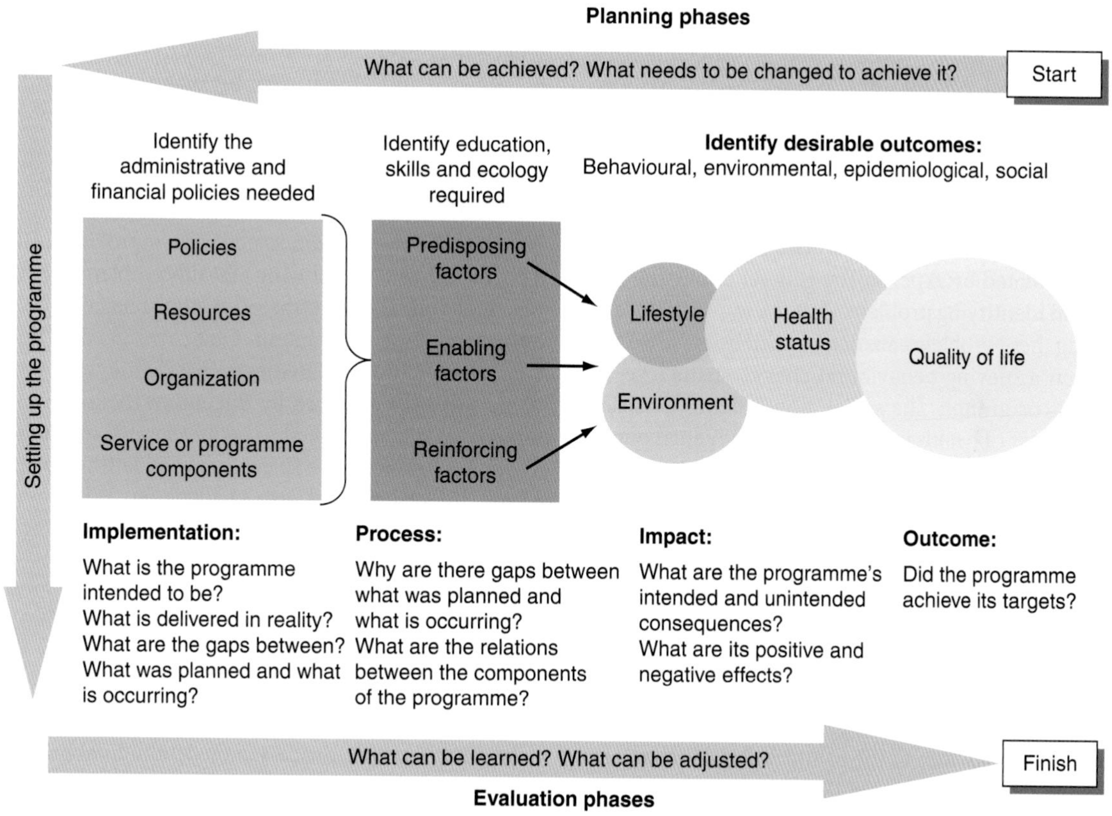

Fig. 22.3 PRECEDE-PROCEED planning model (From Green, L.W., Kreuter, M.W., 2005. Health Program Planning: An Educational and Ecological Approach. fourth edn. McGraw-Hill Higher Education, New York.)

Phase 1 Identify desirable outcomes regarding health status and quality of life – the identification of a population's felt concerns and problems relating to their quality of life, e.g., unemployment, crime.

Phase 2 Identify desirable outcomes regarding lifestyle and environment – the identification of a population's health practices, e.g., service utilization, self-care and management, lifestyles and environmental factors.

Phase 3 Identify required education, skills and ecology, e.g., beliefs, values and attitudes that affect motivation to change; skills and resources; social factors, e.g., income; social norms and social support.

Phase 4 Identify the administrative and financial policies that are needed. How well does the implementation of the programme meet these needs?

Phase 5 Implementation of the intervention follows logically from the previous phases. The management and administration of the intervention are also considered at this stage. Administrative diagnosis includes assessment of resources and organizational relationships, and the production of a timetable.

Phase 6 The impact and outcomes of the programme are used in the evaluation of the intervention, although Green and Kreuter (2005) stress that this should be an integrated activity addressed throughout the planning process.

http://www.lgreen.net/precede.htm). For example, it is unusual to begin the process of planning with an agenda as open as 'quality of life'. Priority topics, target groups or settings are more often identified at the outset. For example, public health white papers in England have typically focused on specific diseases. So in practice PRECEDE often begins at the behavioural diagnosis rather than the needs assessment phase.

The PRECEDE-PROCEED model may be criticized on several grounds. PRECEDE as a health education planning model mirrors the medical world. The planning process is dominated by experts. The general public may be involved in identifying problems, but the ways and means of tackling these problems are determined by experts. The focus is on achieving behavioural change at the level of individuals or groups. The social, political and environmental context of health is systematically screened out of the model in phases 2 and 3. To some extent this may be explained by PRECEDE being a health education rather than a health promotion planning model. A model developed specifically for health education cannot be expected to apply to other forms of health promotion, but for most people education, even if it does not include changing the environment, does include clarifying values, beliefs and attitudes, facilitating self-empowerment and supporting autonomy. Using the PRECEDE-PROCEED model subordinates these activities to the primary aim of behaviour change. It could be argued that PRECEDE-PROCEED is a model dominated by social psychology and behavioural perspectives rather than educational perspectives, and that the label is therefore misleading. PRECEDE-PROCEED is, however, a highly structured planning model which ensures that certain issues are considered. If the objective is behaviour change, then PRECEDE-PROCEED is a useful model to follow.

Stage 1: What Is the Nature of the Problem?

A range of issues is important in the 'diagnosis' stage of planning. In Green and Kreuter's model (2005) shown in Fig. 22.3, this step is about understanding why a problem should be addressed, how it arises, what are the contributory factors and for whom it is a problem. As we saw in Chapter 20, priorities do not always arise out of needs that may be identified in community profiles or needs assessments, but may be defined on the basis of national or local epidemiological data reporting trends in illnesses and deaths. Equally, the causes identified from epidemiological data may not accord with what people

themselves identify as the causes of problems. As we also saw in Chapter 20, it is important to identify what can be changed. If the problem or issue is incorrectly understood and diagnosed, then everything that flows from it will be ill conceived. Case Study 22.1 considers the issue of violence and how it may be 'diagnosed' in order to identify appropriate interventions.

Stage 2: What Needs to Be Done? Set Aims and Objectives

Aims are broad goals concerned with improving health in a particular area or reducing a health problem, for example, reducing the amount of alcohol-related ill health, and are statements of intent. Objectives need to be specific, and should be statements that define what participants will have achieved by the end of the intervention. Objectives therefore need to be measurable in some way. There is a balance to be struck between setting objectives which are realistic but also challenging. When writing objectives it is recommended that they are SMART:
Specific
Measurable
Achievable
Realistic
Time-bound

Health promotion objectives can refer to educational, behavioural, policy, process or environmental outcomes. Learning Activity 22.4 asks you to draft some objectives for an educational intervention with healthcare professionals about alcohol use.

- Educational objectives may be divided into three categories, and are usually expressed in relation to the learner:

  knowledge objectives concerning increased levels of knowledge

  affective objectives concerning changes in attitudes and beliefs

  behavioural or skills objectives concerning the acquisition of new competencies and skills.

  These will lead to short-term outcomes.
  Medium term outcomes will have:

- Behavioural objectives, including changes in lifestyles and increased take-up of services, for example, reducing the amount of binge drinking or the prevalence of drink-driving.

- Policy objectives, including the development or implementation of policy, for example, implementing alcohol-free policies in workplaces.

CASE STUDY 22.1

Violence as a Public Health Issue

There are 2.5 million violent incidents in England and Wales each year. These result in 300,000 emergency department attendances and 35,000 emergency admissions into hospital. There are considerable health-related consequences of violence and it has been estimated that violence costs the National Health Service £2.9 billion every year (Bellis et al., 2012). This figure underestimates the total impact of violence on health, for example, exposure to violence as a child can increase risks of substance abuse, obesity and illnesses such as cancer and heart disease in later life (Hughes et al, 2017) and may well be an underestimate of the scale of, for example, knife incidents.

Serious violence is strongly associated with inequalities. The poorest fifth of people have hospital admission rates for violence five times higher than those of the most affluent fifth (DHSC, 2019). The range of contributory factors is shown in the following figure in this case study (Bellis et al., 2012, p. 27).

A review by the Scottish Violence Reduction Unit (Russell, 2021) identified effective interventions that include the following:

- School and education programmes to mitigate adverse childhood experiences (ACEs) and potentially prevent violence in intimate partner and dating relationships.
- School programmes to build resilience to criminal exploitation in gang recruitment.
- Intensive support for those involved in violence including those carrying knives.
- Identifying safe spaces in the community, for example, chicken shops and their staff.
- Creating employment and education opportunities.

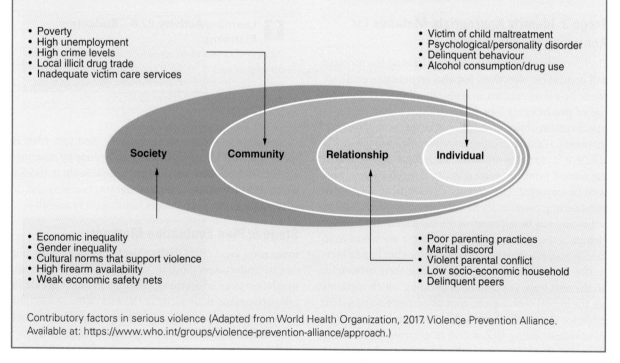

- Poverty
- High unemployment
- High crime levels
- Local illicit drug trade
- Inadequate victim care services

- Victim of child maltreatment
- Psychological/personality disorder
- Delinquent behaviour
- Alcohol consumption/drug use

Society Community Relationship Individual

- Economic inequality
- Gender inequality
- Cultural norms that support violence
- High firearm availability
- Weak economic safety nets

- Poor parenting practices
- Marital discord
- Violent parental conflict
- Low socio-economic household
- Delinquent peers

Contributory factors in serious violence (Adapted from World Health Organization, 2017. Violence Prevention Alliance. Available at: https://www.who.int/groups/violence-prevention-alliance/approach.)

- Process objectives include the achievement of health promotion principles, for example, participation and intersectoral collaboration.
- Environmental objectives include changing the environment to make it more health promoting, for example restricting the advertising and sale of alcohol.

Learning Activity 22.4   Setting Health Education Objectives

What might be appropriate objectives for a project on the early identification of alcohol-related problems by GPs and practice nurses?

Objectives also reflect perspectives about the determinants of health and values about what are the most important things to achieve. These perspectives and values may be your own or may be derived from your organization and Learning Activity 22.5 asks you to consider how the goals set for an intervention may reflect views about the determinants of the issue.

 Learning Activity 22.5   The Role of Determinants in Planning

Consider the different aims that may be included in a drug prevention strategy:
1. To reduce the risks associated with drug use and enable clients who do choose to use drugs to do so safely.
2. To reduce levels of harmful drug use.
   What values and views about the determinants of drug use are reflected in these different aims?

Stage 3: Identify Appropriate Methods for Achieving the Objectives

Decisions about how to go about addressing the problem will depend on objectives, but also on available evidence of effective interventions, available funding and the expertise of practitioners (see Chapter 21). Certain methods match certain objectives but would be quite inappropriate for others. For example, participative small group work is effective at changing attitudes, but a more formal teaching session would be more effective if specific knowledge is to be imparted. Community development is effective at increasing community involvement and participation, but would not be appropriate if local government policy change is the objective. The mass media are effective in raising people's awareness of health issues but largely ineffective in persuading people to change their behaviour. So the next stage in planning is deciding which methods are the logical choice given your objectives and based on evidence about what works. You may find you have to compromise owing to constraints of time, resources or skills, but this compromise should concern the amount of input or the use of complementary methods. It should not mean that you end up using inappropriate methods which are unlikely to achieve your objectives.

Stage 4: Identify Resources and Inputs

When objectives and methods have been decided, the next stage is to consider whether any specific resources are needed to implement the strategy. Resources include:

- financial: for example, investment; specific funding stream(s)
- people: for example, workforce/capacity/capability; community capacity and networks; end users
- estates: for example, buildings, sites and can also be 'places' or geographies/communities
- technology: for example, information and communications technology systems.

Funding is an important issue for larger-scale interventions which require additional inputs over and above existing services and staff. For larger-scale interventions you may need to prepare a budget, which is a statement of expected costs. This includes direct costs, which relate to the project, and fixed costs, which occur anyway. Learning Activity 22.6 focuses on budgetary planning and asks you to begin to identify key costs when planning an intervention.

 Learning Activity 22.6   Budgetary Planning

What would you need to include in a budget plan for training sessions for GPs and practice nurses on the early identification of problematic alcohol use, discussed in Learning Activity 22.4?

A budget control system regularly monitors what is spent and what remains. This is usually done by monitoring the amount of money allocated, the amount of money spent and the variance between the two (underspend or overspend) under each budget heading every month.

Stage 5: Plan Evaluation Methods

Evaluation must relate to the objectives you have set, but can be undertaken more or less formally. For example, in relation to an educational session you might decide to ask participants their views at the end of the session, or spend some time noting your own perceptions of what went well and what could be improved next time. Or you might design a more formal means of evaluation, for example, a questionnaire for participants to fill in anonymously, which is timetabled into the session. Project evaluation is discussed in more detail in Chapter 23.

Stage 6: Set an Action Plan

This is a detailed written plan which identifies tasks, the person responsible for each task, resources which will be used, a timescale and means of evaluation. You might also include interim indicators of progress to show if you are proceeding as planned. Many factors can threaten the sustainability of a project. Being clear about the external factors underlying the structure of the project, and what assumptions are being made, is a key requirement of most project plans, especially where large sums of money are being allocated. For example, projects may depend on achieving community involvement or successful funding bids.

A Gantt chart (set out as an example in Fig. 22.4) is a useful tool at this stage. A Gantt chart plots tasks and the people responsible for these tasks against a timescale in which these activities need to be undertaken. It portrays in a graphical form the interdependence of project tasks and how each single task contributes to the whole. The evaluation and review of the training sessions and the final report record the project outcomes and assess whether objectives have been met. It is useful to have a time lag between completing the project and the final review in order to assess long-term as well as immediate outcomes.

Stage 7: Action or Implementation of the Plan

It is often useful to keep a log or diary to note unexpected problems and how you dealt with them, as well as unintended benefits. This information can then be fed into the evaluation process. You will also want to plan for the documentation and dissemination of the project findings, whether this is in the form of a report, a newsletter or a presentation.

Log frames (logistical frameworks) are widely used in international development projects to identify the activities of a programme and any inherent risks that might delay completion. A log frame is not the same as the logic model described earlier. A logical framework takes the form of a table. The rows describe the four different results the project aims to achieve or contribute to: objectives, outcomes, outputs and activities. The columns describe the verifiable indicators, the means of verification (i.e. what information is used to provide verification), and the assumptions and external factors that may influence the project. Log frames can be useful to ensure that activities are monitored, outcomes evaluated, and means and ends are brought together. Critics argue that they are potentially inflexible and time-consuming to produce. Learning Activity 22.7 asks you to try to produce a log frame for a project about alcohol.

QUALITY AND AUDIT

Assessing the quality of practice through quality assurance, quality management or audit is an important aspect of professional practice. It helps to improve standards, identify cost-effective activities, demonstrate worth to outside agencies and ensure that activities meet stakeholders' requirements. In the UK a strategic process to identify and understand healthcare needs has been in place since 1990. Its purpose is to decide how to spend available resources and to secure and monitor appropriate services, engaging in activities that lead to improved population health, reduced health inequalities and improved access, quality, experience and outcomes of care for service users. Currently the process is conducted by clinical commissioning groups (CCGs), which assess local needs, determinants of health and inequalities. This introduction of commissioning of services and placing of contracts has highlighted the need for specification of quality. There has also been an increased emphasis on audit of public sector activities, and clinical audit is well established. Targets have been set, for example, a reduction in accident and emergency and ambulance attendance waiting times, and in infections acquired in hospital. Such targets are not popular with everyone, and have been criticized as distorting clinical priorities. Setting targets is about measuring performance in relation to a level of service or activity level.

Quality is less concerned with number crunching than with how the activity is perceived by recipients. There is now more emphasis on quality through specifications such as 'commissioning for quality and innovation' or CQUINS. Continuous quality improvement, total quality management and the use of external standards all aim to improve services and also provide answers to the variability in programme development. Quality in healthcare relates to:

- safe care (avoidance of harmful interventions)
- effectiveness (care which conforms with best practice)
- enhancement of the patient/user experience.

The core principles of quality interventions in health promotion have been defined (Speller et al., 1997) as follows:

- equity – that users have equal access to and/or equal benefit from services
- effectiveness – that services achieve their intended objectives

	March	April	May	June	July	August	September	October
Marketing and publicity	H and A							
Recruit participants		A						
Plan sessions				H	H			
Accreditation			H and A					
Pre-course needs assessment questionnaire				H and R				
Prepare materials, collect resources					H and A			
Check venue, timing, refreshments						A		
Action: training sessions							H	
Post-course sessions								H and R
Evaluation report								H and R

Three workers are involved:

H is a health promotor.
A is an administrative officer.
R is a researcher.

Fig. 22.4 Gantt chart

💡 Learning Activity 22.7   Using a Log Frame for a Project to Reduce Binge Drinking

Complete the log frame below.

Project	Indicators of achievement	Means of verification	Important risks and assumptions
Objectives			
To reduce the harmful effects of binge drinking among young women			
Outcomes			
To raise awareness of using safe taxi companies to get home			
Outputs			
Purse cards with taxi numbers			
Posters in bar and club toilets			
Tannoy announcements in bar and club toilets			
Activities			
Working with specified taxi companies to recruit women drivers			
Working with bar and club owners			

- efficiency – that services achieve maximum benefit for minimum cost
- accessibility – that a service is easily available to users in terms of time, distance and ethos
- appropriateness – that a service is what the users require
- acceptability – that services satisfy the reasonable expectations of users
- responsiveness – that services adapt to the expressed needs of users.

Quality expresses a notion of 'fit for the purpose', but also conveys a notion of excellence. Quality assurance or audit is a systematic process through which desirable levels of quality are described, the extent to which these levels are achieved is assessed and follow-up action is taken to achieve optimum levels of quality. Quality assurance is an ongoing process of continual assessment and improvement of practice, and therefore differs from evaluation, which focuses on outcomes at a specific point in time. A quality system may include elements of quality assurance and quality management.

Quality improvement approaches can be traced back to attempts to improve production quality control in industry from the 1920s. The Plan, Do, Study, Act (PDSA) is a widely adopted model for continuous improvement, in which changes are tested in small cycles, shown in Fig. 22.5.

Co-design and co-production are concepts that have grown in profile. They mean working in partnership with users and patients and using their experience to identify 'touch points' in their journey and where improvements in services could be made.

Audit is a systematic process of scrutinizing a service or programme in order to improve performance. Audit may focus on a particular aspect, for example, organization and management or training. Part of the purpose of an audit is to build a picture, providing evidence of gaps and areas for improvement by comparing what is done with agreed best practice. A key part of an audit is to see if a service meets the needs of its users, so it may involve gathering and acting on local people's views. Audit may involve an internal review or scrutiny by an independent external auditor (e.g., the Audit Commission or Office for Standards in Education, Children's Services and Skills [OFSTED] inspectors of schools).

Model for improvement

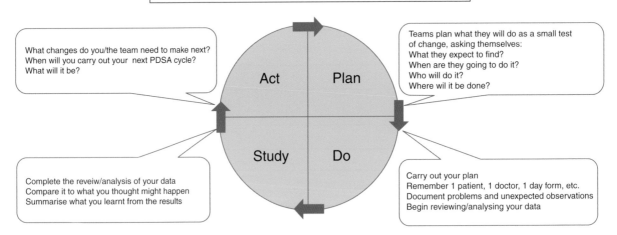

1. What are we trying to accomplish?
2. How will we know that a change is an improvement?
3. What changes can we test that will result in an improvement?

What changes do you/the team need to make next?
When will you carry out your next PDSA cycle?
What will it be?

Act

Plan

Teams plan what they will do as a small test of change, asking themselves:
What they expect to find?
When are they going to do it?
Who will do it?
Where wil it be done?

Study

Do

Complete the reveiw/analysis of your data
Compare it to what you thought might happen
Summarise what you learnt from the results

Carry out your plan
Remember 1 patient, 1 doctor, 1 day form, etc.
Document problems and unexpected observations
Begin reviewing/analysing your data

Fig. 22.5 Quality improvement: Plan, Do, Study, Act (From Clinical Excellence Commission and New South Wales Government, 2020. Model for improvement & PDSA cycles. New South Wales Government. Available at https://www.cec.health.nsw.gov.au/Quality-Improvement-Academy/quality-improvement-tools/model-for-improvement-and-pdsa-cycles.)

■ CONCLUSION

There are sound reasons for adopting a planning model to structure health promotion interventions. Recognizing that health is a complex socially determined concept means that activities to promote health require careful planning, and often collaboration and working together with different agencies. Activities at different levels all benefit from planning, although the factors which need to be considered will vary according to the level of planned intervention.

A systematic approach will ensure that what is done:

- is relevant to agreed strategic objectives
- involves key stakeholders at the important stages of the project
- is relevant to the real problems and issues of target groups/beneficiaries
- has feasible objectives and can be realistically achieved
- measures and verifies successes
- ensures that benefits generated by projects are likely to be sustainable.

Planning provides a standard framework in which projects/programmes/interventions are developed, implemented and evaluated. The planning cycle ensures that the results of a project are fed back into new projects and programmes. Many health promotion projects fail because they are ill conceived, have simple educational or behavioural objectives which fail to analyse causes, take a narrow reductionist view of health and/or do not take account of existing evidence.

In reality, planning health promotion is a more complex process than planning models suggest. This is because rational decision-making is only one factor in determining what happens. Many other factors are also important, including historical precedent, enthusiasms of key people and the political context. So it is unlikely that any health promotion intervention proceeds exactly along the lines indicated by a planning model, but this does not mean models are not useful. Models help structure activities and can act as a checklist to ensure that important stages are not missed out. They are there to be modified in the light of experience, not to act as straitjackets.

Chapter 23 goes on to discuss the evaluation stage. Evaluating interventions and being able to determine to what extent health promotion is successful in achieving its objectives is the key to establishing health promotion as a central plank of health work.

REFLECTION ON PRACTICE

- What factors would you take into account when planning a health promotion intervention? How could you assess the quality of your health promotion work?
- Think about an intervention, project or programme in which you have taken part. What is the relative importance of the following in its shaping: needs, evidence, theory, resources?
- What examples can you identify of patient or user involvement in the design of projects or interventions?

SUMMARY

This chapter has clarified the terminology used in the planning process and discussed the reasons for planning health promotion interventions. Planning happens at different levels, and an account of this has been given. Two planning models which have been developed specifically for health promotion have been discussed in greater detail. The assessment and evaluation of planning have been discussed through reference to quality assurance and audit cycles.

FURTHER READING AND RESOURCES

Davies, M., Kepford, J., 2006. Planning a health promotion intervention. In: Davies, M., Macdowall, W. (eds.), Health Promotion Theory. Understanding Public Health Series. OUP, McGraw Hill, Maidenhead.
A useful short summary of some key factors to take into account.

Ewles, L., Simnett, I., 2017. Promoting Health: A Practical Guide, seventh edn. Baillière Tindall, Edinburgh.
Chapter 5 gives further details and a practical guide to Ewles and Simnett's model.

Green, J., Tones, K., Cross, R., Woodall, J., 2019. Health Promotion. Planning and Strategies, fourth edn. Sage, London.
Chapter 4 provides a readable and detailed discussion of systematic approaches to planning, and discusses various planning models.

Taylor, V. (ed.), 2012. Leading for Health and Wellbeing. Sage, London.
Chapter 7 focuses on leading at a local level including performance management. Chapter 8 focuses on project management.

FEEDBACK TO LEARNING ACTIVITIES

22.1. Fig. 22.1 suggests that the planning cycle begins with a needs assessment through which the programme's focus and any specific target groups may be identified. The underlying causes and contributory factors that led to the problem, and the areas that will need to be addressed, are then identified.

22.2. Learning Activity 22.2 asks you to identify the steps in planning a working group to develop an alcohol strategy:

1. *Who would you involve?* Identifying likely partners and developing a team. This is likely to include elected councillors, licensed victuallers, magistrates, police service and voluntary agencies dealing with alcohol-related problems.
2. *What would influence the goals?* An analysis of the current situation would identify the issues that present the greatest demand on resources, or possibly the issue that is most amenable to change.
3. *What might be achievable outcomes? Where do we want to go?* Objectives might include:
   - reducing the promotion of alcohol
   - reducing alcohol-related antisocial behaviour
   - protecting young people from alcohol-related harm.
4. *Activities or interventions. How do we get there?* Possible activities might be an awareness workshop for local councillors, banning advertisements for alcohol on local authority premises, promoting health practitioners' awareness via sessions for GPs and practice nurses on early identification and referral, use of local by-laws to prevent drinking in public, and sessions in youth clubs and community centres.
5. *What factors may affect what we want to achieve? What may stop us getting there?* The local council may not be supportive of a proactive policy on licensing. The alcohol industry may be a powerful economic force locally.

22.3. Learning Activity 22.3 asks you to consider the objectives for a specific project to train GPs and practice nurses in the early identification of problems in alcohol use:

- An objective of reducing problem drinking is unrealistic and too long term for a single intervention project.

Continued

- Unidisciplinary training has the advantage of practitioners understanding each others' roles and being less competitive, but most issues benefit from a multidisciplinary approach, as this enables mutual understanding of the extent of the problem.
- Criteria to evaluate the success of the project could include data on staff involvement in the project, for example, take-up of training and number of accredited staff by the end of the project. Data on reducing problem drinking in the practice population, although the ultimate goal of the project, are more problematic to collect (e.g., does one rely on self-reports, or require independent corroboration through measures such as blood and liver function tests?). Even if reduced problem drinking is verified, attributing this to the project is also problematic. Ideally, there needs to be a control population to ensure any positive results are attributable to the project.

22.4. A training session might have the following educational objectives:

1. Increasing participants' knowledge of the range of harmful effects and symptoms associated with problematic alcohol use.
2. Increasing participants' knowledge of the extent of problematic alcohol use and its association with social and demographic factors, for example, gender, age, employment status, occupation.
3. Investigating participants' attitudes towards alcohol and cultural depictions of alcohol use. Identifying the range between social drinker and alcoholic, with the many stages in between. Recognizing social, media and peer pressures to drink, which contribute to many people's problematic usage of alcohol.

4. Enabling participants to use an assessment tool effectively to identify problematic alcohol use.
5. Enabling participants to use the stages of change model to identify problem drinkers and appropriate interventions.

22.5. The first aim is harm reduction, where the focus is on the prevention of harm rather than the prevention of drug use itself, and on people who continue to use drugs. It recognizes the complex interplay of social factors that influence vulnerability to drug-related harm, including poverty, social inequality and discrimination. The activities may include needle exchanges, peer education and counselling. The second aim is simply a disease-reduction approach, where the focus may be on education or enforcement activities controlling supply.

22.6. Direct costs include:

- staff costs – salaries, superannuation, employer's national insurance payments, annual increments
- capital costs, for example, computers
- costs of specific activities, for example, rental of community centre for training, buying resources to use in the training
- telephone, postage, photocopying
- travel and subsistence
- training and conferences to support staff development.

  Fixed costs include overheads to cover, for example, accommodation, heating, lighting, telephone rental.

22.7. Learning Activity 22.7 asks you to complete a log frame or plan for a project to reduce binge drinking, showing the objectives, expected outcomes, outputs and activities:

Project	Indicators of achievement	Means of verification	Important risks and assumptions
Objectives To reduce the harmful effects of binge drinking among young women	Reduction in hospital admissions to accident and emergency and other wards due to the effects of alcohol	Hospital statistics	That the harmful effects of binge drinking are health related (as opposed to safety related, e.g., driving under the influence of alcohol) That hospital admission will be sought by women under the influence of alcohol
Outcomes To raise awareness of using safe taxi companies to get home	Increase in use of safe taxi companies by women under the influence of alcohol	Taxi records	That young women have available resources (money) to use taxis, and that there are no public transport options for the journey home

Project	Indicators of achievement	Means of verification	Important risks and assumptions
Outputs			
Purse cards with taxi numbers	Publication and distribution of cards advertising taxis	Data confirming publication and distribution of cards	That women will use the cards to order taxis, and that they have the money to pay for taxis
Posters in bar and club toilets	Production and placement of posters in bar and club toilets	Spot checks in bars and clubs to verify placement of posters	That women will read the posters and act on the information displayed in them
Tannoy announcements in bar and club toilets	Playing tannoy announcements in bar and club toilets	Monitoring tannoy announcements in bar and club toilets	That women will hear and process the information given in the announcements
Activities			
Working with specified taxi companies to recruit women drivers	Data on the sex of taxi drivers employed by taxi companies	Taxi companies' records on the sex of their drivers	That women will feel safer with women taxi drivers, and be more likely to use taxi companies which can provide women drivers on request
Working with bar and club owners			

REFERENCES

Bellis, M.A., Hughes, K., Perkins, C., Bennett, A., 2012. Protecting people, promoting health: a public health approach to violence prevention for England. Public Health England.

Department of Health and Social Care (DHSC), 2019. Preventing serious violence: summary. Available at: https://www.gov.uk/government/publications/preventing-serious-violence-a-multi-agency-approach/preventing-serious-violence-summary.

Green, L.W., Kreuter, M.W., 2005. Health Program Planning: An Educational and Ecological Approach, fourth edn. McGraw-Hill Higher Education, New York.

Hughes, K., Bellis, M.A., Hardcastle, K.A., Sethi, D., Butchart, A., et al., 2017. The effect of multiple adverse childhood experiences on health: a systematic review and meta-analysis. Lancet Public. Health 2, e356–e366.

Russell K, 2021. What works to prevent youth violence: a summary of the evidence. Available at: https://Users/willsj/Downloads/works-prevent-youth-violence-summary-evidence.pdf.

Speller, V., Evans, K., Head, M., 1997. Developing quality assurance standards for health promotion in the UK Health Promotion International. Perspectives 12, 215–224. Available at: https://dera.ioe.ac.uk//37355/1/works-prevent-youth-violence-summary-evidence.pdf.

23

Evaluating Health Promotion Interventions

LEARNING OUTCOMES

By the end of this chapter you will be able to:
- understand the importance of evaluation in project management
- critically assess the challenges of evaluating complex interventions
- understand the differences between process, impact and outcome evaluation
- identify appropriate methods to evaluate projects
- discuss how evaluation can build an evidence base for health promotion.

KEY CONCEPTS AND DEFINITIONS

Acceptability Adequate to satisfy a need, requirement or standard.

Complex intervention An intervention comprising multiple components which interact to produce change.

Economic evaluation A study which addresses questions of efficiency by standardising outcomes in terms of their dollar/GBP value to assess their value for money, cost-effectiveness and cost-benefit.

Equity The state of being just or fair.

Evaluation The assessment of the worth or value of something.

Fidelity The consistency of what is implemented with the planned intervention.

Impact The immediate effect.

Outcome An end result or consequence.

Outcome evaluation A study which determines whether the programme/intervention caused demonstrable effects, identifying for whom, how, and in what circumstances the outcomes were achieved.

Process evaluation A study which aims to understand the functioning and delivery of an intervention by examining implementation, impact and contextual factors.

IMPORTANCE OF THE TOPIC

Evaluation is an integral aspect of all planned activities, enabling an assessment of the value or worth of an intervention. Evaluation also performs several other roles. For practitioners, evaluation helps develop their skills and competencies. For funders, evaluation demonstrates where resources can be most usefully channelled. For lay people, evaluation provides an opportunity to have their voices heard. There are additional reasons why evaluating health promotion is a key aspect of practice. As a relatively new discipline, there is great pressure on health promotion to prove its worth through evaluation of its activities. In addition, there is a drive to ensure that all practice is evidence-based. In a situation where resources will always be limited, demonstrating the cost-effectiveness of interventions is important. There are thus many factors leading to a demand for evaluation of health promotion practice.

Evaluating health promotion is not a straightforward task. Health promotion interventions often involve different kinds of activities, a long timescale and several partners who may each have their own objectives. Health promotion may be seen as belonging within the health services, where the dominant evaluation model is quantitative research centred on experimental trials, with randomized controlled trials (RCTs) as the preferred evaluation tool. Health promotion has had to argue its case for a more holistic evaluation strategy encompassing qualitative methodologies and taking into account contextual features.

The focus of this chapter is on evaluating health promotion interventions. This chapter considers what is meant by evaluation, the range of research methodologies used in evaluation studies, its rationale, how it is done and its role in building the evidence base for health promotion.

DEFINING EVALUATION

Evaluation is a complex concept with many definitions that vary according to purpose, disciplinary boundaries and values. A comprehensive definition is 'the systematic examination and assessment of features of a programme or other intervention in order to produce knowledge that different stakeholders can use for a variety of purposes' (Rootman et al., 2001, p. 26). This definition is useful, because it also flags up the importance of the purpose of evaluation and that there can be many different reasons to evaluate. Evaluation can provide information on:

- the extent to which an intervention meets its aims and goals
- the manner in which the intervention was carried out
- the cost-effectiveness of the intervention.

It is important to be clear at the outset about the purpose of evaluation, as this will determine what information is gathered and how it is obtained and this is the focus of Learning Activity 23.1. Evaluation uses resources which might otherwise be used for programme planning and implementation, so a clear purpose is necessary to legitimate and protect this use of resources.

> ### 🔲 Learning Activity 23.1 The Role of Evaluation
>
> You have a limited budget (from lottery money) and a tight timescale to deliver a community health promotion intervention designed to improve nutrition. Stakeholders include the funders, local schools, social housing and sheltered accommodation providers, community associations, primary healthcare staff, social care staff and the community. Your proposed plan of action includes an evaluation, and you have suggested earmarking 5% to 10% of your budget and time for this purpose. A group of some

of the stakeholders has approached you requesting that you omit the evaluation and concentrate all your resources on the intervention. How would you respond? What arguments might you use to defend the proposed evaluation?

WHY EVALUATE?

From a practitioner's perspective, evaluation is needed to assess results, determine whether objectives have been met and find out if the methods used were appropriate and efficient. These findings can then be fed back into the planning process in order to progress practice. Evaluations of interventions are used to build an evidence base of what works, enabling other practitioners to focus their inputs on where they will have most effect. From a lay perspective, evaluation helps to clarify expectations and assess the extent to which these have been met. Evaluation may also help determine what strategies had most impact, and why. Without evaluation, it is very difficult to make a reasoned case for more resources or expansion of an intervention. Even when a programme is rolling out an established and effective intervention, specific local features may have an unanticipated impact that will only become apparent in an evaluation. There are sound reasons for evaluating all interventions, although more innovative projects will require more substantial and costly evaluation.

The rationale for evaluation includes the following reasons:

- to assess how resources were deployed (*effort*)
- to assess whether what has been achieved was an economically sound use of resources (*efficiency*)
- to measure impact and outcomes, and whether the intervention was worthwhile (*effectiveness*)
- to assess the intervention's or programme's contribution to equity (*equity*)
- to judge the adequacy, feasibility and sustainability of the delivery of the intervention or programme (*feasibility*)
- to assess the overall benefits of the intervention (*efficacy*)
- to inform future plans
- to justify decisions to others.

Evaluation uses resources that could otherwise be used to provide services. Given that services are always in demand, there needs to be a strong rationale for devoting resources to evaluation rather than service provision.

New or pilot interventions warrant a rigorous evaluation, because without evidence of their effectiveness or efficiency, it is difficult to argue that they should become established work practices. Other criteria that can be used to determine if evaluation is worth the effort relate to how well it can be done. If it will be impossible to obtain cooperation from the different groups involved in the activity, it is probably not worthwhile trying to evaluate. If evaluation has not been considered at the outset, but is tacked on as an 'afterthought', the chances are that it will be so partial and biased as to not be worth the effort.

Evaluation is only worthwhile if it will make a difference. This means that the results of the evaluation need to be interpreted and fed back to the relevant audiences in an accessible form. All too often, evaluations are buried in inappropriate formats. Work reports may go no further than the manager, or academic studies full of jargon may be published in little-known journals.

> ### Learning Activity 23.2   What to Evaluate
>
> A well-man clinic is introduced in a primary health-care practice. The aim is to monitor the health of middle-aged men and provide information and advice enabling them to adopt healthier lifestyles, so that in the longer term health risks such as high blood pressure or smoking are reduced. Over a period of time, the practice nurse invites all men aged 50 to 65 to attend a half-hour session where she checks vital statistics (weight, blood pressure), asks about lifestyle (e.g., diet, smoking, alcohol and drug use, sexual activity, exercise), and gives individually tailored information and advice about adopting a healthier lifestyle. This intervention takes up a significant proportion of her time and workload.
>
> How would you evaluate this programme?

WHAT TO EVALUATE

Health promotion objectives may be about changes in individual lifestyles or service use, or changes in the environment. A range of possible objectives associated with smoking-reduction interventions, each of which would need evaluation, might include:

- increased knowledge for example, regarding the harmful effects of passive smoking
- changes in attitudes, for example, less willingness to breathe in others' smoke

- changes in behaviour, for example, stopping smoking
- acquiring new skills, for example, learning relaxation methods to reduce stress
- introduction of healthy policies, for example, funding to enable general practitioners to prescribe nicotine replacement aids for people on low incomes
- modifying the environment, for example, making no smoking the norm in public places, monitoring sales and displays, banning tobacco for oral use
- reduction in risk factors, for example, reduction in the number of smokers and amount of tobacco smoked per person
- increased use of services, for example, increased take-up rates for smoking-cessation clinics and the number of calls made to quit-smoking telephone helplines
- reduced morbidity, for example, reduced rates of respiratory illness and coronary heart disease
- reduced mortality, for example, reduced rates of lung cancer.

Although all these factors relate to health they are quite separate and there is no necessary connection between, for example, increased knowledge and behaviour change. It is therefore inappropriate to evaluate a given objective (e.g., increased physical activity) by measuring other aspects of an intervention (e.g., number of leaflets taken at a health fair or number of people reporting that they would like to exercise more). It is important to choose appropriate indicators for an intervention's stated objectives. This issue is discussed further in Chapter 22, which emphasizes the use of a logic model to identify appropriate indicators.

PROCESS, IMPACT AND OUTCOME EVALUATION

Evaluation is always incomplete because it is impossible to assess every element of an intervention. Instead, decisions are taken about which evaluation criteria to prioritize, and also sometimes which objectives are to be assessed. A distinction is often made between process, impact and outcome evaluation. Process evaluation (also called formative or illuminative evaluation) is concerned with assessing the process of programme implementation. Outcomes can be immediate (impacts), intermediate or long term (outcomes). Impact and outcome evaluations are both concerned with assessing the effects of interventions.

Chapter 22 identified that evaluation may refer to various features of an intervention or project.

- *Effectiveness* or the extent to which an intervention achieves its intended outcomes. Does the intervention work? Are any changes achieved as a result of the intervention or project? Does the intervention or project work better than alternatives?
- *Efficacy* or the extent to which an intervention achieves maximum benefit for minimum cost. Does the project provide value for money? Is the project more cost-effective than other interventions?
- *Acceptability* or the extent to which an intervention meets needs. Do people respond to, or take up, the service? Are people satisfied with what is offered?
- *Equity* or the extent to which it ensures equal access and ability to benefit. Does the intervention enable equal access for those in need? Do people with greater needs gain greater benefits?
- *Quality* or is the project or intervention delivered in the best possible way? Is it sustainable? Is it feasible? What are the barriers to implementation?

Process Evaluation

Process evaluation may adopt the perspective of participants and/or practitioners and/or other stakeholders such as funders. Stakeholders' perceptions and reactions to health promotion interventions and their facilitating or inhibiting factors may be sought. More objective data, such as whether targets were met and timescales and budgets adhered to, can also be included. The aims of process evaluation are practical – can the intervention be repeated, if it is repeated will another organization or practitioner deliver it in the same way (fidelity), can it be refined, and if it is ineffective is that due to its implementation or the intervention itself?

Fig. 23.1 shows the purposes of a process evaluation which aims to explore the following aspects of an intervention:

- Implementation: the intervention's structures, resources and processes, and the quantity and quality of what is delivered (its reach, acceptability, integrity, quality).
- Impact: if, and how, the activities and responses of participants or recipients will lead to change.
- Context: how external factors influence the functioning of the intervention.

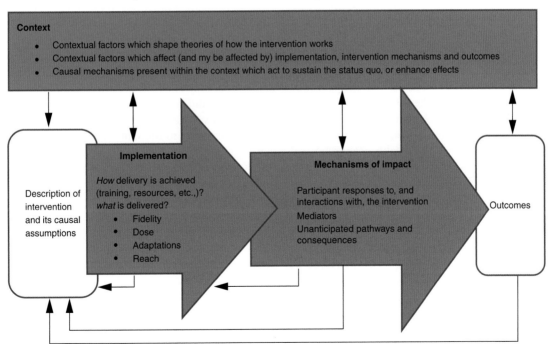

Fig. 23.1 Process evaluation (From Medical Research Council, 2019. Process evaluation of complex interventions, p. 11. Available at: https://mrc.ukri.org/documents/pdf/mrc-phsrn-process-evaluation-guidance-final/.)

Process evaluation employs a wide range of methods including interviews, diaries, observations, secondary analysis of routine data and content analysis of documents. These methods tell us a great deal about particular programmes and the factors responsible for their success or failure, but they are unable to predict what would happen if a programme was replicated in other areas. We need to understand how health promotion interventions are interpreted and responded to by different groups of people, and whether the intervention itself is health promoting, and for this we need process evaluation.

Impact and Outcome Evaluations

Evaluation of health promotion programmes usually focuses on effects and whether any changes are achieved as a result of an intervention. Outcomes are measurable changes which may occur immediately or in the medium or longer term. An example of an immediate outcome is self-reported behaviour changes resulting from a training programme. Outcomes in the medium term include the adoption of lifestyle changes. Long-term impact is usually expressed as increases/reductions in, for example, body mass index, or system changes, for example, provision of exercise facilities in workplaces.

Evaluations face the challenge of identifying what changes have happened as part of normal life, and what changes are attributable to the intervention. Learning Activity 23.3 considers this challenge of when to evaluate to identify outcomes from a project or intervention. A common expectation is that health promotion will contribute to a reduction in morbidity and mortality. Yet any such effect is likely to be small, and may not be apparent for some years. The timing of an evaluation will affect what data can be collected, and how confident we can be that any identified effects are due to the intervention.

Learning Activity 23.3　When to Evaluate: Impact and Outcomes of a Cardiovascular Disease Reduction Programme

A programme to reduce cardiovascular disease may have the following six effects:

1. Improves people's knowledge of the risk factors for coronary heart disease and stroke.

2. Increases people's motivation and intention to take up risk factor screening opportunities
3. Persuades more people to attend screening clinics.
4. Increases media coverage of coronary heart disease and stroke.
5. Increases people's behaviour changes, for example, smoking cessation and adoption of regular exercise.
6. Reduces premature mortality rates from cardiovascular disease.

Which of these outcomes could be evaluated immediately, after 6 months, after 12 months or after 5 years?

Outcomes or changes can be hard to attribute to an intervention. Consider, for example, a school-based programme to educate young people about alcohol. A measurable change might be participants' health-related behaviour (e.g., alcohol consumption and patterns of drinking) before and after the programme. However there are bound to be changes in students' behaviour over 1 year, irrespective of any health promotion programme. So it would be better to compare the students to another group of similar students who did not receive the programme, to see if the same changes occur in both groups. The second or control group of students is necessary to avoid the danger of attributing all behaviour change to the health promotion programme and therefore overestimating its influence. Pre- and post-studies and experimental studies are the most reliable ways to determine effects. Going back a year later to the same students and getting new information from them will, however, take up time and resources, as will obtaining a matched group of students to use as a control group. Results using data on outcomes are often expressed numerically, which increases credibility.

In the previous chapter on planning (Chapter 22), you were introduced to logic modelling. A logic model distinguishes between outputs (the activities of a project) and outcomes. Learning Activity 23.4 asks you to clarify this and define each term.

Learning Activity 23.4　Outcome Versus Output

What is the difference between an outcome and an output?

EVALUATION RESEARCH METHODOLOGIES

Evaluation covers many different activities undertaken with varying degrees of rigour and reflectiveness. At its simplest level, evaluation describes what any competent practitioner does as a matter of course – the process of appraising and assessing work activities, for example, 'How did that consultation go?' or 'Did the patient understand what I said?'. This includes informal feedback and the reviewing of health promotion interventions. Evaluation also refers to a more formal or systematic activity where assessment is linked to intentions. Evaluation takes place at different levels, and may be of a defined project or intervention, or a series of interventions. Depending on what you want to know, evaluation may focus on:

- assessing effectiveness, for example, RCTs, non-randomized studies, or case control studies
- understanding the change process, for example, a process evaluation using qualitative methods can provide insight into why an intervention succeeds or fails
- understanding what is implemented and any facilitators or barriers to implementation
- assessing cost-effectiveness – an economic evaluation using cost–benefit or cost-effectiveness analysis.

> **Learning Activity 23.5   Evaluation Research Methodologies**
>
> A hospital nurse has set up a project to help cardiac patients to stop smoking. The intervention involved the identification of a key worker who was allocated time to interview patients to assess their smoking behaviour and draw up individual plans. After discharge, patients were followed up by a weekly telephone call for 6 weeks.
>
> How could this project be evaluated so that any success in terms of smoking cessation in the target group could be shown to be due to the project?
>
> What would be the strengths and limitations of the methods you identify?

Evaluation is often more formally conducted as research using a variety of different methods. The classic scientific method of proof, the experiment, relies on controlling all factors apart from the one being studied, and can best be achieved under laboratory conditions. However, this is clearly impossible to achieve and

unethical where people's health is concerned. The RCT is the second most rigorous scientific method of proof, and involves the random allocation of people to an intervention or control group. Random allocation means that the two groups should be matched in terms of factors such as age, gender and social class, which are known to affect health. Any changes detected in the intervention group are then compared to those found among the control group. Changes which occur in the intervention group but not the control group can then be attributed to the health promotion programme.

In the well-man clinic example in Learning Activity 24.2, an RCT study as illustrated in Fig. 23.2 would involve randomly allocating all men in the target group to either the intervention group (invited for screening) or the control group (not invited). The two groups would then be compared after the intervention had taken place. If the intervention group showed statistically significant improvements in health status or health-related behaviour over and above those recorded for the control group, the intervention would be deemed to be effective.

The degree of scientific rigour necessary to conduct an RCT is hard to achieve in real-life situations. Most health promotion programmes have spin-off effects, and indeed are designed to do so. It is impossible to isolate different groups of people or to ensure that programmes do not 'leak' beyond their set boundaries. However, the RCT design does mean that changes detected in the input group may be ascribed to the health promotion programme with a greater degree of confidence.

Evaluation research may also use qualitative methods to focus on understanding the processes involved in change. Methods such as observation, interviews and focus groups provide details on what is happening in interventions and which features have been effective, and seeks to explain the mechanisms leading to the change.

Evaluating Complex Interventions

Many health promotion interventions are complex, involving multiple stakeholders and many different programme components, and have an effect at an individual, organizational, service or population level. Health promotion goals may include not just direct effects but triggering changes that will impact on the context and magnify the effects. It is important to understand the whole range of effects, what aspects of the intervention trigger which effects, and how and why the effects vary among recipients of the intervention, between sites and over time.

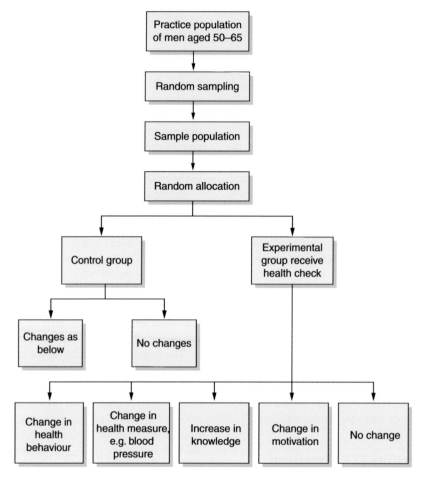

Fig. 23.2 A randomized controlled trial to assess a well man clinic

Pawson and Tilley (1997) describe this process as looking inside the black box to explore what is happening at the inputs/outcomes interface. Outcome and process evaluations need to take place simultaneously. Pawson and Tilley's (1997) realist approach to evaluation provides a means of doing this, and may be summarized as:

context + mechanisms = outcomes.

In other words, an evaluation seeks to understand the following:

- How does an intervention lead to the outcome, and what is the mechanism by which change is produced?
- What factors account for why change takes place, and are there factors that explain the intervention's differential effects?

The realist approach is described further in Case Study 23.1. The realist approach is one of the 'theory-driven' approaches to evaluation. It assumes evaluation follows the classic scientific methodology of beginning with hypotheses and then using empirical evidence to support or falsify theories. There are five steps in the theory-of-change approach to evaluation.

1. Identify long-term goals and the assumptions behind them.
2. Backwards mapping to reveal the necessary preconditions to achieve goals.
3. Identify the initiative's interventions that will lead to the desired changes.
4. Develop outcome measurement indicators to assess the initiative.
5. Write a narrative to explain the logic of the initiative.

As complex interventions contain a number of components, so there are several dimensions of complexity in evaluating such programmes:

- the interactions between the components of the intervention/s
- the number of groups or organizational levels targeted by the intervention
- the number and variability of outcomes
- the degree of flexibility or tailoring of the intervention.

CASE STUDY 23.1
Realist Evaluation

Realist evaluation is an approach that aims to find out the factors influencing outcomes and why an intervention works differently in different contexts (Pawson and Tilley, 1997). (Pawson explains realist evaluation at https://www.youtube.com/watch?v=xJSehOBa75I.) Realist evaluation is important as it helps us understand how an intervention can be consistently replicated. A realist evaluation tries to understand what works, for whom, in what respects, to what extent, in what contexts and how. The evaluation's principal task is to extract and test the theories of change that describe how the intervention is expected to lead to its effects and what mechanisms will generate what outcomes. A programme which 'works' needs to operate successfully at a number of different levels.

For example, the evaluation of health education programmes would need to take into account the following:

- Ideas – are the programme ideas persuasive, is the information fresh and interesting?
- Individuals – are the teachers/presenters effective; are the audience/students interested?
- Institution – programmes can be delivered in schools, colleges or prisons by tutorials, lectures, virtual learning environments or social media. Does the medium make a difference?
- Infrastructure – supposing that the subject has advanced in skills and learning, does the surrounding culture, economy and environment value the learning?

The evaluation design begins by formulating hypotheses about potential programme mechanisms. The next part of the design is to formulate hypotheses about the contexts that might make a difference to the action of the mechanisms. The different hypotheses make predictions on 'for whom and in what circumstance the programme will succeed (or fail)'.

Evaluating Cost-Effectiveness

Part of the reason for evaluation is to determine whether the desired results were achieved in the most economical way, and whether allocating resources to health promotion can be justified. There are many different ways of calculating the economic pluses and minuses of health promotion. Cost–benefit analysis is a way of calculating whether, and to what extent, something is worth doing. Cost–benefit analysis relies on pricing both the inputs and the beneficial outcomes of a health promotion programme. An attempt is then made to calculate the cost of each beneficial outcome. This is known as a cost–benefit ratio. Putting a price on health outcomes or benefits is a very difficult exercise. One approach to this problem is to compare the cost–benefit ratio for a health promotion intervention with the cost–benefit ratio for some other health intervention. It is often assumed that prevention is cheaper than cure and that health promotion saves money, but this is not necessarily the case. Some of the challenges in assessing cost-effectiveness of an intervention are outlined in relation to smoking in Case Study 23.2.

Once a decision has been made to implement an intervention, economic analysis can help to determine the most efficient way of resourcing it. Efficiency refers to the maximum benefit that can be derived from the least cost. Cost-effectiveness is a comparison in monetary terms of different methods used to achieve the same outcomes. Cost-effectiveness analysis addresses *technical* efficiency in the sense that it can tell us the best way to do something, but not whether or not that something is worth doing (Cohen and Flood, 2022). Opportunity costs refer to what is sacrificed or foregone when resources are allocated to something, for example, a health promotion project.

Economic appraisal is an important element in evaluation because there are always competing claims for limited resources. Using economics to make health-related decisions might seem a distasteful idea, and people may shy away from attempts to put a value on people's health, well-being or life. But the reality is that people, societies and governments are constantly making choices and decisions that are influenced by economic considerations. It is therefore important to make the decision-making process transparent, and to include economic principles and concepts in evaluation studies. A review of evidence used to support the decisions made by NICE found that the majority of public health interventions are highly cost-effective (Owen et al., 2012).

CASE STUDY 23.2
Cost-Effectiveness of Smoking Cessation

Numerous studies have examined the cost-effectiveness of cessation as well as for individual types of treatment or management. National Institute of Health and Care Excellence (NICE) (2019) have an economic modelling report on interventions and services at https://www.nice.org.uk/guidance/ng92/evidence/economic-modelling-report-pdf-4790596573.

Smoking cessation saves money by:
- the National Health Service not having to treat people with smoking-related diseases
- not having to pay sickness benefit and disability pensions to people with smoking-related diseases
- increased production in industry because fewer employees are off sick.

Other benefits that are less easy to cost include:
- less exposure to second-hand smoke
- the effect of smoking cessation on reducing the uptake of smoking among children and young people.

Smoking cessation costs the government money in the following ways:
- paying retirement pensions for a longer time as people live longer
- paying unemployment benefits for people in the tobacco production and retail industries who become unemployed due to a fall in demand
- loss of government revenue from tobacco taxation
- costs of pharmacotherapies.

HOW TO EVALUATE: THE PROCESS OF EVALUATION

There are several steps in an evaluation, as shown in Table 23.1.

What to Measure

Deciding what to measure to assess the effects of health promotion is not easy. In theoretical terms, the many meanings and definitions of the concept 'health' result in a lack of consensus about how best to evaluate it. For those who subscribe to the medical model of health, data concerning morbidity, disability and mortality are appropriate measures to use for evaluation purposes. For those who adopt a more social model of health, a much broader range of measures (including for example, measures of socio-economic status or environmental quality) will be appropriate. For people who have prioritized an educational approach, measures of knowledge and attitude change will be paramount.

The golden rule must be to measure the objectives set during the planning process (for more details on objectives, see Chapter 22 on programme planning). Although this sounds straightforward, in practice it can be difficult, and a surprising number of evaluation studies violate this principle. Different stakeholders might have different objectives, and the evaluation needs to take this into account. The objectives set may relate to areas where there is a lack of consensus over appropriate measurement. For example, process objectives such as increased multiagency collaboration, or increased community involvement, are difficult to measure. To collect relevant data would require a special effort because they are not measured routinely. Changes in people's attitudes or beliefs are particularly problematic to measure.

The success of a health promotion intervention is not solely about achieving behavioural changes or reductions in disease rates. For example, a needle-exchange scheme should not be judged solely by a reduction in the rate of human immunodeficiency virus (HIV) infection among drug users. Other markers of success, such as the take-up rate, are also important. In many cases, expecting a clear change in morbidity from a behaviour change would be unrealistic. Although there is a link between needle sharing and HIV infection, there are other risk factors, and expecting risk reduction from this initiative might be unwise.

As we saw in Chapter 22, by using a logic model you will have a theory of change which explains how and why a set of activities – be they part of a project or a comprehensive initiative/complex intervention – is expected to lead to early, intermediate and long-term outcomes over a specified period. The research evidence and knowledge from practitioners and participants will have informed the programme. For example, the evaluation of an antenatal education programme with the overall goal of preparing new parents for parenthood and giving children a good start in life will have a range of outcomes to measure, including the following:
- Short term: knowledge; confidence and levels of trust; behaviours during pregnancy, for example, diet, smoking
- Intermediate: birth outcomes, for example, reduction in clinical interventions, birth weight, mood
- Longer term: reduction in mothers' postnatal depression rates, improvements in children's cognitive development and later educational achievement.

TABLE 23.1   Designing an Evaluation

Manage:
Who are the stakeholders?
What do they want?
How will you find out?
What is the mechanism for reporting to them?

Define and frame:
What is the purpose of the evaluation?
E.g.,: contribute to the broader evidence base, inform decision
    making aimed at improvement, ensure accountability, ensure
    diverse perspectives are included, demonstrate value for
    money or a return on investment.
What is the theory of change that explains how the
    intervention activities lead to the expected outcomes?
What 3–5 questions need to be answered by the evaluation?
Should there be an advisory group?

Describe:
What quantitative data needs to be collected?
By whom? When? How?
What qualitative data needs to be collected?
By whom? When? How?
How will you cost the programme/intervention?
How will you assess the quality of the programme/
    intervention?
How will you assess the impact of the programme/
    intervention across different population groups and show
    that you are addressing health inequalities?

Understand outcomes:
Are there elements of your programme/intervention that are
    unique or distinctive? If so, which elements?
What aspects of your local context might influence outcomes?
How will you demonstrate the association or relationship
    between any outcomes and the programme/intervention?

Synthesis and presentation:
What will the evaluation look like? What might be its
    structure?
To whom will it be presented?
How often will you report on your evaluation?

The logic model will:

- Make explicit hypothesized links between determinants of health and health outcomes, for example, whether knowledge about pain during childbirth is associated with less use of pain relief, or whether preparation for parenthood is associated with greater parental input, such as reading in early childhood, leading to educational achievement.
- Examine an intervention's theoretical plausibility and mechanisms of action.

- Identify key effect mediators or moderators, such as the capability of the person delivering antenatal education.
- Specify intermediate outcomes and potential harms, including differential take-up and effects among population subgroups.

A programme may have several objectives, some of which are easier to measure than others. It then becomes tempting to measure the easiest objectives and extrapolate from these findings. But if the objectives are of different categories (e.g., behavioural, environmental and attitudinal), it is not legitimate to do this.

 Learning Activity 23.6   Indicators of Success

A programme has been launched with the objective of reducing child accidents. Key stakeholders include community and hospital-based health practitioners, community groups (parents' and neighbourhood groups) and local authority staff, including environmental health officers and health and safety officers. Various indicators have been suggested as suitable means of evaluating the programme including:

- take-up of campaign literature
- awareness of the campaign
- sales of child-safety equipment
- making changes to the home environment to improve safety, for example, installing stair gates
- making changes to the local environment, such as traffic-calming measures
- reduction in the number of severe accidents to children that require hospitalization.

For each indicator discuss the following questions:
Is it appropriate?
Is it feasible?
Who would measure it?

A balance needs to be struck between setting the threshold for success too high, leading to interventions that are unjustly deemed to be ineffective, and setting the threshold too low, leading to a judgement that health promotion is not worth the effort. Striking the correct balance involves knowing what changes are likely to take place in the absence of the intervention, and then setting a realistic goal of what additional change is feasible and represents an efficient use of resources. Learning Activity 23.7 asks you to consider and discuss an evaluation of a smoking-cessation programme and whether, given its outcomes, it would be deemed a success.

 Learning Activity 23.7   What Constitutes Evidence of Success?

A smoking-cessation programme including clinics for those wishing to give up smoking is launched. A clinic run by a health promoter attracts 20 clients who attend all six sessions. An evaluation 6 months later finds that 25% of the participants have stopped smoking. Is this a success?

When to Evaluate

The timing of an evaluation is a challenge because it can affect results. If an evaluation is seeking to determine the outcomes of an intervention a longer timescale is desirable. However this presents problems. Health promotion is a long-term process, and contexts and settings are constantly changing, so it can be difficult to be sure that any changes detected are due to the health promotion input and not to any other factor. Health-related knowledge, attitudes and behaviour are constantly changing, regardless of health promotion programmes. Societies and environments are also changing in response to many different factors. One solution to this problem might be to evaluate sooner and use a shorter timescale; but to do so might mean that longer-term sustained outcomes are missed. The best solution is to evaluate over different time periods, but this requires more resources.

Who Evaluates

Success means different things to different groups of people, or stakeholders, all of whom have their own agendas and interests. Different stakeholders have varying levels of power to impose their evaluation agendas on others. Different groups of people engaged in health promotion interventions will each have invested something, but may well be looking for different results. For example, funders of a project may be looking for efficiency or results which can be interpreted as cost-effective. Practitioners may be looking for evidence that their way of working is acceptable to clients and achieves the set objectives. Managers may be looking for evidence of increased productivity, measured by performance indicators. Clients may be looking for opportunities to take control over some health-related aspects of their lives. It is therefore important to be clear at the outset about whose perspectives are being addressed in any evaluation. A starting point is simply to acknowledge that different vested interests are involved, and to try and identify them. Ideally an evaluation would represent the views of different stakeholders by collecting data from each group. This process is called pluralistic evaluation (Smith and Cantley, 1985). Using the process of methodological triangulation, which employs a wide range of data sources, an overall picture may be constructed. Pluralistic evaluation is more complete than evaluation using one group's views, although the findings may be complex and lack clarity. Pluralistic evaluation can also be used to build capacity and empower clients and service users as well as practitioners. In practice, pluralistic evaluation may appear too complex and costly. Evaluation is often carried out by external researchers or insider practitioners. The former tend to be larger scale in remit and potentially more objective.

 Learning Activity 23.8   Internal or External Evaluation?

A dental health project has been launched and needs to be evaluated. There are two choices, either an 'in-house' evaluation conducted by the people involved in running the project, or an external evaluation conducted by outside researchers. What are the pros and cons of each option?

HOW TO EVALUATE: GATHERING AND ANALYSING DATA

The scale of the evaluation should be proportionate to the size or significance of the programme. For programmes that have significant investment, are innovative, large scale or of long duration evaluation may involve a series of projects and related activities. The process of evaluation involves making decisions about what methods to use to gather and analyse relevant data.

Gathering Data

Practical difficulties arise when trying to obtain data and when trying to combine different forms of data to provide an overall picture. Some relevant data are already available and accessible, for example, morbidity and mortality rates. Other data already exist and may be obtained, for example, policy documents or health surveillance data. However, some data will need to be collected and in areas such as attitude change or empowerment there are no easy or accepted means of doing this.

A wide range of data, both qualitative and quantitative, may be used in evaluation studies. Guiding principles when selecting methods of data collection are to use appropriate and feasible tools. 'Appropriate' means gathering data that will help meet the objectives of the evaluation. 'Feasible' means gathering data within budgetary and time constraints. Process evaluation often uses qualitative data, whereas outcome evaluation is more likely to use quantitative data. However, both qualitative and quantitative data may be applicable in various ways at different times.

The medical model of research dominant within healthcare settings prioritizes the RCT as the most rigorous form of quantitative methodology. However, as we have seen in this chapter, RCTs may be inappropriate for evaluating health promotion interventions, where the context is an important and acknowledged element, and stakeholders need to be able to understand, contribute to and oversee the process.

Evaluation seeks to assess process and effect, and it is therefore vital to have baseline data to use for comparison purposes. Unless baseline data is collected, it will be impossible to state that impacts or outcomes are due to the intervention. Planning needs to take account of this, and allocate sufficient resources to allow for the collection of pre- and post-intervention data.

Analysing the Data

There are various ways of analysing data, depending on whether the data is quantitative or qualitative, what kind of intervention or study was carried out, and what resources and expertise is available. There are many excellent textbooks that discuss data analysis in depth (e.g., Bowling, 2014), and the reader is referred to these for a more detailed discussion of methods. However, data analysis is not just a question of methodological awareness and expertise. Values also impact on data analysis processes. The assumption is that faced with a certain set of findings, everyone would agree on their significance or meaning, but this is not necessarily the case. There may also be disputes about which findings are relevant or significant. Data analysis should be an inclusive and capacity-building exercise for all participants, enabling everyone to have a say about what data is significant, and why.

WHAT TO DO WITH THE EVALUATION: PUTTING THE FINDINGS INTO PRACTICE

Evaluation helps build a basis of research to demonstrate which health promotion interventions succeed in meeting objectives, and how best they can be implemented.. Evaluation therefore identifies effective health promotion practice which others can adopt.

Evidence-based practice is firmly established in medicine and nursing, where RCTs of alternative treatment protocols are used to establish which form of treatment is most effective for most people. In health promotion, creating evidence-based practice is more problematic, and is discussed in Chapter 21. Evidence-based health promotion has been defined as 'a public health endeavour in which there is an informed, explicit, and judicious use of evidence that has been derived from any of a variety of science and social science research and evaluation methods' (Rychetnik et al., 2004). It is more challenging and Learning Activity 23.9 asks you to consider and discuss why evidence-based practice in health promotion is more difficult to achieve.

 Learning Activity 23.9   Evidence-Based Health Promotion

Why might it be difficult to establish evidence-based health promotion practice?

Predictability, repeatability and falsifiability are the criteria by which results are assessed in evidence from medicine, and these are based on widely recognized scientific principles. Predictability is said to be met when a properly implemented intervention will bring about an expected outcome every time. Repeatability, sometimes referred to as replicability, means the intervention can be repeated and achieve the same results wherever and whenever it is carried out. To be falsifiable, the intervention must be capable of being disproved as an effective intervention. Once implemented, the intervention is validated if rigorous evaluation research demonstrates that it works. The intervention is falsified if it is shown to be ineffective or harmful. As we have seen in this chapter, such conditions are almost impossible to meet in the real world and, as realist evaluation approaches show, context is a key influence on outcomes.

In biomedical sciences it is easier to argue that if x (the exposure/intervention) precedes y (the effect), and there is a statistical association between x and y, and if a reduction of x will lead to a reduction of y and there is not a z confounding the association, then causation is imputed. Health promotion operates in an environment where numerous cultural, social, economic and political factors interact. Given a complex context where the links among the elements of an intervention are interrelated, causality cannot be confirmed.

This does not mean that there is no evidence on which to base health promotion work. Meta-analyses or systematic reviews of research studies pool together findings from different studies in effectiveness reviews. Effectiveness reviews are a means of building up a knowledge base that can tell us what are reasonable

expectations of success in health promotion. An independent national body in the UK, the NICE, is devoted to providing evidence-based guidance on the promotion of good health and the prevention and treatment of ill health. These sources of evidence are discussed in Chapter 21. Nevertheless, as discussed in Chapter 21, practitioners do not always plan projects and interventions based on evidence and Learning Activity 23.10 asks you to reflect on this.

 Learning Activity 23.10   Certainty and Uncertainty

Think of an intervention that you have developed or implemented. How confident were you that you were right to do so?

Often decisions are made even when we are not certain of the outcomes. We may believe, but not know for a fact, that something is true., These are the assumptions that the logic models discussed in Chapter 22 are supposed to highlight. Fig. 23.3 illustrates this, showing how confidence and certainty impact on decision-making, and how their absence means much of what is done may be just muddling through. Learning Activity 23.11 asks you to discuss if projects or interventions should take place if there is no evidence of its effectiveness.

 Learning Activity 23.11   In the Absence of Evidence

Should an intervention not be undertaken if there is no evidence base to support it?

This chapter has advocated the importance of evaluating what we do to provide 'proof' of making a difference, and to make decisions explicit and transparent. But it has also shown how logic and theory can provide plausible explanations of what might work, alongside existing evidence. Simply relying on existing evidence has limitations:

- it can be restrictive, devaluing expert opinion and ignoring the context
- the scientific model demands good-quality (well-reported) studies, not necessarily good-quality interventions
- the scientific model relies on the experiment to demonstrate effectiveness, but there are other considerations for health promoting interventions, such as efficiency, acceptability, quality and equity.

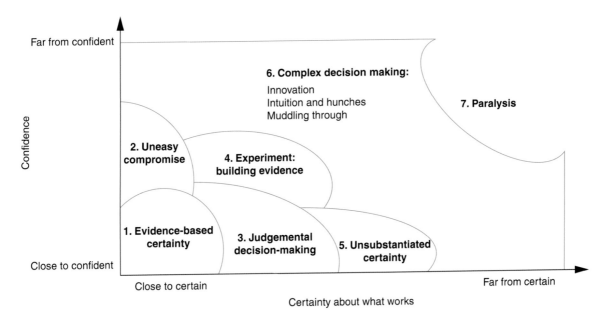

1. There is evidence clearly linking actions to outcomes, e.g., guidelines.
2. There is some evidence but disagreement or lack of evidence as to its acceptability or applicability.
3. There is a lack of certainty about the effect of actions and a lack of evidence.
4. There is confident decision-making based on theoretical plausibility and assumptions but no evidence.
5. We need to be seen to be doing something!
6. The majority of decisions are made here – a lack of evidence so decisions are made based on other considerations.
7. Nothing is done because there is no evidence.

Fig. 23.3 Certainty and uncertainty in decision-making (Adapted from Stacey, R.D., 2002. Strategic Management and Organisational Dynamics: The Challenge of Complexity, third edn. Prentice Hall, Harlow.)

Dissemination of findings is important to publicize good practice and flag up interventions that were not as successful as had been anticipated. Knowing what does not work is as valuable as knowing what does, but there is a great emphasis on producing and publicizing positive results. As Hawe et al. (1994) argue, health promoters may avoid evaluation so as not to appear to be failing, but stigma should not be attached to programmes that fail, only to programmes that fail to learn from these experiences or programmes that fail to evaluate.

Putting findings into practice can take many forms. The results of evaluation should ideally feed into an ongoing cycle of action and reflection, allowing more knowledgeable and reasoned interventions to take place. Evaluation may also enable stakeholders to progress with activities and gain more support to do so.

Numerous studies of knowledge translation (e.g., Clar et al., 2011) cite difficulties with getting evidence into practice:

- lack of time
- lack of availability of research results
- information overload and lack of comprehensibility
- lack of relevance.

This leads policy makers and practitioners to rely on:
- single studies
- experts
- policy statements.

Making research and evaluation findings more accessible to policy makers, increasing opportunities for interaction between policy makers and researchers, addressing structural barriers such as research receptivity in policy agencies and a lack of incentives for academics to link with policy makers, and increasing the relevance of research to policy are all ways in which there can be greater synergy between research, evaluation and practice. Local government is often distant from academic research and opportunities to learn and evaluate can be easily lost. Public Health Intervention Responsive Studies

Teams (PHIRST) are being set up across the UK to link universities with local government to provide timely evidence to underpin policy and practice through the evaluation of selected projects that have generalizability. The evaluation approach is embedded in a model of co-production and design to ensure joint ownership of the research design, outcomes and dissemination.

CASE STUDY 23.3
Assessing Impact of Research

Within UK academia the Research Evaluation Framework (REF) evaluates the impact of research beyond academia as well as academic excellence, defining impact as 'an effect on, change or benefit to the economy, society, culture, public policy or services, health, the environment or quality of life, beyond academia'.

The impact on policy from an evaluation could be evidenced as shown below:

Type of Impact	Example
Shaping the policy agenda	• The framing of discussion changes • New items appear • Increased attention • Media debate
Development of policy	• Better understanding of the nature of a problem (causes, effects and scale) • Develop policy solutions (what has worked elsewhere; costs/benefits) • Capacity building (developing skills, processes, resources)
Change in policy Implementation	• Change in policy direction • Withdrawal of a policy • Improvement in technology or process • Quality, accessibility or cost effectiveness has been improved • Identification of new services • New networks or coalitions

Adapted from a guide to writing policy briefings in Antonopoulou, V., Chadwick, P.1, McGee, O., Sniehotta, F.F., Lorencatto, F., et al., 2021. Research Engagement with Policy Makers: A Practical Guide to Writing Policy Briefs. NIHR Policy Research Unit, pp. 23–26.

CONCLUSION

Evaluation contributes to the accountability and development of evidence-based health promotion practice and is an important aspect of the health promoter's work. It involves evaluating health promotion activity with which you are involved. The purpose of an evaluation is to know what works and to understand the nature of the change/outcomes. There are often pressures to adopt unrealistic measures of success, such as reduced mortality rates or demonstrable cost benefits. Most health promoters are engaged in more modest activities which seek to achieve changes in knowledge, behaviour, attitudes, service take-up or the policy process. These are therefore more appropriate outcomes to use for evaluation purposes.

Evaluation is a practical activity which feeds into the theoretical debate about the nature and purpose of health promotion. This debate cannot be confined to professionals, or those who hold managerial or financial power. It must include the public, who are the targets of health promotion activity. This is why pluralistic evaluation, which enables participants to have a voice in determining effectiveness, is so important.

Evaluation is not a simple activity, and it consumes resources which might otherwise be spent on practising health promotion. The decisions about whether, when and how to evaluate are therefore important. The question of evaluation should be considered at the outset of any planned health promotion intervention. If it is to be done, it should be done in the best possible way. If this is not feasible, then it is better to admit this and not attempt to evaluate. Ongoing monitoring may be the best one can do. This is acceptable, but there is a distinction between routine monitoring of activities through the use of performance indicators and a more thoroughgoing evaluation. It is important not to confuse the two, and to be clear about which it is you are doing.

REFLECTION ON PRACTICE

• Think of a health promotion activity you have undertaken. What factors would you wish to consider in its evaluation?

SUMMARY

This chapter has looked at how evaluation is defined, the different kinds of research methodologies used in evaluation research, and why health promotion needs to be evaluated. Different kinds of evaluation have been identified, including process, impact, outcome and whole-systems evaluation. The process of evaluation, including principles and stages, has been outlined. The importance of demonstrating the cost-effectiveness of health promotion and the role of evaluation in building an evidence base for health promotion have been discussed.

FURTHER READING AND RESOURCES

Evaluation Support Scotland https://evaluationsupportscotland. org.uk/ and Better Evaluation https://www.betterevaluation. org/.
These two organizations provide guides to evaluation and outline different approaches. In Australia the New South Wales government have also produced a guidance document for evaluation at https://www.dpc.nsw.gov.au/tools-and-resources/evaluation-toolkit/

Green, J., South, J., 2006. Evaluation. Open University Press, Maidenhead.
A very readable account of the theoretical underpinnings and practicalities of doing evaluation. The real-life challenges and complexities of evaluation are discussed in depth.

Medical Research Council, 2019a. Process evaluation of complex interventions. Available at https://mrc.ukri.org/ documents/pdf/mrc-phsrn-process-evaluation-guidance-final/.

Medical Research Council, 2019b. Developing and evaluating complex interventions. Available at https://mrc.ukri.org/ documents/pdf/complex-interventions-guidance/.
These two guidance handbooks are clearly written and provide an analytical and practical guide to evaluation.

Rootman, I., Goodstadt, M., Hyndman, B., McQueen, D.V., Potvin, L., et al. (eds.), 2001. Evaluation in Health Promotion: Principles and Perspectives. WHO, Denmark. Available at: http://www.euro.who.int/__data/assets/ pdf_file/0007/108934/E73455.pdf.
A very thorough and comprehensive account of the theoretical and methodological issues relating to the evaluation of health promotion interventions.

Thorogood, M., Coombes, Y., 2010. Evaluating Health Promotion Practices and Methods, third ed Oxford University Press, Oxford.
A useful guide that helps to explore the processes of implementation and evaluation methods.

NICE produces guidance documents and effectiveness reviews on a variety of topics, including public health and health promotion issues such as obesity and nutrition, exercise and smoking cessation. www.nice.org.uk.

FEEDBACK ON LEARNING ACTIVITIES

23.1. Evaluation is an important part of a project or programme. It allows progress to be tracked and implementation issues to be identified, helps to identify whether or not the project was worth doing and enables adaptive management during a project. Evaluation provides accountability to the funders of a project, and also contributes to ongoing learning about why things do or do not work in practice.

23.2. There are many different ways of evaluating the well-man clinic. Monitoring lifestyle behaviours over a period of time could establish whether or not the clinic led to a reduction in unhealthy behaviours. This would be costly, and it would be difficult to follow up the participants. Monitoring vital statistics regularly could establish whether or not health improvements were being made. Monitoring of before and after data might also provide an incentive to maintain healthy changes to lifestyles. Recording the cost of providing the clinic and costing the health improvements gained could provide data about the cost-effectiveness of the intervention. Noting how the sessions have been received by the men, or soliciting their comments or those of peers and colleagues, is part of the evaluation process. Asking the men what they wanted from participating in the programme and whether they achieved their goals would be a participatory form of evaluation. Comparing the socio-economic status of participants and non-participants would help determine if the programme was reinforcing or challenging social and health inequalities.

23.3. An immediate post-programme evaluation may identify the first and second effects, or the impact of the intervention. The third and fourth effects may only be apparent at a later evaluation, for example, after 6 months, and are called outcomes. Twelve months after the programme, the increased attendance at screening clinics may no longer be discernible and attendance figures may have reverted to pre-programme levels. A reduction in the mortality rate may not be discernible for 5 years or more, by which time it will be difficult to attribute it to the health promotion programme. The assessment of the overall success or failure of a programme is therefore influenced by the timing of the evaluation, which in turn is influenced by the amount of funding available. Longer-term evaluation tends to be more expensive, while immediate evaluation costs may be absorbed within programme budgets.

23.4. Outputs are the activities undertaken as part of the intervention or programme (e.g., how many pregnant women attend a smoking-cessation clinic). Outcomes are the changes as a result of an intervention or programme (e.g., the outcome of the programme will be to increase the number of tobacco-free pregnant women).

23.5. An RCT would involve each smoking patient on arrival in the ward being randomly allocated to either the experimental group (who receive the interview) or the control group (who do not receive the interview but get a care plan and general leaflet). Differences in the success rates of the two groups could be attributed to the interview intervention. This evaluation method is scientific and rigorous.

Case study evaluation would interview patients about their involvement in the project and examine their knowledge, attitudes and reported behaviour. This evaluation method is qualitative and less rigorous, but more insightful regarding the process of involvement in the project.

23.6.

23.7. The health promoter may be pleased with these results. People attend clinics often as a last resort, and 6 months is a reasonable time period to assess long-term behaviour change. However, the health promoter's manager may point out that 20% is an average success rate for people trying to quit, regardless of what methods are used. Clinics are time-consuming and 20 people is not a large group: 25% being quitters means five people, four of whom might have quit using other less intensive or expensive methods. So one additional ex-smoker might be the result of the smoking-cessation clinic.

23.8.

Insider Evaluation	
Pros	Knows background to project
	Cheaper
	Acceptable to everyone
Cons	Too involved in project
	No research expertise
	Biased to prove success
Outside Evaluation	
Pros	Unbiased attitude
	Research expertise
	Fresh perspective
Cons	Expensive
	May appear threatening
	Unfamiliar with project

	Appropriateness	Feasibility	Who Would Measure It?
Take-up of campaign literature	No direct link to a reduction in child accidents	Yes	Campaign staff or staff located in venues offering campaign literature, e.g., health visitors
Sales of child-safety equipment	Yes, but also affected by income so does not reflect equity	Yes	Producers or sellers of child-safety equipment
Changes to the home environment, e.g., stair gates	Yes	Uncertain	Health visitors might be able to monitor changes for under-5-year-olds
Changes to the local environment, e.g., traffic-calming measures	Yes	Yes	Environmental health officers or local traffic staff
Reduction in the number of accidents to children	Yes	Minor accidents are not routinely recorded or reported	Health visitors or hospital staff could monitor changes in the number of serious accidents to children
Reduction in the number of accidents requiring hospitalization	Yes	Yes	Hospital staff

23.9. There are several reasons why proving that an evidence base exists for health promotion is problematic. These include knowing when to evaluate, knowing what constitutes success, being able to attribute results to interventions and the inappropriateness of using RCTs.

23.10. Interventions are often implemented even though a practitioner may not be confident about their outcome. This is why logic modelling which includes a theory of change can help to clarify what are the expected outcomes and why these are assumed to arise from the intervention.

23.11. Although we talk of evidence-based practice, often interventions are implemented in the absence of evidence. The challenges of evidence-based practice for health promotion are outlined in Chapter 22 which describes how any decision about what to do is made up of a balanced consideration of:
- what we know (evidence)
- what we think might plausibly work (theory)
- what we think we ought to do (principle)
- what we think we can do (resources).

Where it is available, external evidence can inform, but can never replace, the expertise of individual practitioners. It is this expertise that decides whether the external evidence is applied to the target group of an intervention at all, and, if so, how it should be used for achieving effectiveness. In other words, for an effective intervention, other critical areas in addition to evidence need to be taken into consideration – for example, the needs and expectations of direct service recipients, the interests of other key stakeholders and the competency of a practitioner in planning and evaluation. More confidence in decision-making may come from the decision being evidence based, and knowing that what you do is based on sound and robust research.

But practitioners can also feel more confident and secure in their decisions if they believe that the values underpinning the intervention are just, and a cognitive processing of theory suggests that the intervention 'makes sense' – that it should plausibly work.

REFERENCES

Bowling, A., 2014. Research Methods in Health: Investigating Health and Health Services, fourth edn. Open University, Maidenhead.

Clar, C., Campbell, S., Davidson, L., Graham, W., 2011. What are the effects of interventions to improve the uptake of evidence from health research into policy in low and middle-income countries? Systematic Review. Dfid, UK. Available at: https://assets.publishing. service.gov.uk/media/57a08ab3ed915d3cfd0008c2/ SR_EvidenceIntoPolicy_Graham_May2011_ MinorEditsJuly2011.pdf.

Cohen, D., Flood, C., 2022. Health economics. In: Naidoo, J., Wills, J. (eds.), Health Studies: An Introduction, fourth edn. Springer, Singapore.

Hawe, P., Degeling, D., Hall, J., 1994. Evaluating Health Promotion: A Health Worker's Guide. Maclennan and Petty, Sydney.

Owen, L., Morgan, A., Fischer, A., Ellis, S., Hoy, A., Kelly, M., 2012. The cost effectiveness of public health interventions. J. Public. Health 34 (1), 37–45. Available at: http://jpubhealth. oxfordjournals.org/content/34/1/37.full.pdf+html.

Pawson, R., Tilley, N., 1997. Realistic Evaluation. Sage, London.

Rootman, I., Goodstadt, M., Hyndman, B., McQueen, D.V., Potvin, L., et al. (eds.), 2001. Evaluation in Health Promotion: Principles and Perspectives. WHO, Denmark. Available at: http://www.euro.who.int/__data/assets/ pdf_file/0007/108934/E73455.pdf.

Rychetnik, L., Hawe, P., Waters, E., Barratt, A., Frommer, M., 2004. A glossary for evidence based public health. J. Epidemiol. Commun. Health 58, 538–545. Available at: http://jech.bmj.com/content/58/7/538.full.pdf+html.

Smith, G., Cantley, C., 1985. Assessing Health Care: A Study in Organisational Evaluation. Open University Press, Milton Keynes.

Stacey, R.D., 2002. Strategic Management and Organisational Dynamics: The Challenge of Complexity, third edn. Prentice Hall, Harlow.

Note: Page numbers followed by '*b*', '*t*' and '*f*' refer to boxes, tables, and figures respectively.